# Rinderpest and Peste des Petits Ruminants

# Biology of Animal Infections

**Series Editor**
Paul-Pierre Pastoret, Institute for Animal Health, Compton Laboratory, UK
ISSN: 1572-4271

PUBLISHED VOLUMES

**Marek's Disease:** *An Evolving Problem*
Edited by Fred Davison and Venugopal Nair, Institute for Animal Health, Compton Laboratory, UK
ISBN: 0-12-088379-1

**Rinderpest and Peste des Petits Ruminants:** *Virus Plagues of Large and Small Ruminants*
Edited by Thomas Barrett, Institute for Animal Health, Pirbright Laboratory, UK, Paul-Pierre Pastoret, Institute for Animal Health, Compton Laboratory, UK and William P. Taylor, Littlehampton, Sussex, UK
ISBN: 0-12-088385-6

FUTURE VOLUMES

**Bluetongue**
Edited by Peter Mertens, Matthew Baylis and Philip Mellor, Institute for Animal Health, Pirbright Laboratory, UK
ISBN: 0-12-369368-3

**Scrapie**

**Foot-and-Mouth Disease**

**African Swine Fever**

# Rinderpest and Peste des Petits Ruminants
## Virus Plagues of Large and Small Ruminants

**Edited by Thomas Barrett, Paul-Pierre Pastoret and William P. Taylor**

AMSTERDAM • BOSTON • HEIDELBERG • LONDON • NEW YORK • OXFORD
PARIS • SAN DIEGO • SAN FRANCISCO • SINGAPORE • SYDNEY • TOKYO
Academic Press is an imprint of Elsevier

Academic Press is an imprint of Elsevier
84 Theobald's Road, London WC1X 8RR, UK
30 Corporate Drive, Suite 400, Burlington, MA 01803, USA
525 B Street, Suite 1900, San Diego, California 92101-4495, USA

This book is printed on acid-free paper

British Library Cataloguing in Publication Data
Rinderpest and peste des petits ruminants: virus plagues of large and small ruminants.
(Biology of animal infections)
1. Ruminants – Virus diseases
I. Barrett, Thomas II. Pastoret, Paul-Pierre III. Taylor, William P.
636.2'089691

Library of Congress Catalog Data Control Number: 2005932522

ISBN-13: 978-0-12-088385-1
ISBN-10: 0-12-088385-6
ISSN: 1572-4271

For information on all Academic Press publications
visit our web site at http://books.elsevier.com

Typeset by Macmillan, India

Transferred to Digital Print 2007

Printed and bound by CPI Antony Rowe, Eastbourne

Working together to grow
libraries in developing countries

www.elsevier.com | www.bookaid.org | www.sabre.org

ELSEVIER     BOOK AID
             International     Sabre Foundation

# Dedication

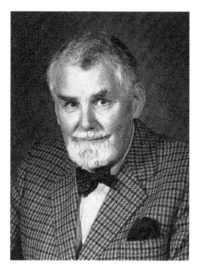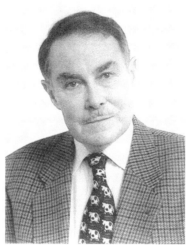

This book is dedicated to the memory of Drs Gordon Scott (1923–2004) and Alain Provost (1930–2002). They were both outstanding figures in the field of tropical veterinary medicine, known especially for their work with rinderpest and peste des petits ruminants viruses. Their tireless research made an invaluable contribution to our understanding of the biology, pathology and epidemiology of these two dreaded diseases.

# Contents

Colour plates appears between pages 206 and 207

# Contributors

**John Anderson**
World Reference Laboratory, Institute for Animal Health, Pirbright Laboratory, Surrey, UK

**Ashley C. Banyard**
Institute for Animal Health, Pirbright Laboratory, Surrey, UK

**Thomas Barrett**
Institute for Animal Health, Pirbright Laboratory, Surrey, UK

**Jean Blancou**
Paris, France

**Mandy Corteyn**
World Reference Laboratory, Institute for Animal Health, Pirbright Laboratory, Surrey, UK

**S. Louise Cosby**
Microbiology, School of Medicine, Queens's University, Belfast, UK

**Adama Diallo**
International Atomic Energy Agency, FAO/IAEA Agriculture and Biotechnology Laboratory, Vienna, Austria

**Marian Horzinek**
Veterinary Faculty, Department of Infectious Diseases and Immunology, Utrecht University, Utrecht, The Netherlands

**Chieko Kai**
Laboratory Animal Research Center, Institute of Medical Science, University of Tokyo, Japan

**Richard A. Kock**
African Union, Interafrican Bureau for Animal Resources, Pan African Programme for the Control of Epizootics (AU–IBAR PACE), Nairobi, Kenya

**Genevieve Libeau**
CIRAD–EMVT, Montpellier, France

**Uwe Mueller-Doblies**
Institute for Animal Health, Pirbright Laboratory, Surrey, UK

**Paul-Pierre Pastoret**
Biotechnology and Biological Sciences Research Council, UK

**Walter Plowright**
Goring-on-Thames, Berkshire, UK

**Bertus K. Rima**
School of Biology and Biochemistry, Medical Biology Centre, The Queen's University, Belfast, UK

**Peter L. Roeder**
Food and Agriculture Organization, Animal Health Service, Animal Production and Health Division, Rome, Italy

**Mark M. Rweyemamu**
Woking, Surrey, UK

**Jeremiah Saliki**
Oklahoma Animal Disease Diagnostic Laboratory, College of Veterinary Medicine, Stillwater, Oklahoma, USA

**William P. Taylor**
Littlehampton, Sussex, UK

**Bernard Vallat**
Office International des Epizooties, Paris, France

**Peter Wohlsein**
Tierärztliche Hochschule Hannover, Institut für Pathologie, Hannover, Germany

**Kazuya Yamanouchi**
Nippon Institute for Biological Sciences, Tokyo, Japan

# Rinderpest: a general introduction

**1**

## PAUL-PIERRE PASTORET
Biotechnology and Biological Sciences Research Council, UK

## Rinderpest

Rinderpest is certainly one of the epizootic diseases for which the most historical information exists (Blancou, 2003). This is no doubt due to the spectacularly high mortality that it causes and the speed with which it spreads, giving it all the hallmarks of an economic and social disaster (Barrett and Rossiter, 1999), which explains why many of the people of Europe, Africa and Asia held painful memories of the incursion of this disease and faithfully recorded the events as recounted in the works of Dieckerhoff (1890), Spinage (2003) and Blancou (2003). Plagues, either affecting humans or animals, have been defined since antiquity by their epidemiological characteristics as proposed by Galen (translated 1936): a disease that affects many people at the same time in the same place is called an epidemic (*epidemon*), but when it is accompanied by many losses, it becomes a plague (*loimos*) (Figure 1.1). During the nineteenth century clinical and pathological descriptions of diseases like rinderpest were added (Fleming, 1871). These were the cornerstones of the classification of plagues until the end of the nineteenth century. Around this time Alexandre Yersin (1863–1943), in collaboration with Louis Pasteur (1822–1895) and independently Shibasaburo Kitasato (1852–1931) with Robert Koch (1843–1910) had isolated the causative agent of the human plague, which turned out to be a bacterium (*Yersinia pestis*).

## The concept of a virus

Rinderpest has always played a major part in the history of veterinary science, but also more broadly in biological science, and animal infectious diseases, most particularly rinderpest, have played a major role in the history of medicine,

ISBN-13: 978-0-12-88385-1
ISBN-10: 0-12-88385-6

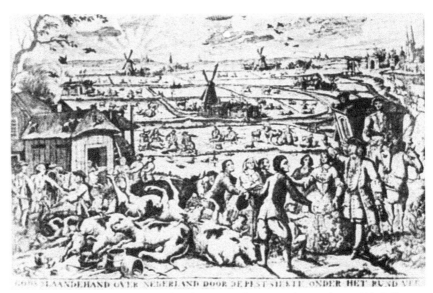

ὅτιπερ ἂν ἅμα πολλοῖς ἐν ἑνὶ γένηται <χρόνῳ τε καὶ> χωρίῳ, τοῦτ᾽ ἐπίδημον ὀνομάζεται, προσελθόντος δ᾽ αὐτῷ τοῦ πολλοὺς ἀναιρεῖν, λοιμὸς γίγνεται.

**Figure 1.1**   An illustration of rinderpest in The Netherlands in the eighteenth century. The original greek text of Galen (129–200) is given along with an english translation: *Translation:* The disease that affects many people at the same time and in the same place is called epidemic (*epidemon*) but when it is accompanied by many losses, it becomes a plague (*loimos*)

helping to defining concepts of infectious agents (Wilkinson, 1984, 1992). The modern history begins with the work of Edward Jenner (1749–1823) on cowpox and smallpox and his contribution to the description of the nervous form of distemper, another morbillivirus infection (Dawtrey-Drewitt, 1931), also called 'maladie de Carré' after the person (Carré, 1870–1938) who first showed that it was caused by a filterable agent (virus).

Pasteur began to work in 1881 on what were later defined as diseases of viral aetiology, and he referred to the rabies agent as '*être de raison*' (being by reason). He still considered rabies to be caused by a microbe, simply one that was smaller than others, contrary to Robert Koch who, in 1890, on the occasion of the Xth international congress of medicine held in Berlin, expressed the opinion that influenza, smallpox, measles and rinderpest were not due to bacterial infection but to another kind of pathogenic agent (Koch, 1891). He speculated that the agents of diseases which bacteriological techniques systematically failed to detect belonged to a completely different group (Figure 1.2).

Following the seminal work of Dimitri Ivanowski (1864–1920) on tobacco mosaic virus (Ivanowski, 1903), later called '*contagium vivum fluidum*' by

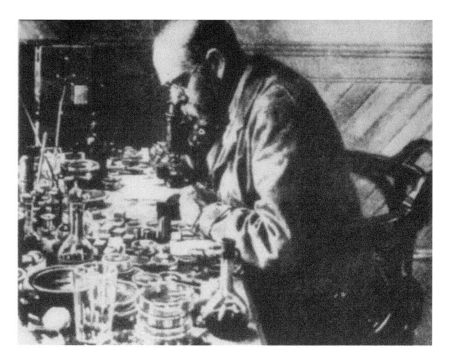

**Figure 1.2**  Robert Koch (1843–1910) looking for Rinderpest (cattle plague) microbes in 1897.

Martinus Beijerinck (1851–1931) (Beijerinck, 1898), Friedrich Löffler (1852–1915) and Pavil Frösch (1860–1928) succeeded in 1897 in demonstrating that an animal infection, foot-and-mouth disease, was caused by a virus and not a bacterium or a toxin. Working in Koch's laboratory, Löffler was associated with many early scientific discoveries before his important work on foot-and-mouth disease. This discovery of the nature of some infectious agents, by then called viruses, was rapidly followed by the discovery that others had a similar character, for example the agent responsible for poliomyelitis in humans.

  The work of Maurice Nicolle (1862–1932) and Mustafa Adil-Bey (1871–1904) showed that rinderpest was also caused by a virus (Nicolle and Adil-Bey, 1902) and this was a great scientific surprise since similar plague-like diseases had not previously been known to be caused by such agents. Now we know that, whereas human plague is caused by a bacterium, rinderpest and peste des petits ruminants are caused by morbilliviruses, classical swine fever (swine plague) by a pestivirus, African swine fever by an asfaravirus, African horse sickness by an orbivirus and fowl plague (avian influenza) by an influenza virus. Nevertheless, this discovery, essential for the advancement of medical thinking at the time, was controversial and Yersin also carried out experiments on the transmission of rinderpest (Yersin, 1898, 1904; Yersin *et al.*, 1899). The work of Geert Reinders (1737–1815) in The Netherlands and Stolte in Germany on inoculation to prevent rinderpest led to the discovery of maternal transmission of immunity (see Chapter 5).

The virus responsible for rinderpest and that of a similar disease of small ruminants, peste des petits ruminants, together with those responsible for measles in humans and distemper in carnivores, pinnipeds and cetaceans, belong to the genus *Morbillivirus* within the family *Paramyxoviridae* (see Chapter 2). Based on antigenic and molecular data, Norrby and colleagues (1985) proposed that rinderpest virus was most probably the ancestor of the morbillivirus group. This conclusion was also based on the fact that populations of susceptible ruminants large enough to maintain the virus in circulation existed before the first ancient civilizations with large enough populations to play the same role for the measles virus, since there is a minimum population size of about 300 000 required to maintain the viruses (Anderson and May, 1983; Black, 1991). Wild ruminant populations today are generally not large enough to maintain rinderpest in circulation and control of the disease in domestic cattle appears to ensure that it will die out in wildlife, as evidenced by the elimination of rinderpest from South Africa and Tanzania, countries that have large wildlife populations (Plowright, 1982; Pastoret *et al.*, 1988).

## Development of prophylactic measures

Rinderpest has always interested the veterinary profession but has also been much studied by the scientific community at large (see Chapter 5). For instance the government of the Cape Colony and of the Free State of Transvaal invited prominent European scientists to come to South Africa in order to help control the alarming situation created by the introduction of rinderpest in 1896 (Figure 1.3). Robert Koch, accompanied by Paul Kohlstock (1861–1900), came from Berlin and participated in research into the cause and prevention of the cattle plague (Koch, 1897). As a result of their work they recommended the use of a mixture of blood and bile from an infected animal as a prophylactic measure to protect naive animals from infection (Figure 1.4). However, Koch's work on rinderpest in South Africa was cut short by his call to India to deal with an outbreak of human plague.

The work initiated by Koch (Koch, 1897) on rinderpest was continued by another group in the Free State of Transvaal comprising Jan Danysz (1860–1928), a Polish bacteriologist, and Jules Bordet (1870–1961), a Belgian medic, both working at that time in the Pasteur Institute in Paris. A young veterinarian from Switzerland, Arnold Theiler (1867–1935) was also involved. Their work was mainly concerned with investigating the use of serotherapy and the production of hyperimmune sera (Danysz and Bordet, 1898), confirming the observations made previously by Semmer in 1893 (see Chapter 11). Later,

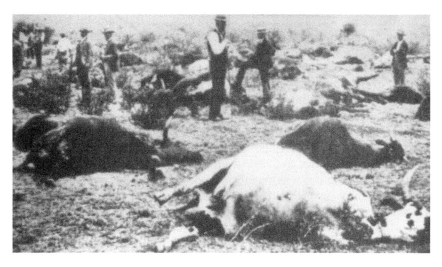

**Figure 1.3** Rinderpest in South Africa. The great African rinderpest pandemic, 1887–1897. This picture was probably taken near Vryburg, Transvaal, in about 1896. (Kindly provided by Sanette Benjamin, Onderstepoort Laboratory, South Africa). This is the most publicised historical photograph of any animal disease in South Africa. Often it is attributed to document the ravages of the disease. In actual fact it documents the 'stamping out' policy instituted to stop the advance of the disease, as evidenced by the presence of two armed members of an 'eradication team'. See Vogel and Heyne (1966) for more details.

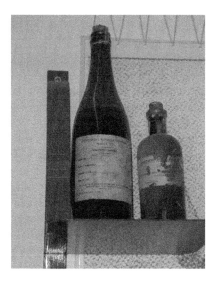

**Figure 1.4** Gall flasks. These flasks were used to collect gall from cattle that had died of rinderpest during the period 1896–1898. Other cattle were then 'vaccinated' with the infected gall. (Exhibited in the Onderstepoort Laboratory, South Africa).

when rinderpest was accidentally reintroduced in Belgium in 1920, Jules Bordet was a member of the Commission in charge of rinderpest control, together with Professor Joseph Hamoir (1872–1924) of the veterinary school of Cureghem in Brussels and Dr Henri de Roo (1861–1930), Chief Veterinary Officer in Belgium who later became the first President of the Office International des Epizooties in Paris.

The reintroduction of rinderpest into Belgium in 1920 was a great concern for France and the French Ministry of Agriculture sent Emile Roux (1853–1933), Director of the Pasteur Institute of Paris (Figure 1.5), and Albert Calmette (1863–1933), Director of the Pasteur Institute of Lille, to Belgium in order to investigate the situation with regard to rinderpest in the country. An international conference was held in Paris in March 1921 to review the situation and, as a consequence, the Office International des Epizooties was created six years later. This body now functions as the equivalent to the World Health Organization (WHO) for animal health (Pastoret, 1986).

## Inoculation–Vaccination against rinderpest

It is remarkable that rinderpest was eliminated from Europe by the end of the nineteenth century by the simple application of sanitary measures (Mammerickx, 2003), thanks to the requirement of close contacts needed for disease transmission, and before the nature of the infectious agent was known. In fact the ability to control rinderpest effectively was often considered to be a measure of the quality of a country's veterinary services. When rinderpest was reintroduced in Belgium it was again eliminated purely by sanitary measures within seven months and without spread to neighbouring countries.

The history of medical prophylaxis (vaccination) against rinderpest also illustrates the evolution of medical thinking (Huygelen, 1997). The Italian Lancisi (1654–1720) wrote very lucidly: 'if such a dreadful disease were to threaten our cattle, I would be in favour of destroying all sick or suspect animals, rather than allowing the contagion to increase simply to gain time in the hope of achieving the honour of discovering a specific remedy, which is often a fruitless quest ...' (Lancisi, 1715; see also Leclainche, 1955; Blancou, 2003; and also Chapter 9).

His contemporaries did not necessarily share this view and Ramazzini was convinced that rinderpest, being a disease similar to smallpox, could be controlled by inoculation (Scott, 1995). This led to a whole series of fruitless inoculation trials. Some clearly stated that it should only be recommended for areas already contaminated, or otherwise run the risk of spreading the disease further. Vicq d'Azyr concluded that: 'inoculation is undesirable since all farm animals die [of it]' (Vicq d'Azyr, 1776, reviewed in Wilkinson, 1992; Cavrot, 1999).

After the discovery by Edward Jenner in 1796 that vaccination could prevent smallpox, pleas for inoculation re-emerged, as exemplified by one from

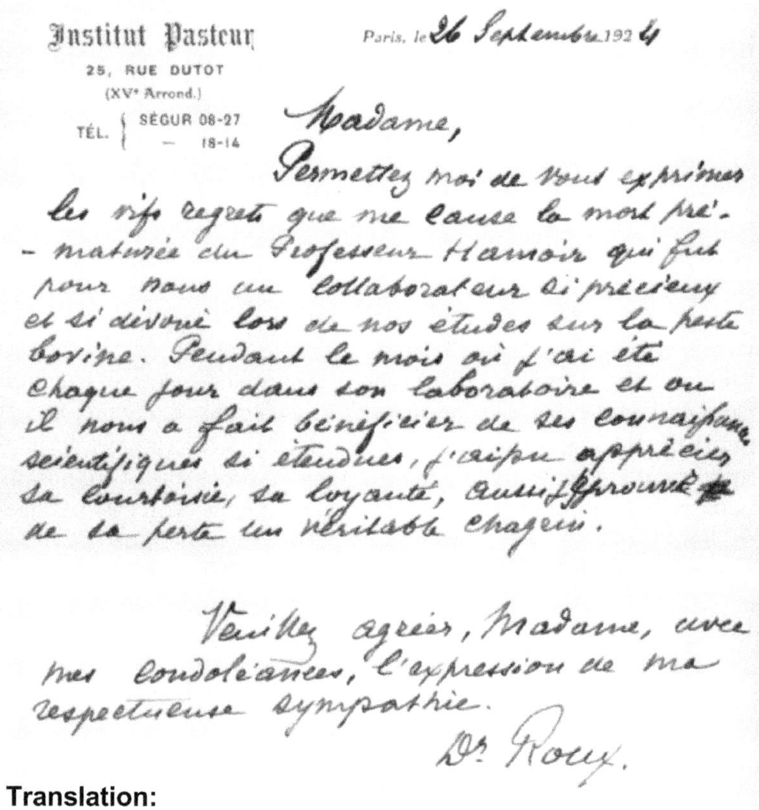

**Institut Pasteur**

25, RUE DUTOT
(XVᵉ Arrond.)

TÉL. { SÉGUR 08-27
       { — 18-14

Paris, le *26 Septembre* 192 *4*

*Madame,*

*Permettez moi de vous exprimer les vifs regrets que me cause la mort pré-maturée du Professeur Hamoir qui fut pour nous un collaborateur si précieux et si dévoué lors de nos études sur la peste bovine. Pendant le mois où j'ai été chaque jour dans son laboratoire et où il nous a fait bénéficier de ses connaissances scientifiques si étendues, j'ai pu apprécier sa courtoisie, sa loyauté, aussi j'éprouve de sa perte un véritable chagrin.*

*Veuillez agréer, Madame, avec mes condoléances, l'expression de ma respectueuse sympathie.*

*Dʳ Roux.*

**Translation:**

Institut Pasteur                               Paris, 26 September 1924

Madam,

Allow me to express my deepest regrets following the untimely death of Professor Hamoir who was for us such a valued and devoted collaborator during our studies on cattle plague. During the month I spent in his laboratory and where we benefited from his broad scientific knowledge, I appreciated his courtesy, his loyalty, I therefore feel a real sorrow at his loss.

Please accept, Madam, with my condolences, the expression of my respectful sympathy.

Dr. Roux

**Figure 1.5**  A letter from Emile Roux (1853–1933) to the widow of Joseph Hamoir (1872–1924) with whom he worked on rinderpest in the veterinary school of Cureghem (Brussels) later to become the Faculty of Veterinary Medicine of the University of Liège. (Courtesy of Prof. Gabriel Hamoir, Liège)

Dr Gottl Rich Frank in 1802:

> Wir müssen also impfen. Das ist eine Wahrheit, die sich uns von allen Seiten aufdringt. Wir müssen impfen, um die Rinderpest zu tödten. Dies ist der einzige sichere Weg auf welchem uns die Hand der Erfahruug leicht und gewiss zum Ziele führt, dies ist der Weg, der die Kunst mit dem höchsten Triumph krönt, dem Triumph, sich die Natur unterwürfig zu machen.

[*Translation:* So we ought to inoculate.* This is the truth, which forces itself upon us from all directions. We ought to inoculate in order to kill Rinderpest. This is the one and only certain way that lends us the hand of experience to achieve this goal swiftly and with certainty. This is the way that crowns the art with the highest of triumphs, the triumph of gaining dominion over nature.]

Attempts were also made using Jenner's vaccine, but finally, in 1865 Henri Bouley (1814–1885) demonstrated the total lack of cross-protection between rinderpest, smallpox and vaccinia thus proving, in the words of Joseph Reynal (1873), 'the utter futility of the doctrine propounding the similarity of these two afflictions'.

These experiments are reminiscent of the unsuccessful attempt by Eusebio Valli (1755–1834) in 1788 to vaccinate humans against human plague by inoculating rinderpest (Giarola *et al.*, 1967). As already mentioned, in 1897 Koch suggested that South African cattle could be protected by subcutaneous injection of blood and bile from an infected animal. This highly dangerous method was soon replaced by the use of immune serum and later by a mixture of immune serum and virulent virus. Subsequently, the technique was improved by serial passages of the bovine virus through goats leading to Edwards' work during the 1920s in India to produce a caprinized vaccine (Curasson, 1932, 1942; Edwards, 1949). Trials with inactivated vaccines also took place (Kakizaki, 1918). Finally, the successful isolation of the virus in cell culture (Plowright and Ferris, 1962; Plowright, 1984) led to the *in vitro* development of an attenuated strain and from this the production of a safe and highly effective vaccine.

## Virus eradication

Smallpox is the first, and to date the only, viral infection to have been eradicated worldwide. This remarkable success was due to several factors, including the availability of an efficacious vaccine (vaccinia virus) the absence of a wildlife reservoir and the fact there was only one serotype of the virus. According to the WHO, eradication of human poliomyelitis and measles may also be possible. The only animal virus diseases which presently share the same

---

*The term *impfen* was then used to describe inoculation, but has evolved into the meaning of vaccination.

characteristics are rinderpest and peste des petits ruminants (see below); there are efficacious vaccines already available for both and the infections seem to be dead-end if transmitted to susceptible wild species (Plowright, 1968; Tillé et al., 1991; Provost, 1992).

Frank Fenner in 1982, in the context of smallpox, listed the characteristics of a disease that allowed its eradication, and these were:

1. It must be an important and 'serious' disease
2. There is the absence of subclinical infection or silent excretion
3. That infected subjects are not contagious during the incubation or pro-dromal period
4. There are no asymptomatic carriers or recurrent access of excretion or disease
5. There is one virus serotype
6. There is an efficacious and stable vaccine available
7. There is seasonal incidence
8. There is no alternative reservoir.

Both rinderpest and peste des petits ruminants fulfil most of these requirements. The Plowright tissue culture vaccine has been used with great success over the past 40 years to vaccinate against rinderpest and has been the major reason behind the success of the global campaigns to eradicate the disease (see Chapter 15). Once rinderpest is eradicated, one could envisage a global programme for the eradication of peste des petits ruminants using a similar strategy.

# A brief history of peste des petits ruminants

The identification of peste des petits ruminants as a separate entity from rinderpest affecting small ruminants in western Africa was another important breakthrough in the history of animal plagues. It was first described in 1942 by Gargadennec and Lalanne working in the Ivory Coast, who identified a disease in goats and sheep similar to rinderpest but which was not transmitted to in-contact cattle. This observation led them to conclude that a disease similar to, but different from, rinderpest existed in small ruminants and they named it 'peste des petits ruminants', now more commonly known as PPR. In 1956 Mornet and collaborators showed that the viruses of rinderpest and PPR were antigenically closely related and in 1979 Gibbs and collaborators classified PPR virus (PPRV) as the fourth member of the morbilliviruses together with rinderpest, measles and distemper viruses, on the basis of its distinct characteristics. In 1962 its causal agent was isolated in sheep cell cultures by Gilbert and Monnier and later the virus was observed by transmission electron microscopy (Bourdin and Laurent-Vautier, 1967).

In many respects PPR has for long lived in the shadow of its big brother rinderpest. Initially, due to the non-availability of an attenuated strain of PPRV, and on the basis of its antigenic similarity with rinderpest virus, trials to vaccinate against PPR were carried out using the rinderpest vaccine (Bourdin *et al.*, 1970). These successful results with the rinderpest vaccine were later confirmed by Taylor and colleagues working in West Africa (Taylor, 1979; Taylor and Abegunde, 1979). In 1989 Diallo and collaborators obtained the first attenuated strain of PPRV by serial passage of the virus in Vero cells which could then be used as a vaccine. In 2004 the entire genomic sequence of PPRV was determined by the group led by Thomas Barrett at the Institute for Animal Health, Pirbright Laboratory (Bailey *et al.*, 2004). We are now at a crucial stage in the rinderpest eradication programme and we must not fail, as we did before in our efforts to eliminate rinderpest from Africa in the 1960s. The predicted global eradication of rinderpest may well result in a renewed interest in PPR as a major disease of farmed ruminants.

# References

Anderson, R.M. and May, R.M. (1983) Vaccination against rubella and measles: quantitative investigations of different policies. *J. Hyg. (Cambr.)* **90**, 259–325.

Bailey, D., Banyard, A., Dash, P., Ozkul, A. and Barrett, T. (2004) Full genome sequence of Peste des Petits Ruminants virus, a member of the Morbillivirus genus. *Virus Res.* **110**, 119–24.

Barrett, T. and Rossiter, P.B. (1999) Rinderpest: the disease and its impact on humans and animals. *Adv. Virus Res.* **53**, 89–110.

Beijerinck, M.W. (1898) Über ein Contagium vivum fluidum als Ursache der Fleckenkrankheit der Tabaksbläter. *Zentralbl. Bakt. Parasitkunde*, Abt. II., **5, 27**.

Black, F.L. (1991) Epidemiology of *Paramyxoviridae.* In: D.W. Kingsbury (ed.), *The Paramyxoviruses*. New York and London: Plenum Press.

Blancou, J. (2003) *Histoire de la surveillance et du contrôle des maladies animales transmissibles.* Paris: Office International des Epizooties.

Bourdin, P. and Laurent-Vautier, A. (1967) Note sur la structure du virus de la peste des petits ruminants. *Rev. Elev. Méd. Vét. Pays Trop.* **20**, 383–6.

Bourdin, P., Rioche, M. and Laurent, A. (1970) Emploi d'un vaccin anti-bovipestique produit sur cultures cellulaires dans la prophylaxie de la peste des petits ruminants au Dahomey. *Rev. Elev. Méd. Vét. Pays Trop.* **23**, 295–300.

Cavrot, C. (1999) *La Participation d'un académicien F. Vicq d'Azyr à la résolution de l'épizootie de 1774.* Nantes: Faculté. de Médecine.

Curasson, G. (1932) *La Peste bovine.* Paris, Vigot Frères.

Curasson, G. (1942) *Traité de pathologie exotique vétérinaire et comparée,* Volume 1. Paris: Vigot Frères, p. 13.

Danysz, J. and Bordet, J. (1898) Rapport sur les recherches concernant la peste bovine. *Bull. Agric.*, 14, 77–88.

Dawtrey-Drewitt, F. (1931) *The notebook of Edward Jenner in the possession of the Royal College of Physicians of London, with an introduction on Jenner's work as a naturalist.by F. Dawtrey-Drewitt.* London: Oxford University Press, pp. 47–9.

Diallo, A., Taylor, W.P., Lefèvre, P.C. and Provost, A. (1989) Atténuation d'une souche de virus de la peste des petits ruminants: candidat pour un vaccin homologue vivant. *Rev. Elev. Méd. Vét. Pays Trop.* **42**, 311–19.

Dieckerhoff, W. (1890) *Geschichte der Rinderpest und ihrer Literatur.* Berlin: Verlag von Th. Chr. Fr. Enslin.

Edwards, J.T. (1949) The uses and limitations of the caprinized virus in the control of rinderpest (cattle plague) among British and near-Eastern cattle. *Br. Vet. J.* **105** (7), 209–53.

Fenner, F. (1982) A successful eradication campaign: global eradication of smallpox. *Rev. Infect. Dis.* **4**, 916–30.

Fleming, G. (1871) *Animal Plagues: Their History, Nature and Prevention.* London: Chapman & Hall.

Galen (AD *c.*129–200) (1936) *Commentaires aux Épidémies d'Hippocrate,* III, 21. Leipzig and Berlin: E. Wenkebach, Teubner, p. 120, II. 11–13 (*Corpus Medicorum Graecorum, V,* 10, 2, 1).

Gargadennec, L. and Lalanne, A. (1942) La peste des petits ruminants. *Bull. Serv. Zootech. Epiz. Afr. Occid. Franc.* **5**, 16–21.

Giarola, A., Cantoni, M. and Magnone, E. (1967) La dottrina esogena delle infezioni dall antichita aigiomi nostri – Xᵉ – Un grande tropicalista ed epidemiologo de '700', Eusebio Valli. *Riv. Ital. di med. e Igiene della Scuola,* XIII, fas II, 191–9.

Gibbs, E.P.J., Taylor, W.P., Lawman, M.P.J. and Bryant, J. (1979) Classification of peste des petits ruminants virus as the fourth member of the genus morbillivirus. *Intervirology* **11**, 268–74.

Gilbert, Y. and Monnier, J. (1962) Adaptation du virus de la peste des petits ruminants aux cultures cellulaires. *Rev. Elev. Méd. Vét. Pays Trop.* **15**, 321–35.

Gottl Rich Frank (Dr) (1802) *Ueber die Rinderpest und die Mittel sie zu heilen und auszurotten.* Berlin, s. 167.

Huygelen, C. (1997) The early history of immunisation against three morbillivirus diseases: measles, rinderpest and canine distemper. *Hist. Med. Vet.* **22**, 21–2.

Ivanowski, D.I. (1903) Über die mosaik-krankheit der tabakpflanze. *Z. Pflanzenkrankh* **13**, 1.

Kakizaki, C. (1918) Study of the glycerinated rinderpest vaccine. *Kitasato Arch. Exp. Med.* **2**, 59–66.

Koch, R. (1891) Uber bakteriologische Forschung. Verhandlungen des X Internationalen Medicinis chen Congresses. Berlin, 4–9 August 1890. Band I. Allgemeiner Theil. Berlin: Verlag von August Hirschwald, pp. 35–47.

Koch, R. (1897) Researches into the cause of the cattle plague. *Br. Med. J.* **i**, 1245–6.

Lancisi, G.M. (1715) *Dissertatio historica de bovilla peste, ex campaniae finibus anno MDCCXIll Latio importata.* Rome: Ex Typographia Joannis Mariae Salvioni.

Leclainche, E. (1955) *Histoire illustrée de la médecine vétérinaire,* Vol. II. Paris: Albin Michel.

Löffler, F. and Frösch, P. (1897) Summarischer Bericht über die Ergebnisse der Untersuchungen zur Erforschung der Maul-und klauenseuche. *Zentralbl. Bakt.,* Abt. I., Orig. **22**, 257.

Mammerickx, M. (2003) La peste bovine, Jules Bordet et le Centre Sérumigène de Cureghem. *Ann. Méd. Vét.* **147**, 197–205.

Mornet, P., Orue, J., Gilbert, Y., Thiery, G. and Sow, M. (1956) La peste des petits ruminants en Afrique occidentale française. Ses rapports avec la peste bovine. *Rev. Elev. Méd. Vét. Pays Trop.* **9**, 313–42.

Nicolle, M. and Adil-Bey, M. (1902) Etudes sur la peste bovine (3ᵉᵐᵉ mémoire). *Ann. Institut Pasteur* **16**, 50–67.

Norrby, E., Sheshberadaran, H., McCullough, K.C., Carpenter, W.C. and Örvell, C. (1985) Is rinderpest virus the archevirus of the morbillivirus genus? *Intervirology* **23**, 228–32.

Pastoret, P.P. (1986) La peste bovine et la profession vétérinaire. In: P.P. Pastoret, F. Mees and M. Mammerickx, De l'art à la science ou 150 ans de médecine vétérinaire à Cureghem. *Ann. Méd. Vét.* pp. 117–22.

Pastoret, P.P., Thiry, E., Brochier, B., Schwers, A., Thomas, I. and Dubuisson, J. (1988) Diseases of wild animals transmissible to domestic animals. *Rev. Sci. Tech. Off. Int. Epizoot.* **7** (4), 705–36.

Plowright, W. (1968) Rinderpest virus. *Virol. Monogr.* **3**, 25–110.

Plowright, W. (1982) The effects of rinderpest and rinderpest control on wildlife in Africa. *Symp. Zool. Soc. Lond.* **50**, 1–28.

Plowright, W. (1984) The duration of immunity in cattle following inoculation of rinderpest cell culture vaccine. *J. Hyg. (Camb.)* **92**, 285–96.

Plowright, W. and Ferris, R.D. (1962) Studies with rinderpest virus in tissue culture. The use of attenuated culture virus as a vaccine for cattle. *Res. Vet. Sci.* **3**, 172–82.

Provost, A. (1992) Global eradication of rinderpest. Discussion document: Expert Consultation on Strategy for the Global Rinderpest Eradication Programme, FAO, Rome, 27–29 October.

Reynal, J. (1873) *Traité de police sanitaire des animaux domestiques.* Paris: Asselin.

Semmer, E. (1893) Über das Rinderpestcontagium und über Immunisierung und Schutzimfung gegen Rinderpest. *Berl. Tierarztl. Wochenschr.* **23**, 590–1.

Scott, G.R. (1995) The history of rinderpest in Britain. Part 1: 809–1799. *State Vet. J.* **6** (4), 8–10.

Spinage, C.A. (2003) *Cattle Plague – A History.* New York: Kluwer.

Taylor, W.P. (1979) Protection of goats against peste des petits ruminants with attenuated rinderpest virus. *Res. Vet. Sci.* **27**, 321–4.

Taylor, W.P. and Abegunde, A. (1979) The isolation of peste des petits ruminants virus from Nigerian sheep and goats. *Res. Vet. Sci.* **26**, 94–6.

Third report of the Commissioners appointed to inquire into the origin and nature etc. of the cattle plague with an appendix. Printed by George Edward Eyre and William Spottiswoode, London, 1866.

Tillé, A., Lefèvre, P.C., Pastoret, P.P. and Thiry, E. (1991) A mathematical model of rinderpest infection in cattle populations. *Epidemiol. Infect.* **107**, 441–52.

Vicq d'Azyr (1776) *Exposé des moyens curatifs et préservatifs qui peuvent être employés contre les maladies pestilentielles des bêtes à cornes.* Paris: Merigot.

Wilkinson, L. (1984) Rinderpest and mainstream infectious disease concepts in the eighteenth century. *Med. Hist.* **28**, 129–50.

Wilkinson, L. (1992) *Animals and Disease. An Introduction to the History of Comparative Medicine.* Cambridge: Cambridge University Press.

Yersin, A. (1898) Expériences sur la peste bovine. *Bull. Économ. Indochine* **2**, 245.

Yersin, A. (1904) Etudes sur quelques épizooties de l'Indochine. *Ann. Institut Pasteur*, **18** (7), 417–49.

Yersin, A., Carré, C., Fraimbault (1899) Traitement de la peste bovine. *Ann. Hyg. Méd Coloniales* **2**, 175–82.

# The morbilliviruses

# 2

## ASHLEY C. BANYARD,* BERTUS K. RIMA†AND THOMAS BARRETT*

*Institute for Animal Health, Pirbright Laboratory, Surrey, UK
†School of Biomedical Sciences, Medical Biology Centre, The Queen's University, Belfast, UK

## Introduction

The members of the genus *Morbillivirus*, classified within the order Mononegavirales, family *Paramyxoviridae*, sub-family *Paramyxovirinae* (Figure 2.1), are responsible for some of the most devastating diseases of humans and animals. Measles virus (MV) is considered the type virus for this genus, the name of which is derived from *morbilli*, the diminutive form of the Latin word for plague (*morbus*). This name was originally used to distinguish measles from smallpox and scarlet fever, which in former times were considered more serious diseases (Carmichael, 1997). In addition to MV, other morbilliviruses that infect terrestrial mammals include rinderpest virus (RPV), which causes cattle plague, peste des petits ruminants virus (PPRV), the cause of sheep and goat plague, and canine distemper virus (CDV), which infects many carnivore species, including domestic dogs, mink and ferrets and can have serious consequences when endangered wildlife species are threatened (Laurenson *et al.*, 1998). Morbilliviruses have also been isolated from a diverse range of marine species and over the past 17 years epizootics of these marine morbilliviruses have caused mass die-offs, mainly of seals and dolphins, in widely dispersed locations (Barrett and Rima, 2002; Barrett *et al.*, 2003). This chapter reviews these viruses in general terms and examines the possible evolutionary relationships between them.

ISBN-13: 978-0-12-88385-1
ISBN-10: 0-12-88385-6

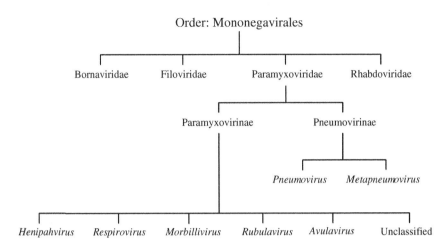

**Figure 2.1**    Classification of the Order Mononegavirales.

## Measles virus

The earliest descriptions of measles date back to Arab writings of the tenth century AD. The fact that Hippocrates did not mention the disease amongst his otherwise careful and accurate description of childhood diseases has been interpreted as evidence that the disease was not present in early human populations. However, at that time measles was often confused with other diseases, such as smallpox and scarlet fever. When MV and other virus diseases such as influenza and smallpox were taken from Europe to the Americas and the Pacific Islands, they wreaked havoc in the indigenous populations, which had no previous exposure to them (Carmichael, 1997). Despite the availability of an effective vaccine, MV remains a major cause of childhood mortality in the developing world, where it is estimated that up to a million children die each year (Sabin, 1992). Vaccination has, however, reduced the number of measles cases by about 75% worldwide, with perhaps as many as 7–8 million childhood deaths occurring annually before the introduction of the current live attenuated vaccines and global eradication campaign coordinated by the WHO (Wild *et al.*, 2000; see also Chapter 14). As well as being a significant human pathogen, MV can infect many primate species, including the great apes, but the virus can only be maintained in human populations. As a result, human encroachment into the habitats of such primate species through tourism or for illegal poaching activities may cause transmission of MV which could further threaten these endangered species.

# Rinderpest

Since the bulk of this volume is devoted to rinderpest only a very brief overview of this virus will be given in this chapter. Rinderpest or cattle plague is one of the oldest recognized diseases of cattle and buffalo, with descriptions dating back to late Roman times (Barton, 1956). The devastation that followed the path of the virus as it swept across the African and Asian continents hitting naive populations of animals and the consequent famines it caused are chronicled historically (Barrett and Rossiter, 1999; see also Chapter 5). The ability to prevent and effectively control rinderpest incursions is considered to be a measure of the effectiveness of a country's veterinary service. The major factor blocking global eradication is the continuation of conflicts in the remaining enzootic region (see Chapter 15). Whilst considered to be a disease of bovids, it has been shown that Asian, but not African, strains of RPV can productively infect sheep and goats, whilst the threat of RPV to general wildlife species is also significant. In experimental infections of sheep and goats the infected animals show only mild clinical signs of disease but are capable of passing the infection to cattle (Ata and Singh, 1967; Anderson *et al.*, 1990).

# Peste des petits ruminants virus

Peste des petits ruminants virus (PPRV) was first identified in West Africa in the early 1940s (Gargadennec and Lalanne, 1942) and was initially thought to be a variant of RPV adapted to small ruminants. Subsequently, however, it was shown to be an antigenically and genetically distinct virus (Gibbs *et al.*, 1979; Diallo *et al.*, 1989). Only limited resources are currently directed to solving the problem of PPR. The disease has become increasingly important economically as a consequence of the success of the rinderpest eradication campaign, PPR being detected more in the absence of RPV, especially in Asia where rinderpest strains were known to infect small ruminants (Anderson *et al.*, 1990). Although PPRV was first discovered in Africa, this may not be its original source, bearing in mind that RPV is of Asiatic origin. The presence of RPV throughout western and southern Asia until the mid-1990s may have concealed the existence of PPRV with subsequent elimination of rinderpest from these areas showing that PPRV is, and had been, present. Easy and rapid differentiation between RPV and PPRV has been made possible by the development of specific and sensitive molecular and serological techniques that can distinguish between these viruses genetically, antigenically and serologically (see Chapter 10). PPRV first appeared as a recognized disease in Asia in the late 1980s and has now been found across the Middle East and the Indian subcontinent, reaching as far as Nepal and Bangladesh (Nanda *et al.*, 1996; Dhar *et al.*, 2002). The wide distribution of PPRV in southern Asia suggests that the virus had been present for some time on the Asian continent before it was first identified in India in 1989 (Shaila *et al.*, 1989, 1996). The full host range of this virus is unknown but several species of antelope have been fatally infected by contact with infected sheep and goats (Furley *et al.*, 1987; Abu Elzein *et al.*, 2004). Indian buffalo (*Bos gaur*) have also been reported to have died from PPRV infections (Govindarajan *et al.*, 1997). Cattle that are seropositive for PPRV have been found in West Africa, with up to 80% prevalence in some herds, but there is no evidence that it can cause disease in bovids (Anderson and McKay, 1994).

The current global situation regarding the endemicity of this disease means that its control is one of the main targets of the FAO's Emergency Preventive System (EMPRES) programme. The attainment of this goal depends on the diagnostic facilities and research programmes carried out at the United Nations Food and Agriculture Organisation's (UN-FAO) national and regional laboratories and at the World Reference Laboratory for Morbilliviruses at the Institute for Animal Health. Sheep and goats are the most seriously affected by PPRV and these are now considered to be economically more important than cattle in the poorer pastoral systems of South-East Asia, South Asia and sub-Saharan Africa. PPRV threatens the production of these two species and thus from an economic and social perspective is of great importance. Only with continued funding from the international community will the control, and possible elimination, of this disease be achieved. Such international support has the potential to impact significantly on the livelihoods of the poor in those countries where the disease is endemic as well as protect those areas currently free of this devastating disease (Perry *et al.*, 2002).

## Canine distemper virus

Canine distemper kills the majority of unvaccinated dogs that become infected and those that survive often suffer long-term neurological sequelae (Appel, 1987). The causative agent of this disease, CDV, was initially thought to be restricted in its host range to members of the *Canidae, Ursidae, Mustelidae* and *Viverridae,* as well as the collared peccary, a member of the order Artiodactyla (Appel *et al.*, 1991). However, more recently CDV has been isolated from members of the Felidae and Hyaenidae, causing mortalities in several species of large cat in American zoos in the 1990s, including lion, leopard and tiger (Appel *et al.*, 1994; Harder *et al.*, 1996) as well as being associated with the deaths of lions and hyenas in the Serengeti Plains in Tanzania (Harder *et al.*, 1995; Haas *et al.*, 1996; Roelke-Parker *et al.*, 1996). At first it was thought that these deaths signalled the emergence of a new cat-adapted biotype of the virus or that co-infection with another virus, possibly feline immunodeficiency virus (FIV), a disease prevalent in African big cats, might have exacerbated the disease in the lions. However, it is now clear that local strains of CDV were responsible for the deaths on the two continents and no correlation could be found between the presence of FIV or any other viruses and the mortality seen in lions (Roelke-Parker *et al.*, 1996). A retrospective study on *postmortem* tissues from large cats that died from unknown causes in Swiss zoos between 1972 and 1992 found that 45% had CDV-specific antigen in their tissues (Myers *et al.*, 1997), indicating that CDV has caused fatal infections in large cats for much longer than was suspected. Failure to recognize the disease earlier in these species was probably due to a lack of awareness of a possible viral aetiology.

Transmission of CDV to zoo animals is most likely to occur through contact with wild carnivores that can freely enter and come into close proximity with them. In one instance a virus sample isolated from a wild racoon was found to be very closely related at the nucleotide level to a virus isolated from a lion held captive in an American zoo. Infection in the Serengeti lions and hyenas was probably due to contact with sympatric dogs infected with the virus (Roelke-Parker *et al.*, 1996). A similar threat is posed by contact with domestic dogs carrying rabies virus to African wild hunting dogs and the Ethiopian wolf, two of the world's most endangered canids (Gascoyne *et al.*, 1993; Laurenson *et al.*, 1998). The populations of unvaccinated domestic dogs in Africa have risen dramatically in recent years providing a ready source of infection for wildlife.

CDV infection is not confined to hosts in the terrestrial environment and has been shown to cause a significant number of deaths in seals (Pinnipedia), which form a sub-order within the order Carnivora. In the winter of 1987–88 the population of Lake Baikal seals (*Phoca sibirica*) suffered an unusual and severe mortality. Nucleotide sequence analysis later confirmed that the agent involved was CDV, rather than phocine distemper virus (PDV) which was then affecting European seals (discussed later in this chapter). The virus was most likely transmitted to the seals through interaction with infected animals on land at haulout sites (Grachev *et al.*, 1989; Visser *et al.*, 1990). Outbreaks of CDV are common in the large number of feral and domestic dogs around the lake and seal hunting brings the seals into close contact with man and dogs. Other possible vectors of the virus for seals included wolves, ferrets, mink and bears that also inhabit areas surrounding the lake.

Similarly, CDV was found in Caspian seals (*Phoca caspica*) during the summer of 1997, and again in 2000 (Forsyth *et al.*, 1998; Kennedy *et al.*, 2000). Although not confirmed, the source of the virus is likely to have been terrestrial carnivores, such as wolves, which prey on seal pups. The seals of the Caspian Sea are now critically endangered and, as well as being threatened by CDV infections, they are at risk from hunting for meat. Furthermore, they have suffered a reduction in breeding efficiency due to high concentrations of toxic pollutants such as DDT in their environment (Allchin *et al.*, 1997). CDV infection has also been documented in captive seals (Lyons *et al.*, 1993; Barrett *et al.*, 2003). A severe die-off of crabeater seals (*Lobodon carcinophagus*) in

Antarctica in the 1950s can, with hindsight, be linked to CDV infection although at the time the deaths were attributed to an uncharacterized acute viral infection. In this case, the infection occurred near a scientific field station that kept unvaccinated sledge dogs (Laws and Taylor, 1957). As there are no terrestrial carnivores in the Antarctic, the dogs were the most probable source of infection. Another explanation could be transmission by direct contact with terrestrial carnivores in New Zealand or South America during seal migrations. Whatever the source, the virus appears to have established itself in the very extensive crabeater seal population as a subsequent serological survey of Antarctic seals showed this species to have a high prevalence of CDV-specific antibodies (Bengtson et al., 1991).

## Phocine distemper virus

Morbilliviruses have also been isolated from marine mammals, including members of the family *Pinnipedia* (seals) and the order *Cetacea* (whales, porpoises and dolphins) (Barrett and Rima, 2002). The first morbillivirus with potentially severe ecological consequences for marine mammals was identified in harbour (*Phoca vitulina*) and grey (*Halichoerus grypus*) seals that died in large numbers off the coasts of northern Europe in 1988 (Osterhaus and Vedder, 1988). This epizootic killed more than 20 000 seals around northern European coasts, the majority being harbour seals. At first, based on clinical and antigenic similarities, the seal virus was thought to be CDV, the main pathological feature being acute interstitial pneumonia (see Figure 2.2). The resulting interest in these novel infections in marine mammals meant that molecular resources were employed to characterize the new virus. It was then quickly shown that this new seal virus was most closely related to, but distinct from, CDV and was classified as a new member of the *morbillivirus* genus and named *phocine distemper virus* (PDV) (Cosby et al., 1988; Mahy et al., 1988; Haas et al., 1991).

The migration patterns of seals allow the virus to be carried over long distances and transmitted to naive seal populations, as was seen in the 1988 epizootic which began on the Danish island of Anholt in the Kattegat before spreading to Sweden, the Netherlands, Norway, Germany, the UK and Ireland (Jauniaux et al., 2001). In 2002 another PDV epizootic occurred in European seals which followed an almost identical course to that of the 1988 outbreak, starting at the end of April and again being first detected on the island of Anholt with a population of approximately 12 000 harbour seals (Barrett et al., 2003). A month later the virus had spread from the initial focus in the Kattegat through the Skagerrak and then into the Dutch Wadden Sea and the North Sea. In the UK, as in 1988, the first PDV-positive harbour seal was identified in The Wash in April. By mid August harbour seal mortalities of epizootic proportions were seen that by mid-September had peaked with almost 400 seals being washed up

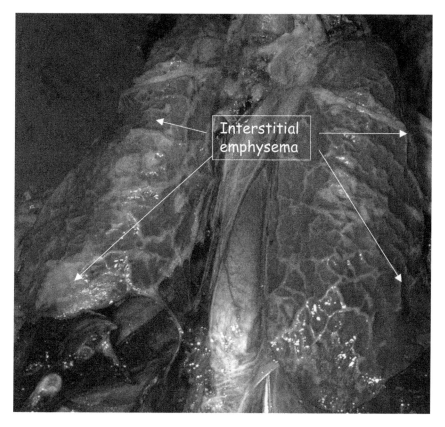

**Figure 2.2** Interstitial pneumonia in a seal necropsied during the 2002 PDV epizootic in Europe.

dead each week. The virus then spread to Scotland, being first identified in a harbour seal found in Dornoch in the Moray Firth. Soon afterwards a small number of dead seals were found in Northern Ireland and along the west coast of Ireland where laboratory tests confirmed the presence of PDV. However, no PDV positives were found in seal samples taken along the Welsh coast (see Figure 2.3). Further PDV-positive harbour and grey seals were subsequently identified in east and west Scotland (including Orkney) in late 2002, although, unlike 1988, no noticeable increase in mortality was apparent. The total death toll in European waters eventually reached over 22 000 seals (Reineking, 2003). The source of virus for the 2002 outbreak of PDV was, as in 1988, most likely due to contact with infected Arctic seals (Dietz *et al.*, 1989). Between these two epizootics a minor disease outbreak occurred in 1998 in seals along the Belgian and northern French coasts and morbillivirus antigen and nucleic acid were detected in tissues from sick animals but molecular analyses showed that these

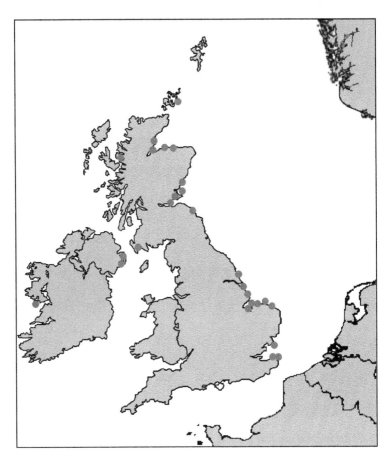

**Figure 2.3**   Locations of PDV-related deaths in seals in the British Isles during the 2002 PDV outbreak.

animals were infected with either a cetacean morbillivirus, discussed in more detail below, or CDV (Jauniaux *et al.*, 2001; El Mjiyad *et al.*, 2002).

The source of the virus in both European epizootics was probably Arctic harp seals (*Phoca groenlandica*), which had been seen further south than usual in the winter before the 1988 epizootic (Dietz *et al.*, 1989). Between the epizootics antibody was detected in the serum of seal pups after the disappearance of maternal antibody indicating that the animals were still exposed to PDV for some time after 1988 though no disease was observed (referred to in Hall, 1995). However, the virus could not, and was not, maintained in the European seals from 1988 to 2002 because of their small population sizes and their scattered distribution. Morbilliviruses such as measles and rinderpest need a constant supply of naive hosts to maintain endemic infection since lifelong immunity to the virus develops in survivors (Black, 1991). The course of the PDV epizootic both in 1988 and 2002, starting off the Danish coast, moving to the Dutch coast and then into English coastal waters before finally moving to Scotland and Ireland, may be explained by the susceptibility, migratory patterns and/or breeding habits of the seals. There is growing consensus among some seal biologists that the grey seal populations may act as key vectors in the transmission of PDV between colonies of harbour seals in European waters, especially where large geographical distances are concerned. Harbour seals are known to frequent and return to specific haulout sites whereas grey seals are known to move much greater distances between haulout sites (McConnell *et al.*, 1999). Virus transmission is unlikely to occur readily in water as close contact between animals is generally required to facilitate aerosol transmission. Therefore, interactions between the different species at haulout sites may be the key to determining how the epizootics progress. Another important factor may be the relative resistance of grey seals to clinical disease with this virus, possibly enabling PDV to circulate without necessarily causing high mortality, or even showing clinical disease.

Retrospective analyses of archival sera obtained from Arctic seals taken long before the first European PDV outbreak in 1988 support the theory that the European PDV infections originated from infected Arctic harp seals as PDV antibodies were found in a high proportion of the archival seal sera from Canadian waters (Henderson *et al.*, 1992; Ross *et al.*, 1992).

Harp seal populations, with an estimated 4 million individuals in Canadian waters alone, are certainly large enough to maintain PDV in circulation. The full host range of PDV is unknown, as are the molecular factors that govern the pathogenic potential of PDV infection in different seal populations, and the virus can cause severe disease in some species whilst other species suffer only mild, subclinical infection (Duignan *et al.*, 1997; Barrett *et al.*, 1998).

Coordinated efforts between the various animal health institutes, governmental agencies, private rescue charities and welfare organizations dealing with marine wildlife diseases meant that the 2002 European PDV epizootic was efficiently dealt with once the virus had been confirmed as causing the seal deaths on Anholt. The various official bodies concerned and the hundreds of volunteers who helped locate the dead seals made monitoring of the epizootic and collection of samples much easier than in the 1988 outbreak, with the networks set up to deal with the previous epizootic being easily re-activated to report on sightings of dead or dying seals and transfer infected animals to quarantine facilities in sanctuaries.

## Cetacean morbilliviruses

Morbilliviruses have been isolated from several cetacean species including the porpoise morbillivirus (PMV) and dolphin morbillivirus (DMV) (Kennedy *et al.*, 1988; Domingo *et al.*, 1990). Large die-offs of cetaceans observed on a number of occasions over the past 15 years have been caused by these viruses. DMV was responsible for the death of thousands of striped dolphins (*Stenella coeruleoalba*) in the Mediterranean sea between 1990 and 1992 (Domingo *et al.*, 1990; Van Bressem *et al.*, 2001), whilst PMV caused mortalities in harbour porpoises along the coasts of the Netherlands and Ireland between 1988 and 1990 (McCullough *et al.*, 1991; Visser *et al.*, 1993) and fatal epizootics in bottlenose dolphins (*Tursiops truncatus*) from the northwestern Atlantic ocean in the late 1980s and the early 1990s (Lipscomb *et al.*, 1996; Duignan *et al.*, 1996). Due to the difficulty in obtaining good quality samples and good estimates of population size from wild cetaceans the effect of these viruses at the population level is unknown. Because of their close sequence relationship, DMV and PMV are considered variants of the same virus (Barrett *et al.*, 1993), much the same as the variation seen with rinderpest and PPR viruses (see Chapter 8), and together are now referred to as cetacean morbillivirus (CeMV) (Bolt *et al.*, 1994). Also they are not confined to one host species and a virus more closely related to PMV has been isolated from dolphins (Taubenberger *et al.*, 1996). There is now serological evidence for CeMV infection in all of the world's major oceans; the north and south-west Atlantic, the east, west and south-west Pacific and the Indian oceans (Van Bressem *et al.*, 1998, 2001).

Questions remain as to the enzootic source of this virus and the likely vector species. Suspicion has fallen on the pilot whale (*Globicephala* spp.) in both categories. Pilot whale populations have many of the characteristics required of a reservoir and vector for CeMV; they move in large groups (pods), have a widespread pelagic distribution and are known to associate with many different cetacean species. Long finned pilot whales are commonly seen in the Western Mediterranean where the 1990 dolphin epizootic was first observed and a high proportion of pilot whales sampled in the mid 1990s showed evidence of infection. Over 90% of pilot whales that were involved in mass strandings between 1982 and 1993 were morbillivirus seropositive (Duignan *et al.*, 1995a, b). Most samples from cetaceans have only been characterized using RT-PCR and limited sequencing data and so it is important to try to obtain more virus isolates from regions remote from Europe to study the extent of variation within this virus type.

## Morbillivirus host range

The factors determining the barriers to host species jumps by morbilliviruses are unknown. CDV appears to be able to jump from species to species successfully (Harder and Osterhaus, 1997). There is also evidence to link CeMV with mortalities in seals (Van de Bildt *et al.*, 2000). However, Mediterranean monk seals were not severely affected during the 1990–1992 epizootic which killed thousands of striped dolphins in that region, despite the fact that CeMV was isolated from the monk seals (Osterhaus *et al.*, 1992). The numbers of this once common species have declined alarmingly in the past 100 years as a result of hunting.

Now the additional pressure of virus infection threatens. A mass die-off of monk seals off the coast of Mauritania in 1997 was associated with CeMV infection (van de Bildt *et al.*, 2000), although an algal bloom might have been an exacerbating or a primary factor in the very high mortality among adult seals at that time (Hernandez *et al.*, 1998). It was estimated that 70% of the population died within the space of one month, a figure representing about one-third of the total world population, leaving only a few hundred animals alive (Harwood, 1998). The monk seals would likely be highly susceptible to PDV or CDV infections (Osterhaus *et al.*, 1992) and another mass die-off, from whatever cause, would certainly be enough to be wipe out the remaining population. Infection without overt disease probably also occurred in manatees (order Sirenia) living off the Florida coast which were found to be serologically positive for CeMV but no unusual mortality that could be virus-related has been reported (Duignan *et al.*, 1995c).

# Evolutionary relationships

The very high level of antigenic relatedness and sequence similarity seen between the different morbilliviruses indicates that they all evolved from a common ancestor. Rinderpest has been proposed as the 'archevirus' of the morbillivirus group since it reacts with a wide range of monoclonal antibodies produced against other morbilliviruses (Norrby *et al.*, 1985). However, this proposal was made when several of the morbiliviruses had not yet been identified and PPRV was thought to be closely related or simply a different manifestation of RPV. The phylogenetic relationships between the different morbilliviruses are shown in Figure 2.4. This tree diagram based on the nucleotide sequence of the nucleocapsid proteins indicates that CeMV, RPV and PPRV are equidistant from each other and that none of the currently circulating morbilliviruses is likely to represent the 'archaevirus'. Similar analyses on the other proteins give the same results. It needs to be stressed however that in the context of rapidly evolving RNA viruses these distances do not imply times since divergence. MV and RPV are closely related but not as closely as CDV and PDV, which together form an outlying group. The evolution of this group of viruses is the subject of a great deal of speculation. Animal populations of the size needed to produce the constant supply of susceptible naive hosts required for a morbillivirus to survive would most likely have been large herds of Asian ruminants, the historic source of rinderpest infection. For MV the minimum population size that satisfies this condition has been estimated to be about 300 000 people, but this may be smaller for animals that produce greater litters every year. MV is genetically closest to RPV and it is possible that, when man settled in sufficiently large communities to maintain a morbillivirus, close contact with infected cattle resulted in rinderpest, or a rinderpest-like infection, being passed to humans. Such a virus may then have evolved to become MV by acquiring pathogenic characteristics for man and other primates and losing them for ruminants.

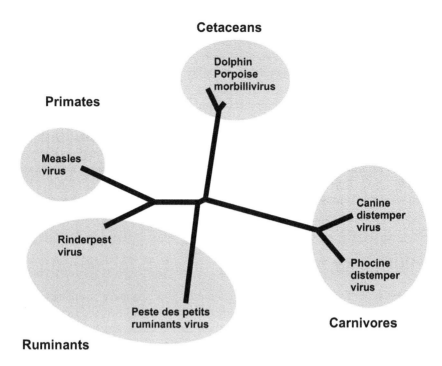

**Figure 2.4**   Phylogenetic tree showing the relationships between the different morbilliviruses based on the coding sequence for the nucleocapsid (N) protein gene. The bar represents nucleotide changes per position. The trees were derived using the PHYLIP DNADIST and FITCH programmes. The branch lengths are proportional to the genetic distances between the viruses and the hypothetical common ancestor that existed at the nodes in the tree.

Accession numbers: measles virus: 9301B strain (AB012948); RPV: Kabete 'O' strain (X98291); CDV: Onderstepoort strain (AF305419); PPRV: Sungri/96 strain (AY560591); PDV: isolate (<u>D10371</u>); DMV/PMV: isolate (AJ608288).

Carnivores of various species preying on infected ruminants may similarly have become infected with the progenitor virus and subsequently this virus could have evolved to produce CDV. The two morbilliviruses of carnivores, CDV and PDV, are very closely related and it is probable that PDV evolved from CDV. Arctic seals may have been infected with CDV several hundreds (or several thousands) of years ago by contact with terrestrial carnivores such as wolves, foxes, dogs and polar bears, which can carry the virus.

PDV and CDV are not exclusively confined to marine and terrestrial mammals, respectively, as evidenced by the many reports of CDV in seals and there is also a report showing that PDV caused a distemper-like infection in mink in Denmark at a farm in the immediate vicinity of diseased seals (Blixenkrone-Møller *et al.*,

1990) and there is evidence for PDV- and CeMV-specific antibodies in a variety of terrestrial carnivores in Canada (Philippa *et al.*, 2004). The fact that the two ruminant morbilliviruses, RPV and PPRV, are not closely related emphasizes that narratives about the direction of evolution of these viruses are highly speculative. Similar arguments also apply to speculation about the origin of CeMV. There appears now to be no natural contact between cetacean species and terrestrial species although contact between terrestrial carnivores and stranded cetaceans is possible. Sequence comparisons with other morbilliviruses suggest that CeMV is most closely related to PPRV at the protein level (Visser *et al.*, 1993; Haffar *et al.*, 1999; Bailey *et al.*, 2005). Interpretation of this, especially as these viruses are considered to be evolving rapidly, is difficult and this similarity may just be due to chance. However, given the great sequence diversity, CeMV is less likely to have evolved directly from either PDV or CDV.

It is possible, with increasing awareness of the importance of these viruses for animal diseases, that other morbilliviruses will be found in the future and techniques are now available which will allow their rapid identification and characterization.

## Control strategies

The existence of only one serotype for each of the morbilliviruses suggests that control of these viruses should be straightforward. However, individual strains are able to cause a wide spectrum of disease in different species as well as between individual animals of the same species. This effectively means that as yet there is no true distinction between mild and pathogenic strains which in turn makes detection and subsequently control of these viruses difficult. Furthermore, viruses carried by humans and domestic animals can threaten wildlife, particularly where highly endangered species are concerned, and control by vaccination of domestic animals and preventing or limiting contact is the most effective way of ensuring that wildlife will be safeguarded. The development of live attenuated vaccines was the key to achieving success in controlling diseases such as MV, CDV and RPV since, as with natural infection, the immunity they induce is long-lived and involves a cell-mediated immune response. However, even with a good vaccine, the control of wildlife diseases is extremely difficult and vaccination of wild animal populations is not only logistically very difficult but is also ethically questionable due to the potential uncontrolled spread of the vaccine virus and the potential disturbance caused which may be very harmful to the animal's well being. Protection of vulnerable animals, such as large cats, ferrets and pandas in zoos and seals in sanctuaries, would probably be more acceptable as the animals are confined and would not, if planned, be released until the excretion of vaccine virus had ceased. In any event, there are no currently licensed vaccines for use in these species.

The close antigenic relationship between morbilliviruses means that strong cross-protection to infection is given by vaccines for other morbilliviruses and an experimental CDV-ISCOM vaccine can protect seals from PDV although duration of the immunity is unknown and may only be short-lived (Visser *et al.*, 1992) another trial with a recombinant vaccinia-distemper vaccine was also carried out (Van Bressem *et al.*, 1991). In any case there is no commercial production of the CDV-ISCOM vaccine and the attenuated CDV vaccines have not been tested for safety in seals, a relevant concern since the CDV vaccine is known to cause death in some wild species (Bush *et al.*, 1976; Carpenter *et al.*, 1976; Sutherland-Smith *et al.*, 1997). During the 2002 epizootic a small trial of a commercially available CDV vaccine was carried out and the results are still awaited. Fortunately, wildlife species quickly recover from such epizootics unless they are critically endangered. When rinderpest was eliminated from most of East Africa the wildebeest populations surged (Sinclair, 1973), similarly buffalo and kudu in Kenya's National parks quickly recovered from the effects of rinderpest in the late 1990s (Kock *et al.*, 1999; see Chapter 7) and following the 1988 epizootic the seal populations recovered their levels within a few years and, it is hoped, the same will happen this time around following the 2002 epizootic.

# References

Abu Elzein, E.M., Housawi, F., Bashareek, Y., Gameel, A., Al-Afaleq, A. and Anderson, E.C. (2004) Severe PPR infection in gazelles kept under semi-free range conditions in Saudi Arabia. *J. Vet. Microbiol.* **51**, 68–71.

Allchin, C., Barrett, T., Duck, C., Eybatov, T., Forsyth, M., Kennedy, S. and Wilson, S. (1997) *Studies on the present status of marine biological resources of the Caspian Sea: Surveys of Caspian seals in the Apsheron Peninsula region and residue and pathology analyses of dead seal tissues.* Bio-resources Network Meeting, Bordeaux, November, Washington, World Bank.

Anderson, E.C., Hassan, A. *et al.* (1990) Observations on the pathogenicity for sheep and goats and the transmissibility of the strain of virus isolated during the rinderpest outbreak in Sri Lanka in 1987. *Vet. Microbiol.* **21** (4), 309–18.

Anderson, J. and McKay, J.A. (1994) The detection of antibodies against peste des petits ruminants virus in cattle, sheep and goats and the possible implications to rinderpest control programmes. *Epidemiol. Infect.* **112** (1), 225–31.

Appel, M.J.G. (1987) Canine distemper virus. In: *Virus Infections of Vertebrates.* Amsterdam: Elsevier Science. Vol. 1, pp. 133–59.

Appel, M.J., Reggiardo, C. *et al.* (1991) Canine distemper virus infection and encephalitis in javelinas (collared peccaries). *Arch. Virol.* **119** (1–2), 147–52.

Appel, M.J., Yates, R.A. *et al.* (1994) Canine distemper epizootic in lions, tigers, and leopards in North America. *J. Vet. Diagn. Invest.* **6** (3), 277–88.

Ata, F.A. and Singh, K.V. (1967) Experimental infection of sheep and goats with attenuated and virulent strains of rinderpest virus. *Bull. Epizoot. Dis. Afr.* **15** (3), 213–20.

Bailey, D., Banyard, A., Dash, P., Ozkul, A. and Barrett, T. (2005) Full genome sequence of peste des petits ruminants virus, a member of the Morbillivirus genus. *Virus Res.* **110**, 119–24.

Barrett, T. and Rossiter, P.B. (1999) Rinderpest: the disease and its impact on humans and animals. *Adv. Virus Res.* **53**, 89–110.

Barrett, T., Forsyth, M.A. *et al.* (1998) Rediscovery of the second African lineage of rinderpest virus: its epidemiological significance. *Vet. Rec.* **142** (24), 669–71.

Barrett, T., Visser, I.K. *et al.* (1993) Dolphin and porpoise morbilliviruses are genetically distinct from phocine distemper virus. *Virology* **193** (2), 1010–12.

Barrett, T.A. and Rima, B.K. (2002) Molecular biology of Morbillivirus diseases of marine mammals. In: C.J. Pfeiffer (ed.), *Molecular and Cell Biology of Marine Mammals.* Florida, Krieger, pp. 161–72.

Barrett, T. Sahoo, P. and Jepson, P.D. (2003) Seal distemper outbreak 2002. *Microbiology Today* **30**, 162–4.

Barton, A. (1956) Plagues and contagions in antiquity. *J. Am. Vet. Med. Assoc.* **129** (11), 503–5.

Bengtson, J.L., Boveng, P., Franzin, U., Have, P., Heide-Jørgensen, M.-P. and Härkönen, T.J. (1991) Antibodies to canine distemper virus in Antarctic seals. *Marine Mammal Sci.* **71**, 85–7.

Black, F.L. (1991) Epidemiology of the paramyxoviridae. In: D. Kingsbury (ed.), *The Paramyxoviruses.* New York, Plenum, pp. 509–36.

Blixenkrone-Møller, M., Svansson, V. *et al.* (1990) Phocid distemper virus – a threat to terrestrial mammals? *Vet. Rec.* **127** (10), 263–4.

Bolt, G., Blixenkrone-Moller, M. *et al.* (1994) Nucleotide and deduced amino acid sequences of the matrix (M) and fusion (F) protein genes of cetacean morbilliviruses isolated from a porpoise and a dolphin. *Virus Res.* **34** (3), 291–304.

Bush, M., Montali, R.J. *et al.* (1976) Vaccine-induced canine distemper in a lesser panda. *J. Am. Vet. Med. Assoc.* **169** (9), 959–60.

Carmichael, A.G. (1997) Measles: the red menace. In: K.F. Kipple (ed.), *Plague, Pox and Pestilence.* London: Wiedenfeld and Nicolson, pp. 80–5.

Carpenter, J.W., Appel, M.J. *et al.* (1976) Fatal vaccine-induced canine distemper virus infection in black-footed ferrets. *J. Am. Vet. Med. Assoc.* **169** (9), 961–4.

Cosby, S.L., McQuaid, S., Duffy, N., Lyons, C., Rima, B.K., Allen, G.M., McCullough, S.J., Kennedy, S., Smyth, J.A., McNeilly, F., Craig, C. and Örvell, C. (1988) Characterization of a seal morbillivirus. *Nature* **336**, 115–16.

Dhar, P., Sreenivasa, B.P. *et al.* (2002) Recent epidemiology of peste des petits ruminants virus (PPRV). *Vet. Microbiol.* **88** (2), 153–9.

Diallo, A., Barrett, T. *et al.* (1989) Differentiation of rinderpest and peste des petits ruminants viruses using specific cDNA clones. *J. Virol. Methods* **23** (2), 127–36.

Dietz, R., Ansen, C.T. *et al.* (1989) Clue to seal epizootic? *Nature* **338** (6217), 627.

Domingo, M., Ferrer, L. *et al.* (1990) Morbillivirus in dolphins. *Nature* **348** (6296), 21.

Duignan, P.J., House, C. *et al.* (1995a) Morbillivirus infection in cetaceans of the western Atlantic. *Vet. Microbiol.* **44** (2–4), 241–9.

Duignan, P.J., House, C., Geraci, J.R., Early, G., Copland, H., Walsh, M.T., Bossart, G.D., Cray, C., Sadove, S., St Aubin, D.J. and Moore, M. (1995b) Morbillivirus infection in two species of pilot whales (*Globicephala* sp.) from the western Atlantic. *Marine Mammal Sci.* **11**, 150–62.

Duignan, P.J., House, C., Odell, D.K., Wells, R.S., Hansen, L.J., Walsh, M.T., St Aubin, D.J., Rima, B.K. and Geraci, J.R. (1996) Morbillivirus in bottlenose dolphins: evidence for recurrent epizootics in the Western Atlantic and Gulf of Mexico. *Marine Mammal Sci.* **12**, 495–515.

Duignan, P.J., House, C., Walsh, M.T., Campbell, T., Bossart, G.D., Duffy, N., Fernandes, P.J., Rima, B.K., Wright, S., Gerachi, J.R. (1995c) Morbillivirus infections in manatees. *Marine Mammal Sci.* **11**, 441–51.

Duignan, P.J., Nielsen, O. *et al.* (1997) Epizootiology of morbillivirus infection in harp, hooded, and ringed seals from the Canadian Arctic and western Atlantic. *J. Wildl. Dis.* **33** (1), 7–19.

El Mjiyad, N., Jauniaux, T., Baise, E. and Coignoul, F. (2002) Cases of morbillivirus infections among seals (*Phoca vitulina*) and fin whales (*Balaenoptera physalus*) stranded on the Belgian and northern French coast from 1997 until 2002. 17th conference of the European Cetacean Society (9–13 March 2003), Las Palmas de Gran Canaria.

Forsyth, M.A., Kennedy, S. *et al.* (1998) Canine distemper virus in a Caspian seal. *Vet. Rec.* **143** (24), 662–4.

Furley, C.W., Taylor, W.P. *et al.* (1987) An outbreak of peste des petits ruminants in a zoological collection. *Vet. Rec.* **121** (19), 443–7.

Gargadennec, L. and Lalanne, A. (1942) La peste des petits ruminants. *Bull. Serv. Zootech. Epiz. Afr. Occid. Franc.* **5**, 16–21.

Gascoyne, S.C., King, A.A. *et al.* (1993) Aspects of rabies infection and control in the conservation of the African wild dog (*Lycaon pictus*) in the Serengeti region, Tanzania. *Onderstepoort J. Vet. Res.* **60** (4), 415–20.

Gibbs, E.P., Taylor, W.P. *et al.* (1979) Classification of peste des petits ruminants virus as the fourth member of the genus Morbillivirus. *Intervirolog,* **11** (5), 268–74.

Govindarajan, R., Koteeswaran, A. *et al.* (1997) Isolation of peste des petits ruminants virus from an outbreak in Indian buffalo (*Bubalus bubalis*). *Vet. Rec.* **141** (22), 573–4.

Grachev, M.A., Kumarev, V.P., Mamaev, L.V., Zorin, V.L., Baranova, L.V., Denikina, N.N., Belikov, S.I., Petrov, S.I., Petrov, E.A., Kolesnik, V.S., Kolesnik, R.S., Dorofeev, V.M., Beim, A.M., Kudelin, V.N., Magieva, F.G. and Sidorov, V.N. (1989) Distemper virus in Baikal seals. *Nature* **338**, 209.

Haas, L., Hofer, H., East, M., Wohlsein, P., Liess, B. and Barrett, T. (1996) Epizootic of canine distemper virus infection in Serengeti spotted hyaenas (*Crocuta crocuta*). *Vet. Microbiol.* **49**, 147–52.

Haas, L., Subbarao, S.M. *et al.* (1991) Detection of phocid distemper virus RNA in seal tissues using slot hybridization and the polymerase chain reaction amplification assay: genetic evidence that the virus is distinct from canine distemper virus. *J. Gen. Virol.* **72** (Pt 4), 825–32.

Haffar, A., Libeau, G. *et al.* (1999) The matrix protein gene sequence analysis reveals close relationship between peste des petits ruminants virus (PPRV) and dolphin morbillivirus. *Virus Res.* **64** (1), 69–75.

Hall, A.J. (1995) Morbilliviruses in marine mammals. *Trends Microbiol.* **3** (1), 4–9.

Harder, T.C., Kenter, M. *et al.* (1995) Phylogenetic evidence of canine distemper virus in Serengeti's lions. *Vaccine* **13** (6), 521–3.

Harder, T.C., Kenter, M., Vos, H., Siebelink, K., Huisman, W., Amerongen, G. van, Orvell, C., Barrett, T., Appel, M.J.G. and Osterhaus, A.D.M.E. (1996) Morbilliviruses isolated from diseased captive large felids: pathogenicity for domestic cats and comparative molecular analysis. *J. Gen. Virol.* **77**, 397–405.

Harder, T.C. and Osterhaus, A.D. (1997) Canine distemper virus – a morbillivirus in search of new hosts? *Trends Microbiol.* **5** (3), 120–4.

Harwood, J. (1998) What killed the monk seals? *Nature* **393**, 17–18.

Henderson, G., Trudgett, A. *et al.* (1992) Demonstration of antibodies in archival sera from Canadian seals reactive with a European isolate of phocine distemper virus. *Sci. Total Environ.* **115** (1–2), 93–8.

Hernandez, M., Robinson, I., Aguilar, A., Gonzalez, L.M., Lopez-Jurado, L.F., Reyero, M.I., Cacho, E., Franco, J., Lopez-Rodas, V. and Costas, E. (1998) Did algal toxins cause monk seal mortality? *Nature* **393**, 28–9.

Jauniaux, T., Boseret, G. *et al.* (2001) Morbillivirus in common seals stranded on the coasts of Belgium and northern France during summer 1998. *Vet. Rec.* **148** (19), 587–91.

Kennedy, S., Kuiken, T. *et al.* (2000) Mass die-off of Caspian seals caused by canine distemper virus. *Emerg. Infect. Dis.* **6** (6), 637–9.

Kennedy, S., Smyth, J.A., Cush, P.F., McCullough, S.J., Allan, G.M. and McQuaid, S. (1988) Viral distemper found in porpoises. *Nature* **336**, 21.

Kock, R.A., Wambua, J.M. *et al.* (1999) Rinderpest epidemic in wild ruminants in Kenya 1993–97. *Vet. Rec.* **145** (10), 275–83.

Laurenson, K., Sillero-Zubiri, C., Thompson, H., Shiferaw, F., Thirgood, S. and Malcolm, J. (1998) Disease as a threat to endangered species: Ethiopian wolves, domestic dogs and canine pathogens. *Animal Conservation* **4**, 273–80.

Laws, D. and Taylor, R.J.F. (1957) A mass dying of crabeater seals, *Lobodon carcinophagus* (Gray). *Proc. Zool. Soc. Lond.* **129**, 315–24.

Lipscomb, T.P., Kennedy, S. *et al.* (1996) Morbilliviral epizootic in bottlenose dolphins of the Gulf of Mexico. *J. Vet. Diagn. Invest.* **8** (3), 283–90.

Lyons, C., Welsh, M.J. *et al.* (1993) Canine distemper virus isolated from a captive seal. *Vet. Rec.* **132** (19), 487–8.

Mahy, B.W.J., Barrett, T., Evans, S., Anderson, E.C. and Bostock, C.J. (1988) Characterisation of a seal morbillivirus. *Nature* **336**, 115.

McConnell, B.J., Fedak, M.A., Lovell, P. and Hammond, P.S. (1999) Movements and foraging areas of grey seals in the North Sea. *J. Appl. Ecol.* **36**, 573–90.

McCullough, S.J., McNeilly, F. *et al.* (1991) Isolation and characterisation of a porpoise morbillivirus. *Arch. Virol.* **118** (3–4), 247–52.

Myers, D.L., Zurbriggen, A. *et al.* (1997) Distemper: not a new disease in lions and tigers. *Clin. Diagn. Lab. Immunol.* **4** (2), 180–4.

Nanda, Y.P., Chatterjee, A. *et al.* (1996) The isolation of peste des petits ruminants virus from northern India. *Vet. Microbiol.* **51** (3–4), 207–16.

Norrby, E., Sheshberadaran, H. *et al.* (1985) Is rinderpest virus the archevirus of the morbillivirus genus? *Intervirology* **23** (4), 228–32.

Osterhaus, A.D. and Vedder, E.J. (1988) Identification of virus causing recent seal deaths. *Nature* **335** (6185), 20.

Osterhaus, A.D., Visser, I.K. *et al.* (1992) Morbillivirus threat to Mediterranean monk seals?, *Vet. Rec.* **130** (7), 141–2.

Perry, B.D., Randolph, T. F., McDermott, J.J., Sones, K.R. and Thornton, P.K. (2002) *Investing in Animal Health Research to Alleviate Poverty.* Nairobi, Kenya, International Livestock Research Institute.

Philippa, J.D.W., Leighton, F.A., Daoust, P.Y., Nielsen, O., Pagliarulo, M., Schwantje, H., Shury, T., Herwijnen, R. van, Martina, B., Kuiken, T., Bildt van de, M.W.G. and Osterhaus, A.D.M.E. (2004) Antibodies to selected pathogens in free-ranging terrestrial carnivores and marine mammals in Canada. *Vet. Rec.* **155**, 135–40.

Reineking, B. (2003) Status Report no. 45. Common Wadden Sea Secretariat. http://www.waddensea-secretariat.org/news/news/Seals/01-seal-news.html#45.

Roelke-Parker, M.E., Munson, L., Packer, C., Kock, R., Cleaveland, S., Carpenter, M., O Brien, S.J., Pospischil, A., Hofmann-Lehmann, R., Lutz, H., Mwamengele, G.L.M., Mgasam, N., Machange, G.A., Summers, B.A. and Appel, M.J.G. (1996) A canine distemper virus epidemic in Serengeti lions (*Panthera leo*). *Nature* **379**, 441–5.

Ross, P.S., Visser, I.K. *et al.* (1992) Antibodies to phocine distemper virus in Canadian seals. *Vet. Rec.* **130** (23), 514–16.

Sabin, A.B. (1992) My last will and testament on rapid elimination and ultimate global eradication of poliomyelitis and measles. *Pediatrics* **90** (1 Pt 2), 162–9.

Shaila, M.S., Purushothaman, V., Bhavasar, D., Venugopal, K. and Venkatesan, R.A. (1989) PPR of sheep in India. *Vet. Rec.* **125**, 602.

Shaila, M.S., Shamaki, D. *et al.* (1996) Geographic distribution and epidemiology of peste des petits ruminants virus. *Virus Res.* **43** (2), 149–53.

Sinclair, A.R.E. (1973) Population increases of buffalo and wildebeest in the Serengeti. *East Afri. Wildl. J.* **11**, 93–107.

Sutherland-Smith, M.R., Rideout, B.A. *et al.* (1997) Vaccine-induced canine distemper in European mink, *Mustela lutreola J. Zoo Wildl. Med.* **28** (3), 312–18.

Taubenberger, J.K., Tsai, M. *et al.* (1996) Two morbilliviruses implicated in bottlenose dolphin epizootics. *Emerg. Infect. Dis.* **2** (3), 213–16.

Van Bressem, M., Waerebeek, K.V. *et al.* (2001) An insight into the epidemiology of dolphin morbillivirus worldwide. *Vet. Microbiol.* **81** (4), 287–304.

Van Bressem, M.F., De Meurichy, J. *et al.* (1991) Attempt to vaccinate orally harbour seals against phocid distemper. *Vet. Rec.* **129** (16), 362.

Van Bressem, M.F., Van Waerebeek, K. *et al.* (1998) Serological evidence of morbillivirus infection in small cetaceans from the Southeast Pacific. *Vet. Microbiol.* **59** (2–3), 89–98.

van de Bildt, M. W., Martina, B.E. *et al.* (2000) Identification of morbilliviruses of probable cetacean origin in carcases of Mediterranean monk seals (*Monachus monachus*). *Vet. Rec.* **146** (24), 691–4.

Visser, I.K., Kumarev, V.P. *et al.* (1990) Comparison of two morbilliviruses isolated from seals during outbreaks of distemper in north west Europe and Siberia. *Arch. Virol.* **111** (3–4), 149–64.

Visser, I.K., Van Bressem, M.F. *et al.* (1993) Characterization of morbilliviruses isolated from dolphins and porpoises in Europe. *J. Gen. Virol.* **74** (Pt 4), 631–41.

Visser, I.K., Vedder, E.J. *et al.* (1992) Canine distemper virus ISCOMs induce protection in harbour seals (*Phoca vitulina*) against phocid distemper but still allow subsequent infection with phocid distemper virus-1. *Vaccine* **10** (7), 435–8.

Wild, F.T., Vidalain, P.O., Servet-Delprat, C. and Rabourdin-Combe, C. (2000) Vers l'éradication de la rougeole?, *Méd./Sci.* **16**, 87–93.

# Molecular biology of the morbilliviruses

# 3

## THOMAS BARRETT,* ASHLEY C. BANYARD* AND ADAMA DIALLO[†]

*Institute for Animal Health, Pirbright Laboratory, Surrey, UK
[†]International Atomic Energy Agency, FAO/IAEA Agriculture and Biotechnology Laboratory, Vienna, Austria

## Introduction

Rinderpest virus (RPV), a member of the *Morbillivirus* genus within the family Paramyxoviridae, shares structural, biological, antigenic and molecular features in common with the other members of the group (see Chapters 1, 2 and 10). Members of the *Paramyxoviridae* are indistinguishable in the electron microscope where the virions are seen as pleomorphic particles with a lipid envelope enclosing a ribonucleoprotein (RNP) core. This RNP core contains the genome, a single strand of negative polarity RNA, encapsidated by the nucleocapsid protein giving it a characteristic 'herring bone' appearance. The RPV virions have a maximum diameter of 300 nm while those of the other ruminant morbillivirus, peste des petits ruminants virus (PPRV), are larger and have a mean diameter of 400–500 nm (Bourdin and Laurent-Vautier, 1967; Gibbs *et al.*, 1979). The most extensively studied morbillivirus at the molecular level is the human pathogen measles virus (MV), although similar studies are also being carried out on RPV, PPRV and canine distemper virus (CDV). This chapter will attempt to summarize this work in the context of what is known about the molecular biology of the paramyxoviruses and other negative strand RNA viruses.

## Genome organization

All morbilliviruses share the same genome organization although their RNA lengths differ slightly, each being just under 16 kb in length. Their genomes are

ISBN-13: 978-0-12-88385-1
ISBN-10: 0-12-88385-6

organized into six contiguous, non-overlapping, transcriptional units which encode the six structural proteins, namely the nucleocapsid (N), the phospho (P), the matrix (M), the fusion (F), the haemagglutinin (H) and the large (L) proteins, the latter being the viral RNA-dependent RNA polymerase (RdRp). In addition, all morbilliviruses encode two non-structural proteins, V and C, using alternative expression strategies from the P gene transcription unit. This genome organization is similar to other members of the *Paramyxovirinae* with only the Pneumovirinae having a different gene order (Figure 3.1).

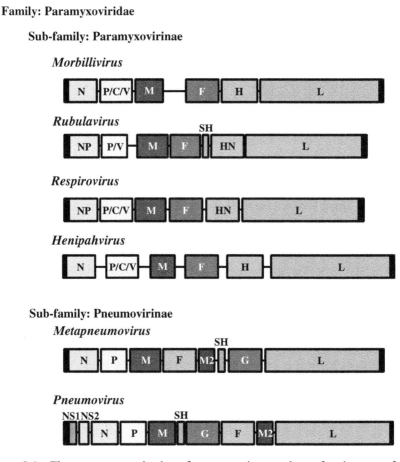

**Figure 3.1** The genome organization of representative members of each genus of the family Paramyxoviridae. For some members of the pneumoviruses, the M2 and L ORFs overlap. Gaps between each ORF are also shown although not to scale. Each ORF is denoted by an abbreviation for the protein as detailed in the text. For the rubulaviruses and the pneumoviruses and metapneumoviruses an SH (small hydrophobic) gene is present. The pneumoviruses also have separate NS (non-structural) genes located upstream of the N protein gene. (Adapted from Lamb and Kolakofsky, 2001)

All paramyxovirus genomes contain sequences at their terminal extremities that act as promoters for transcription and replication. At the 3' of the genome RNA there is a leader region of 52 nucleotides that precedes the N gene start and a similar length untranslated region (UTR) before the N gene open reading frame (ORF) that contain promoter functions. These regions contain all the *cis*-acting signals necessary for primary transcription as well as for the production of a full-length positive sense RNA genome copy required for the production of new genome RNA. At the 5' end there is a 37 nucleotide trailer region whose complement, as well as the complement of the UTR at the end of the L gene, performs a similar function at the 3' end of the antigenome RNA. These regions, and the possible mechanisms by which they interact with the RdRp complex, are discussed in more detail in the next section. Each morbillivirus transcription unit ends in a sequence rich in U residues, followed by an intergenic motif (IG) and a conserved sequence (UCCU/C) at the start of the next. The 3' leader region is also separated from the N gene start by an IG trinucleotide, usually GAA in the genome sense. This IG triplet is conserved at each of the gene junctions differing only at the H/L junction and at the junction of the L gene and the trailer region. At the H/L gene junction the IG sequence is GCA for MV, RPV and the PPRV Côte d'Ivoire/89 strain although the GAA motif is again seen in the PPRV vaccine and a recent PPRV isolate from Turkey (Turkey/2000) (Crowley *et al.*, 1988; Baron and Barrett, 1995; Bailey *et al.*, 2005; A. Diallo, unpublished results). At the junction between the L protein and the trailer region the GAA is replaced by GAU for PPRV and GUU for CDV, PDV and DMV.

Several members of the Paramyxoviridae, including all members of the morbillivirus genus, have a strict genome length requirement. Minigenome systems expressing reporter genes flanked by genome and antigenome promoters first indicated the existence of the 'rule of six'. Studies with Sendai virus (SeV), using both copy-back and internally deleted DI particles, showed that minigenome replication was only efficient when the length of the RNA genome analogue was exactly divisible by 6. This finding was explained by the fact that each N protein monomer associates with exactly 6 nucleotides and that efficient transcription and/or replication can only occur if the RNA genome is encapsidated by the N protein in its entirety (Calain and Roux, 1993). Subsequently, this rule was also shown to apply to the morbilliviruses (Sidhu *et al.*, 1995) and the respiroviruses (Dimock and Collins, 1993; Durbin *et al.*, 1997). However, it does not apply in all members of the *Paramyxoviridae* as work with rubulaviruses has shown that while the rule of six is required for efficient transcription and/or replication, it is not an absolute requirement (Kolakofsky *et al.*, 1998). Initial work on hPIV2 also suggested that the rule of six did not apply to this virus; however, recent studies have shown that recombinant hPIV2 viruses recovered from non-polyhexameric-length antigenomic cDNAs contain a biased distribution of length-correcting mutations (Skiadopoulos *et al.*, 2003). Members of the *Pneumovirinae* also do not conform this rule where terminal extensions to GP and/or AGP regions were found to have no obvious effect on minigenome activity (Collins *et al.*, 1991;

**Table 3.1** Details of full-length genome sequences available for members of the morbillivirus genus

| Virus | Length | Database Accession Number | Reference |
|---|---|---|---|
| Rinderpest | 15 882 | Z30697 | Baron *et al.*, 1996 |
| Peste des petits ruminants | 15 948 | AJ849636 | Bailey *et al.*, 2005 |
| Canine distemper | 15 702 | AF378705 | Von Messling *et al.*, 2001 |
| Phocine distemper | Unknown | na | na |
| Dolphin morbillivirus | 15 882 | AJ608288 | Rima *et al.*, unpublished |
| Porpoise morbillivirus | Unknown | na | na |

Samal and Collins, 1996). Full-length genome sequences are now available for most members of the morbillivirus genus (Table 3.1).

# Virus promoters

All negative strand RNA viruses contain untranslated regions that allow attachment of the RdRp polymerase complex at the 3′ ends of their genomes and antigenomes that are known as promoter regions. The 3′ genome terminus, as mentioned above, contains the 52 nucleotide leader region followed by a trinucleotide GAA and the 3′ UTR of the N gene. This stretch of 109 nucleotides before the N ORF start codon acts as a promoter for both the synthesis of virus mRNA and the production of a full-length positive sense antigenome RNA copy, the template for virion RNA synthesis, and as such is referred to as the genome promoter (GP). The promoter for the synthesis of genome-sense RNA is the complement of the 5′ UTR after the L protein stop codon and includes the trailer region which then becomes the 3′ end of the antigenome and is commonly referred to as the antigenome promoter (AGP). The limits of sequence required within the promoter regions of a number of paramyxoviruses have been partially defined using artificial replication systems including naturally occurring defective-interfering (DI) particles and artificially constructed genome analogues or 'minireplicons' expressing reporter genes (Harty and Palese, 1995b; Whelan and Wertz, 1999a, b; Tapparel and Roux, 1996; Tapparel *et al.*, 1998; Hoffman and Banerjee, 2000; Mioulet *et al.*, 2001). Minireplicons, sometimes called minigenomes, are plasmid constructs containing the GP and AGP elements flanking a reporter gene, usually either chloramphenicol-acetyl transferase (CAT) or β-galactosidase (β-gal) gene, whose expression can be easily measured and related to promoter efficiency.

Recent attempts to define critical residues within the GP and AGP of the respirovirus SeV have identified two distinct domains required for their efficient functioning, suggesting that the promoters are at least bipartite in nature. A highly conserved sequence at the 3′ RNA termini forms one element while sequences in the 3′ UTR of the N protein transcription unit form the other. This bipartite model for the promoters is reflected to some extent in all other paramyxoviruses. Within the *Paramyxoviridae*, the first promoter element consists of a conserved stretch of 16–25 nucleotides at the 3′ RNA termini. The 3′ and 5′ regions of each RNA species shares a high level of sequence complementarity, reflecting similarities in the GP and AGP functions, although terminal complementarity as such is not thought to contribute to promoter efficiency or function (Hoffman and Banerjee, 2000). The second promoter element, present in both the GP and the AGP, is a series of three hexamer motifs present at positions 79–84, 85–90, and 91–96 with respect to the genome ends (Tapparel *et al.*, 1998; Vulliémoz and Roux, 2001). The relative positioning of these elements has been shown to be critical for SeV as displacing them even by six nucleotides abolished promoter function. Working on the rule of six model of replication, these motifs are located in hexamers 14, 15 and 16 from the 3′ end. Image reconstruction of negatively stained electron micrographs of SeV nucleocapsids show that the nucleocapsid is a left handed helix consisting of 13 N monomers per turn, with each N monomer contacting 6 nucleotides. This structure predicts that the three hexamer motifs (CXXXXX) in the second promoter element lie on the same face of the helix, exactly above the first three hexamers at the 3′ terminus (Lamb and Kolakofsky, 2001). It is therefore likely that these two regions in the GPs and AGPs of paramyxoviruses directly interact with each other to form a functional promoter unit (Figure 3.2). A similar arrangement is found in the promoters of other paramyxoviruses (Murphy and Parks, 1999). In the case of RPV, scanning mutagenesis analyses of the 3′ end of the genome have identified nucleotides in the GP that are essential for promoter function; these include nucleotides 1, 3, 4, 10, 19 in the first promoter element and nucleotides 85 and 91 in the second promoter element. Changes to the first hexamer motif (position 79) in the GP also greatly reduce promoter activity but conservation at this site was not an essential requirement for replication (Mioulet *et al.*, 2001). Studies using PPRV minigenome constructs have also shown that the second 'hexamer motif' promoter element in the AGP is essential for replication (Bailey *et al.*, unpublished data).

While the GP has two functions, being required for both transcription of virus mRNAs and transcription of a full-length positive sense virus genome replicative intermediate, the AGP performs only a single function, the production of full-length negative sense genomes. The AGP is a much stronger promoter fine tuned for replication, a fact that has been demonstrated experimentally through analysis of the amount of full-length genome and antigenome sense RNAs produced during infection *in vitro*. Udem and Cook (1984) reported a ratio of two- to three-fold excess of genomic over antigenomic RNA for CDV and for other paramyxoviruses this can be up to 5- to 10-fold higher (Whelan and Wertz, 1999a). For other members of the Mononegavirales much greater ratios have been reported, a 50:1 ratio being found in rabies virus (RV), showing just how strong a promoter the AGP can

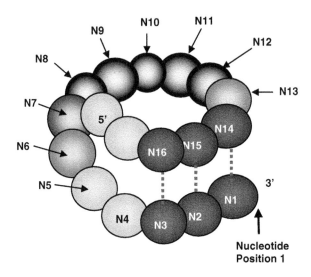

**Figure 3.2** Proposed structure for the nucleocapsids of paramyxoviruses. The 3′ genome terminus starts at position 1, with each N protein encapsidating 6 nucleotides. The first three protein hexamers and the three hexamers containing the conserved C residues in the respiroviruses and the morbilliviruses are more darkly shaded. The spatial arrangement of the SeV nucleocapsid structure suggests that the three conserved C residues at positions 79, 85, and 91 (present in hexamers N14, N15 and N16, respectively) lie directly above and interact with N subunits 1, 2 and 3 as indicated by the dashed lines. The N mRNA starts at nucleotide position 56, present in N hexamer unit 10. (Adapted from Lamb and Kolakofsky, 2001)

be compared to the comparatively weak GP (Finke and Conzelmann, 1997; Whelan and Wertz, 1999a). Interestingly, for vesicular stomatitis virus (VSV), extending the length of the conserved regions at the 3′ and 5′ ends by mutagenesis, enhances replication activity while at the same time transcription is downregulated (Whelan and Wertz, 1999a). Moreover, the presence of a replication enhancer sequence (RES) in the AGP of VSV has been postulated and also could be a factor determining asymmetric transcription by the viral genomic and antigenomic RNPs (Li and Pattnaik, 1997). Similar enhancer elements have not been identified in morbilliviruses.

## Transcription

After virus fusion with the cell membrane the nucleocapsid is released from the envelope and transcription begins in the cytoplasm (Plate 1–see colour plate section). Here, the virus-encoded RdRp, a component of the infecting RNP, initiates transcription of mRNAs. How the RdRp accesses the template RNA is unclear as the association of the nucleocapsid protein with the RNA is strong; it can resist even the high salt conditions required for caesium chloride (CsCl) density gradient purification. Access is thought to be made possible either by a reversible transition in the protein-RNA association or by local displacement of N during transcription, as occurs in the separation of the two strands of DNA during its transcription (for review, see Kolakofsky et al., 1998). A third possibility, which is suggested to be the case for VSV, is that N associates with the RNA at the sugar–phosphate backbone thus leaving the Watson–Crick positions free to act as a template for transcription by the RdRp (Iseni et al., 2002).

In all paramyxoviruses the RdRp can only attach at the GP on virion RNA. From there transcription begins and the RdRp proceeds sequentially along the genomic RNA in a 'stop–start' mode, each transcription unit being defined by the IG and the conserved gene start and stop signals that flank it. In transcription mode access of the RdRp to downstream transcription units is, therefore, entirely dependent upon completion and release of a newly synthesized copy of the mRNA from the preceding unit. If the RdRp becomes detached from the RNP template during transcription, which often occurs at the IG regions, it must return again to the GP to reinitiate mRNA synthesis. This leads to a transcriptional gradient being set up whereby less mRNA is transcribed the further a gene is distant from the GP. A progressive decline in synthesis of mRNA occurred as the distance from the GP increased with a 20–30% attenuation of transcription across each gene junction. This has been shown experimentally with VSV where, using reverse genetics, the positions of the transcription units along the genome were changed relative to the GP (Wertz et al., 1998, Wertz and Ball, 2002). This is a way of controlling the amount of protein produced and results in the 3′ proximal gene coding for the N protein being the most abundantly transcribed while the L protein gene (RdRp), which is only required in catalytic amounts, is furthest from the GP and the least abundantly transcribed.

Similar transcriptional gradients have been shown to occur in MV infected cells, where, if the frequency of N mRNA production is taken as 100%, percentages of 81%, 67%, 49%, 39%, respectively for P, M, F and H are found (Horikami and Moyer, 1995). No estimation was made for the L mRNA since the quantity of this messenger is too low to be measured accurately. In the stop–start mode the IG sequence is not normally transcribed as it acts as a signal to the polymerase indicating the end of the transcription unit and, if this signal is correctly recognized by the polymerase, only monocistronic mRNA is synthesized. However, the transcription of negative strand RNA genomes is not always completely accurate and both monocistronic and polycistronic mRNAs are produced, although only the first cistron is ever translated from a bicistronic mRNA (for review, see Horikami and Moyer, 1995; Wong and Hirano, 1987). Before genome sequences were determined these transcriptional aberrations were used to map the gene order for these negative strand viruses.

All messenger RNAs are transcribed as naked RNAs and are capped at their 5′ ends and polyadenylated at their 3′ ends by the virus encoded polymerase so they are stable and efficiently translated by the host ribosomes. Experiments carried out with VSV show that the conserved trinucleotide (AGG) at the start of the mRNAs is critical for efficient gene expression and contains essential signals for the correct processing of the nascent mRNA and in its absence the majority of transcripts are prematurely terminated (Stillman and Whitt, 1998, 1999). This conserved trinucleotide probably also forms part of the signal for capping and methylation of the messenger RNA. The conserved tract of four U residues, which always precedes the IG, signals the polyadenylation of the mRNA transcripts. These U-rich sequences are integral to the polyadenylation signal and are the point where 'stuttering' of the RdRp allows hundreds of A residues to be added to the ends of mRNAs on only a very short template. This polyadenylation signal may have other functions, at least in VSV, as not only does it indicate the end of the upstream mRNA, but it appears necessary for efficient transcription of the downstream transcription unit (Hinzman *et al.*, 2002). Other studies suggest that the number of U residues reflects the variable lengths of the mRNA poly-A tails and it has been hypothesized that this variation in U tract-length may affect the efficiency of transcription termination in the paramyxoviruses (Rassa *et al.*, 2000). These mechanisms have not been investigated in detail for the morbilliviruses.

It remains unclear whether the transcription process in all single-strand negative sense RNA viruses starts from the first nucleotide at the 3' end of the genome or at the start of the N transcription unit. Initiation at the 3'end would require the synthesis and release of leader-complementary RNA which would then be followed by transcription of the different virus mRNAs (see review by Banerjee, 1987). Free leader RNA has been identified in MV nucleocapsid transcription products *in vitro* (Horikami and Moyer, 1995) but this RNA has not been found in MV-infected Verocells (Billeter *et al.*, 1984; Crowley *et al.*, 1988; Castaneda and Wong, 1989). Based on these observations, Castaneda and Wong (1990) suggested that transcription of the MV genome might start directly at the N protein start *in vivo*. It is possible that this strategy is valid for some, if not all, other non-segmented negative strand viruses and indeed it has been shown that VSV transcription and replication are initiated at different sites; the replicase complex initiates at the first nucleotide at the 3' end while transcription is initiated directly at the start of the N transcription unit (Chuang and Perrault, 1997; Whelan and Wertz, 1999b, 2002). The mechanism by which the polymerase complex makes the choice between initiation sites, however, is still not clear. It could be determined by modifications either to the RdRp or the template or by a combination of both (Barr *et al.*, 2002). The involvement of cellular factors has also to be considered since *in vitro* transcription of the MV genome is known to be stimulated by cytoplasmic cell extracts (Moyer *et al.*, 1990).

During transcription the paramyxoviruses exhibit what would seem to be an evolutionary adaptation to maximize coding capacity. Here, the P gene uses two different mechanisms to generate more than one protein from its transcription unit and so, unlike the other five transcription units, is not equivalent to one gene. As well as the full length P protein, synthesized from the first initiation codon, a second protein, the C protein, is also translated. This results from leaky ribosomal scanning whereby the first AUG initiation codon is ignored, translation instead starting at the second initiation codon, 19 nucleotides downstream of the first (Bellini *et al.*, 1985). This 'leaky scanning' occurs because neither initiator AUG codon is in the ideal Kozak consensus sequence context (A/GXXAUGG) required for efficient translation of the protein (Kozak, 1984). The second non-structural protein encoded from the P gene is derived from the P transcription unit by a novel mechanism. The mRNA for this protein is generated by a process known a co-transcriptional editing whereby one or more non-templated G residues are added to approximately 50% of the P mRNAs at a highly conserved editing site (3' AAUUUUUCC-CGUGUC 5'). As the polymerase hits this editing site, approximately half-way along the P ORF, it is thought to 'stutter' on the short stretch of U residues upstream of the G insertion site (after the CCC sequence) and inserts a pseudo-templated G residue (Cattaneo *et al.*, 1989b; Mahapatra *et al.*, 2003). This insertion causes a translational frameshift and the V protein, a C-terminally truncated cysteine-rich form of the P protein, is generated (Schneider *et al.*, 1997). In rare cases it is thought that this mechanism can cause the insertion of two extra G residues, generating a further smaller and poorly characterized protein, the W protein. Morbilliviruses, with the possible exception of PDV, generally insert only one G residue into the P mRNA and for MV, RPV, CDV and PPRV the ratio of P and V mRNA produced is roughly a 1:1. However, Blixenkrone-Møller *et al.* (1992), found that 10% of P gene transcripts in PDV infections contain two extra G residues with the proportion of P and V mRNAs (1 G insertion) being 5:3 (for reviews see Kolakofsky *et al.*, 1998; Hausmann *et al.*, 1999).

While the morbilliviruses have developed a strategy to maximize the coding capacity/potential of the P ORF, they have also retained a long UTR of 870–1000 nucleotides between the M and F protein ORFs which seems to offer no advantage to the virus. The M ORF ends about 400 nucleotides before the poly U tract, the IG is conserved and then the F ORF start codon for MV lies 580 nucleotides after the IG region. This region, between the ORFs of the M and F proteins, has a high GC content. The UTR at the end of the M ORF has not yet been shown to play a significant role in the virus life cycle, but the long F UTR has been shown to enhance the production of the F protein in a transient expression system (Evans *et al.*, 1990). For MV and RPV, deleting the 5' UTR of the F gene had little effect on virus growth *in vitro* (Radecke *et al.*, 1995; Liermann *et al.*, 1998; Barrett, unpublished data), although another mutant MV with a deletion in this area did not grow well in an *in vivo* murine model (Valsamakis *et al.*, 1998). This suggests that this region may be more important *in vivo*, perhaps through interactions with host cell proteins somehow regulating viral transcription, replication or translation.

## Replication

At some point after infection the viral RdRp stops transcribing mRNAs and instead generates a full-length antigenome RNA. This full-length positive sense RNA, like the negative sense genome RNA, is always encapsidated by the N protein since both the GP and AGP sequences contain RNA encapsidation signals. As a consequence the synthesis of full-length antigenome RNA and N protein production must be linked (Gubbay *et al.*, 2001), although the precise trigger for the switch from the transcriptive mode to replication is not clearly understood. In the 1980s a self-regulatory model was proposed (Blumberg and Kolakofsky, 1981; for review see Banerjee, 1987). In this model, which was widely accepted for many years, the unassembled N protein plays the major role in switching the RdRp between its transcriptase and replicase functions. This model envisaged a mechanism whereby the RdRp starts copying the genomic RNP into mRNA and, in the absence of sufficient N for binding nascent RNA, recognizes the transcription control sequences at the leader–N junction and releases the leader and initiates the synthesis of N mRNA. The RdRp would then transcribe the genes in tandem, recognizing all of the *cis*-acting stop, polyadenylation, IG and start sequences, to produce a full complement of mRNAs. Once a sufficient concentration of N was achieved, these signals would be masked, perhaps by RNA encapsidation with the N protein, driving the switch in RdRp activity/function to its replicative mode to begin synthesis of an antigenome RNA, subsequently used as the template for the production of new genome sense RNA. This theory accords with the observation made by Wertz *et al.* (1998) that if the N protein transcription unit is moved further down the genome less N protein is produced with a consequent decrease in replication. However, increasing the amount of N protein produced in a minireplicon system for respiratory syncytial virus (RSV) does not enhance the rate of replication relative to transcription (Fearns *et al.*, 1997) and more recent work has led to revision of the model since it is increasingly clear that the switch mechanism is more complicated.

It is now thought more likely that transcription and replication require different sets of accessory proteins to interact with the RdRp to form either a transcriptase or a replicase complex. Gupta *et al.* (2003) and Kolakofsky *et al.* (2004) proposed the existence of two different forms of the RdRp, one which is used for transcription and the other for replication. It has long been understood that both L–P and N–P complexes are essential for the replication process and that association of P with N maintains the latter in a soluble form ready to encapsidate newly synthesized viral RNA, but not cellular RNAs, as the N–P complex requires an encapsidation signal to bind the RNA (Horikami *et al.*, 1992; Spehner *et al.*, 1997). In the Gupta model, the transcriptase complex is formed by an RdRp associated with an L-P$_{oligomer}$ and possible host cell factors and differs from the replicase which is formed from a tripartite association with the additional involvement of an N-P$_{oligomer}$. In the Kolakofsky model the transcriptase complex is proposed to consist of the RdRp with an L-P$_{oligomer}$ and a free P$_{oligomer}$ which will bind directly to the genomic RNA while in the replicase complex the L-P$_{oligomer}$ is associated with an N-P$_{oligomer}$. In both models the N protein plays a major role in determining the replicase activity.

The M protein may also be involved in the regulation of RdRp activity and the inhibitory effect of M on VSV transcription has been known for many years (see review by Banerjee, 1987). This inhibition has also been shown to occur in MV and in rabies virus (RV) (Suryanarayana *et al.*, 1994). The inhibitory effect of M seems to be independent of its role in virus assembly and budding, the amino acid residue at position 58 in the RV M protein being critical for this function (Finke and Conzelmann, 2003). The exact mechanism underlying M protein inhibition is not yet fully understood but, if the transcriptase complex is functionally different from the replicase complex, it might target the transcriptase directly and leave the replicase unaffected. This inhibition by M has not been investigated for the other morbilliviruses.

# Virus structural proteins

## The N protein

The N protein is the major viral structural protein in the non-segmented negative strand RNA viruses. Differently phosphorylated forms of RPV N are produced with some virus strains (Diallo *et al.*, 1987) but no biological significance has been attributed to variations in N protein phosphorylation in morbilliviruses. However, for the rhabdovirus (RV), both RNA transcription and replication are reduced if the N protein is not phosphorylated (Yang *et al.*, 1999; Wu *et al.*, 2002). Sequence data are now available for all the morbillivirus N proteins. They consist of 525 amino acid residues in RPV, MV and PPRV but only 523 amino acids in CDV, DMV and PMV and migrate with apparent molecular weights of between 60 and 68 kDa in polyacrylamide gels. Sequence comparison of the different N proteins reveals amino acid identities varying from 67 to 74% between the different morbilliviruses but alignment of the sequences has defined four regions with different degrees of conservation: region I (amino acid residues 1 to 120) is quite well conserved with 75–83% identity across the group, region II (amino acid residues 122–145) shows only a low sequence identity at about 40%, region III (amino acid residues 146–398) is the most conserved with 85 to 90% identity and finally region IV, which is the C-terminal fragment (amino acids 421–523/525), is the least conserved part of the protein (Diallo *et al.*, 1994). The nascent N protein when expressed alone, either in mammalian, insect or bacterial cells, quickly associates into nucleocapsid-like aggregations to form a more condensed form of the protein (Mitra-Kaushik *et al.*, 2001). These N-protein aggregations can be detected in both the cytoplasm and the nucleus of the transfected cells. The signal required for nuclear transport is located in the first 80 amino acids as demonstrated for CDV by Yoshida *et al.* (1999). However, this signal sequence is not conserved throughout the morbilliviruses and is probably altered in the PPRV attenuated strain Nigeria 75/1 since neither its native N nor the corresponding recombinant protein are found in the nucleus of infected cells (A. Diallo, unpublished data).

The region involved in N protein self-assembly has been mapped to what is termed the $N_{core}$ (Bankamp *et al.*, 1996; Liston *et al.*, 1997) and is well conserved within the morbillivirus genus, probably reflecting its vital function in nucleocapsid assembly. Changes in residues 228S and 229L in MV N lead to impaired self-association (Karlin *et al.*, 2002). While normal N protein can encapsidate RNA, the mutated MV N protein with impaired N–N association is unable to package RNA, suggesting that correct self-polymerization of MV N protein may create a structure involved in RNA-binding. The C-terminal variable fragment IV ($N_{Tail}$), which is about 12 kDa, is exposed on the surface of the protein and is easily cleaved by trypsin digestion. On removal of the $N_{Tail}$ from the protein, the $N_{core}$ still retains the ability to form nucleocapsid-like structures (Giraudon *et al.*, 1988). The C-terminal residues (488–499) are involved in binding to the P protein (Bankamp *et al.*, 1996; Longhi *et al.*, 2003; Bourhis *et al.*, 2004). The C-termini of morbillivirus N proteins also interact with cellular regulatory proteins such as heat shock protein Hsp72, interferon regulator factor IRF-3, and a novel cell surface receptor (tenOever *et al.*, 2002; Zhang *et al.*, 2002; Laine *et al.*, 2003), interactions which may be vital for efficient replication and which could explain features such as restriction in host cell tropism.

## The P protein

The P is one of the three protein components of the RNP and acts as a co-factor for the RdRp. It is a multifunctional protein, which binds both the N and L proteins and acts as a chaperone to keep the N in a soluble form for binding to the RNA. The P proteins are much smaller (54–55 kDa) than the values determined from polyacrylamide gels where they migrate at 72–86 kDa (Diallo *et al.*, 1987; Bolt *et al.*, 1995). This aberrant migration can be attributed to the post-translational phosphorylation of the protein which is rich in serine and threonine. PPRV has the longest P protein with 509 amino acids while the DMV P is the shortest with 506 amino acids. MV, RPV, CDV and PDV all have P proteins of 507 amino acids. The P is one of the least conserved virus proteins, RPV and PPRV sharing only 51.4% amino acid identity (Mahapatra *et al.*, 2003) with the region extending from position 21 to 306 containing many unconserved residues. Of the three serine residues (positions 49, 38 and 151) identified as potential phosphorylation sites in the RPV P protein, only that at position 151 is conserved in all morbilliviruses (Kaushik and Shaila, 2004).

The C-terminal region of paramyxovirus P proteins contains the domain that interacts with the exposed C-terminus of the N protein (Ryan and Portner, 1990; Huber *et al.*, 1991). Harty and Palese (1995a) have mapped the N binding sites of MV P to two regions, one present in the N-terminal 100 amino acids, the other being more precisely defined as residues 459–507 at the C-terminus. Using the yeast two-hybrid system it was shown that an N-terminal 60 amino acid region and a C-terminal amino acid region (316–346) are simultaneously involved in an N–P interaction in RPV (Shaji and Shaila, 1999). A more distant C-terminal region of the P protein interacts with L protein in the case of SeV (Smallwood *et al.*, 1994). Furthermore, reflecting the fact that this region has important functions, the C-terminal half of P is more conserved than the N-terminal half, residues 311–418 being the most conserved. The active form of P protein is a tetramer and oligomerization of the protein rather than its phosphorylation, as previously suggested (Kaushik and Shaila, 2004), is absolutely required for its replication/transcription activity in the RdRp complex *in vitro* (Rahaman *et al.*, 2004). While the N protein of morbilliviruses is found both in the cytoplasm and in the nucleus, when complexed with the P protein, it is found exclusively in cytoplasm (Huber *et al.*, 1991; Gombart *et al.*, 1993).

It has been suggested that the C-termini of both the N and P proteins of MV belong to a class of intrinsically disordered proteins that fold to a defined structure only upon binding to their partners (Johansson *et al.*, 2003; Longhi *et al.*, 2003; Bourhis *et al.*, 2004). This class of unfolded, or intrinsically unstructured proteins, have little or no ordered rigid structure under physiological conditions and are usually involved in key biological processes such as cell cycle control, transcription and translation regulation, transport, etc. (Wright and Dyson, 1999; Iakoucheva *et al.*, 2004). This gives the advantage of increased plasticity since they can bind many distinct targets, although with a low affinity. Because the domains involved in the N–P interactions are naturally unstructured, the complex they form is not very stable, allowing a dynamic and rapid transition between two states, and formation and breakage of links to facilitate the progress of the polymerase in copying the template RNA and encapsidating the nascent RNA during replication (Johansson *et al.*, 2003). The P protein may also be required to facilitate the proper folding of the L-protein, since in SeV the P protein must be co-expressed with L to keep it stable (Horikami *et al.*, 1992) and mutation(s) in the L binding domain produce P proteins which are inactive in replication (Tuckis *et al.*, 2002).

## The M protein

It is well established that epithelial cells are polarized, having distinct apical and basolateral domains which are different in structure, for example lipid and protein composition, and possibly function (Rodriguez-Boulan and Nelson, 1989). It has been shown in MV that maturation and release of virus particles occur at the apical surfaces of epithelial cells although the two viral glycoproteins are found mainly at the basolateral surfaces (Blau and Compans, 1995; Maisner *et al.*, 1998; Naim *et al.*, 2000; Moll *et al.*, 2001; Riedl *et al.*, 2002). The M protein serves as a bridge between the external surface viral proteins (H and F) and the internal nucleocapsid and as such plays an important role in the formation of new virus particles which are released from the infected cell by a process of budding from the cell surface (for review, see Simons and Garoff, 1980; Peeples, 1991). The M protein is known to direct the glycoproteins to the apical surfaces of polarized cells and any that escape capture by M accumulate on basolateral surfaces due to a tyrosine-dependent sorting signal located in their cytoplasmic tails. MV viruses bearing a tyrosine point mutation in this sorting signal are unable to propagate by formation of syncytia in polarized cells *in vitro* and *in vivo* (Moll *et al.*, 2004). Blood cells such as macrophages which disseminate the virus in the host are likely to be infected upon contact with the basal surface of epithelial cells by direct cell–cell fusion, which is an alternative way for MV to infect cells (Naim *et al.*, 2000; Moll *et al.*, 2001).

The M protein is located inside the viral envelope and is the most conserved protein within the group with identities ranging from 91%, between CDV and PDV, to 76%, between RPV and PDV/CDV, while RPV and PPRV share 84% identity. When conservative substitutions are taken into account, the similarities of the different morbillivirus proteins is higher (Table 3.2). Only a stretch of 20 residues lying between positions 195 and 214 varies significantly between morbilliviruses (Haffar *et al.*, 1999). A pivotal role is played by M in ensuring efficient incorporation of nucleocapsids into virions for HIPV. Here, a process whereby the M protein interacts with the F and H proteins through their cytoplasmic tails and with the RNP complexes in the cytoplasm brings these virus components together at the cell surface to form new virus particles (Coronel *et al.*, 2001).

**Table 3.2**  Percentage similarity of the RPV Kabete 'O' strain to other morbilliviruses

| Virus | Genome | N | P | C | V | M | F | H | L |
|---|---|---|---|---|---|---|---|---|---|
| Peste des petits ruminants | 66.98 | 79.66 | 58.65 | 54.02 | 54.61 | 89.82 | 82.74 | 59.14 | 83.44 |
| Measles | 70.50 | 82.70 | 65.35 | 65.34 | 64.55 | 92.26 | 85.98 | 67.33 | 87.73 |
| Canine distemper | 63.58 | 75.38 | 53.57 | 52.91 | 44.67 | 83.93 | 78.75 | 46.26 | 81.05 |
| Dolphin morbillivirus | 65.91 | 79.69 | 57.91 | 55.29 | 50.50 | 89.29 | 84.52 | 57.14 | 83.29 |

The genome column represents comparisons made at the nucleotide level for the full-length genomes. Columns N, P, C, V, M, F, H and L represent comparisons of the eight viral proteins at the amino acid level. Similarity scores were calculated using the BESTFIT program of the Wisconsin GCG package (Accelrys). RPV: Kabete 'O' strain (X98291); MeV: 9301B strain (AB012948); CDV: Onderstepoort strain (AF305419); DMV (AJ608288); PPRV: Tu00 strain (AJ849636).

Budding of morbilliviruses may occur at specialized membrane regions for which the M protein has more affinity; for example lipid raft microdomains are the potential locations for MV assembly (Manie *et al.*, 2000; Vincent *et al.*, 2000; Chazal and Gerlier, 2003) and it is possible that the apical domains are richer in these membrane structures. Actin filaments, responsible for cellular transport, also are required for virus budding and it has long been known that destruction of actin filaments prevents MV budding (Stallcup *et al.*, 1983). Actin is highly concentrated in apical microvilli in epithelial cells (Riedl *et al.*, 2002) and if, as is probable, the M protein binds to this protein it may also explain the preferential budding of MV at apical surfaces. The outcome of this process is the release of virus particles at the apical domain of epithelial cells which will then be excreted by the host to infect neighbouring cells or a new host.

The M protein or, more precisely, defects in its synthesis, are hypothesized to contribute to the molecular basis of a fatal complication of MV infection, subacute sclerosing panencephalitis (SSPE). This disease is the result of virus persistence in the brain after the acute phase of the disease when the host's immune responses have cleared the infection from other organs. The invariably fatal outcome of SSPE has meant that a considerable effort has been put into understanding its pathogenesis and the molecular events leading to persistent infection in the brain. The SSPE-associated N, P and L mRNAs found in the brain have very few mutations. In contrast, the F and H genes, as with the M, contain mutations which are also believed to influence the development of disease. These defects in sequence arise through biased hypermutation and such defects prevent completion of the viral replication cycle thus enabling establishment of a non-productive persistent infection in the brain. The low levels of virus replication in the brain may allow defects to build up in genes that are not essential for replication or these mutations may be explained by the release from the selective pressure normally exerted on viral genes. In SSPE pathogenesis, the virus only needs to replicate and spread from cell to cell, without the necessity to produce infectious progeny. In fact altered transcription gradients have been observed in SSPE infections where transcription of the non-essential glycoproteins and M protein are more steeply downregulated (Cattaneo *et al.*, 1988; Cattaneo *et al.*, 1989a; Schneider-Schaulies *et al.*, 1991; Suryanarayana *et al.*, 1994; Ecker *et al.*, 1995). A similar pathogenesis has been suggested to cause the canine syndrome 'old dog encephalitis' (ODE), although studies on this disease have been limited to pathological observations (ter Meulen and Martin, 1976; Rima *et al.*, 1987; Billeter *et al.*, 1994).

Using reverse genetics technology it has been possible to rescue MV which lacks an M protein. Although the titre of the M-minus virus is dramatically reduced *in vitro*, it is more efficient in inducing cell-to-cell fusion than normal virus and it appears that the presence of M somehow downregulates the efficiency of fusion in infected cells (Cathomen *et al.*, 1998; Spielhofer *et al.*, 1998).

## The F protein

The morbilliviruses produce two glycoproteins which are embedded in the viral envelope and protrude as spikes, the F and the H protein spikes. The F protein enables the virus to penetrate the cell by mediating the fusion of the viral and cellular membranes at the cell surface at neutral pH. For this process to happen, cooperation with the H protein is also required as the H acts as a fusion promoter (Moll *et al.*, 2002; Plemper *et al.*, 2002). The nucleotide sequences of the F gene of all morbilliviruses consist of 2200 to 2400 nucleotides depending on the virus. One interesting feature which characterizes morbillivirus F mRNAs, is the existence of long 5′ UTR, which in MV is 580 nucleotides long. This region is very variable and has a high G-C content. It is predicted to be rich in secondary stem loop structures and contains either one (MV) or up to five (PDV) potential initiator AUGs preceding what is believed to be the actual initiator codon used for F protein translation (Figure 3.3).

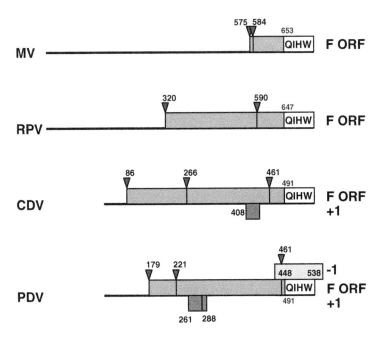

**Figure 3.3** Diagrammatic representation of the structure of the 5′ UTRs in different morbilliviruses. MV has two AUG initiator codon before the presumed signal peptide sequence. Others have several other in-frame initiator codons preceding this sequence while CDV and PDV also have out of frame AUGs. According to the rules for signal peptidase recognition signals (von Heijne, 1988) cleavage of the signal peptide should occur at the amino acid preceding the QIH motif.

The protein encoded by the F mRNA is translated to produce an $F_0$ protein which consists of 537–552 amino acids depending on the virus. Alignment of the $F_0$ from different morbilliviruses reveals high conservation along the whole length of the protein sequence apart from two variable hydrophobic domains (Evans *et al.*, 1994; Meyer and Diallo, 1995). The first is located near the N-terminus and ends at the conserved motif QIHW. This hydrophobic region is predicted to be the signal peptide sequence required for directing the protein to the rough endoplasmic reticulum (RER) for translation and which is removed from the mature protein by the cellular signal peptidase during translation. Without the signal sequence all mature morbillivirus $F_0$ proteins consist of 527 amino acids. The second variable region is located towards the C-terminus and is predicted to anchor the protein in the membrane; the only requirement for this function appears to be that their sequences be hydrophobic in nature. This leaves the extreme C-terminus on the cytoplasmic side of the membrane where it can interact with the M protein. This orientation in the membrane classifies the F as a type I glycoprotein.

The fusion domain is the third hydrophobic domain in the F protein but, unlike the other two, is highly conserved in all paramyxoviruses. The translated protein, the $F_0$ protein, is inactive in fusion and must be activated by a proteolytic cleavage to form $F_1$ and $F_2$ subunits, which remain linked to each other by disulphide bonds. This places the hydrophobic fusion domain at the N-terminus of the $F_1$ protein. Cleavage of $F_0$ is not required for virus assembly but is critical for the infectivity and pathogenesis in all paramyxoviruses (Watanabe *et al.*, 1995a). In morbilliviruses cleavage occurs at the carboxyl side of the pentapeptide Arg-Arg-X1-X2-Arg (X1 being any amino acid but X2 must be either arginine or lysine). This sequence conforms to the minimal consensus sequence Arg-X-X-Arg recognized by furin endopeptidase which is present in the *trans*-Golgi network. Inhibition of the furin-catalysed cleavage of $F_0$ prevents syncytia formation in MV infected cells and reduces the infectious titre virus by three to four orders of magnitude (Watanabe *et al.*, 1995b). A similar result is obtained when the last Arg residue in the motif is replaced by another amino acid such leucine, indicating the necessity to maintain the site recognized by the cellular endopeptidase (Alkatib *et al.*, 1994a).

The F protein, like all membrane-associated proteins, is glycosylated by cellular enzymes during its passage to the cell surface. The $F_0$ proteins of morbilliviruses have three potential N-linked glycosylation sites (Asn-X-Ser/Thr) which are all located on the $F_2$ subunit of the mature protein. Their positions are exactly conserved within the genus and it appears that all are utilized (Meyer and Diallo, 1995). Studies with MV have confirmed the critical role of these oligosaccharide side chains for transport of the protein to cell surface and in the maintenance of its fusogenic activity. They are also essential for maintaining the $F_2$ subunit in its optimum conformation (Alkatib *et al.*, 1994b; Cathomen *et al.*, 1995; Bolt *et al.*, 1999).

Morbillivirus F proteins have a leucine zipper motif, located just before the anchor sequence, which was thought at one point to facilitate oligomerization of the molecule, the F protein spikes being homotrimers (Bolt, 2001; Plemper *et al.*, 2001). However, mutagenesis of the four leucine residues in this motif have no effect on the oligomerization state, or on transport of the protein to the membrane but does affect its fusion function (Buckland *et al.*, 1992). How the leucine zipper motif contributes to the fusion function of the protein is not yet clear as it is located far from the protein fusion domain in the primary sequence.

## The H protein

The H protein enables the virus to bind to the cell receptor, the first step in the process of infection. These proteins vary in length from 604 amino acids for DMV to 617 amino acids for MV while the RPV and PPRV H proteins have 609 amino acid residues. The H protein has only one long hydrophobic domain near the N-terminus (positions 35–58), which acts as a signal peptide but, unlike the signal peptide in the F protein it is not cleaved from the mature protein as it also functions to anchor the protein in the membrane. The N-terminal 34 amino acids remain on the cytoplasmic side of the membrane while the C-terminus is extruded to the outside. This arrangement, with an N-terminal anchor and a C-terminal external domain, classifies H as a type II glycoprotein. The mature protein is a disulphide-linked homodimer which probably associates into tetramers in the spike (Plemper *et al.*, 2000; Vongpunsawad *et al.*, 2004).

Like the F protein the H protein is also translated on ribosomes of the RER and folding to form the correct antigenic epitopes on MV H, as well as oligomerization, occurs as it passes through the RER. It then moves to the cell surface through the Golgi complex (Hu *et al.*, 1994; Blain *et al.*, 1995; Plemper *et al.*, 2001). This folding is mediated through a transient association of H with cellular chaperone proteins such as calnexin and GRP78 and misfolding of the MV H may result in its retention by the chaperones in the RER and inefficient migration to the cell surface (Bolt, 2001). Reduced transport to the cell surface impairs its fusion promotion ability (Plemper *et al.*, 2000). Oligosaccharide side chains are added to the polypeptide in the lumen of the ER, the number of potential N-glycosylation sites on H varying between and within each virus. These side chains are required to move the protein along the exocytic pathway to the cell membrane as well as influencing the antigenicity of the molecule (Hu *et al.*, 1994). The degree of glycosylation may also affect virulence as has been shown for the haemagglutinin-neuraminidase (HN) protein of Newcastle Disease virus (NDV) (Panda *et al.*, 2004).

The H protein, like the P protein, is not well conserved in morbilliviruses. The most distantly related viruses, RPV and PDV, share only 32% amino acid identity and this only rises to about 50% when the two ruminant morbil-liviruses, RPV and PPRV, are compared. This high degree of sequence variation most probably reflects the role of H in binding to host cell receptor(s) and this means that it is also the main target of the host's humoral immune responses and neutralizing antibodies are mainly directed against the H protein. The amino acid changes in H that are potentially linked to the host's adaptive evolution in MV are located in B-cell epitopes and at sites linked to its interactions with the cell receptor (Lecouturier *et al.*, 1996; Hsu *et al.*, 1998). B-cell epitopes capable of inducing neutralizing antibodies have been mapped on the H protein to exposed $\beta$-sheets on the proposed three-dimensional structure (Langedijk *et al.*, 1997; Sugiyama *et al.*, 2002). Recombination by reverse genetics has shown that, while the H proteins of MV and CDV and those of RPV and CDV are interchangeable (Nussbaum *et al.*, 1995; von Messling *et al.*, 2001; Brown *et al.*, 2005b), those of RPV and PPRV are not (Das *et al.*, 2000).

A number of paramyxovirus glycoproteins have been shown to have both haemagglutinating and neuraminidase activities. However, for the morbilli-viruses, strains of MV adapted to grow in tissue culture were the only example within the genus of haemagglutinating activity, amino acid residues at positions 451 and 481 being critical for the maintenance of this activity (Lecouturier *et al.*, 1996). More recent studies have shown that PPRV also has haemagglutination capabilities (Seth and Shaila, 2001) and in terms of activity, is the only morbillivirus H protein that resembles the haemagglu-tinin-neuraminidase (HN) protein of viruses of the other paramyxovirus genera as it also has neuraminidase activity (Langedijk *et al.*, 1997; Seth and Shaila, 2001). The RPV H protein has been shown to have limited neu-raminidase activity but it cannot agglutinate red blood cells (Langedijk *et al.*, 1997).

Virus receptor proteins on cell surfaces have only been clearly identified for MV. These are CD46, used by tissue culture-adapted vaccine strains, and signal lymphocyte activating molecules (SLAM), which can be used by both vaccine and wild-type viruses (Hsu *et al.*, 1998; Tatsuo *et al.*, 2000; von Messling *et al.*, 2001). However, there is evidence that all morbilliviruses can interact with SLAM and this may be a universal morbillivirus receptor; for example CDV can infect cells more readily if they are expressing dog rather than human SLAM (Seki *et al.*, 2003).

## The L protein

The RdRp (L protein) is the largest of the virus proteins and is also the least abundant. It migrates with an apparent molecular weight of about 200 kDa and is composed of 2183 amino acids in MV, RPV, PPRV and DMV. Considering the size of the L protein it is surprisingly conserved between morbilliviruses, the percentage identity between the L proteins of RPV and PPRV being 70.7%. CDV and PDV L proteins share the highest percentage of homology with 89.7% of amino acids in common while PPRV L and CDV L share only 57% (Bailey *et al.*, 2005). Comparison of the L protein sequences of morbilliviruses identified three relatively conserved domains separated by less conserved 'hinge regions' (McIlhatton *et al.*, 1997). Reverse genetics has enabled foreign epitopes, and even a functional GFP, to be inserted at the second hinge region for both MV and RPV while attempts to introduce foreign sequence at the first hinge failed (Duprex *et al.*, 2002). Insertion of the GPF ORF in frame with the L protein sequence produces a green fluorescent virus (Plate 2) which grows to an equivalent titre to that of the parent virus in Vero cells; however, this insertion greatly attenuates the virus for cattle (Brown *et al.*, 2005a).

Because of its size, the RdRp is assumed to carry all the activities necessary for genomic RNA transcription and replication, as well as being able to cap, methylate and polyadenylate viral mRNAs. All deletion/site mutation studies carried out so far on the protein of different non-segmented negative-sense RNA viruses indicate that the three conserved domains perform the diverse functions of the protein (Malur *et al.*, 2002; Cartee *et al.*, 2003). The first domain, residues 1 to 606, has the sequence KEXXRLXXKMXXKM at position 535–549, which is thought to be the RNA binding motif. The second domain, residues 650–1694, contains the sequence GDDD, flanked by hydrophobic regions, which is thought to be the functional site of RdRp (Blumberg *et al.*, 1988) while the third domain, residues 1717–2183, has kinase activity and it may act also act as an ATP binding site.

The L protein can only function as an RdRp when it is associated with its co-factor, the P protein. Horikami *et al.* (1994) mapped the binding site for the P protein of MV to the N-terminal 408 amino acids of the L protein, part of domain I. The sequence ILYPEVHLDSPIV, at positions 9 to 21 of morbillivirus L proteins, is partially conserved within the paramyxoviruses and mutations/deletions involving the sequence ILYPE reduces the binding of P protein to L in the human parainfluenza virus type 3 (hPIV3) L protein and also reduces its transcription function (Malur *et al.*, 2002).

# Virus non-structural protein functions

## The C protein

In addition to the six structural proteins, paramyxoviruses can produce a range of non-structural proteins in infected cells. These are encoded in the P transcription unit in alternative reading frames. The first of these, the C protein, is generated by translation initiation at a second AUG within the P ORF and is read in a different frame to the P protein and so bears no antigenic relationship to it. The C protein is a small basic protein with a molecular weight of 19–21 kDa. In both RPV and PPRV the C protein is composed of 177 amino acids, three residues longer than those of CDV and PDV. The MV C protein with 186 amino acids is the longest whilst DMV, with only 160 amino acid residues, is the shortest. Sequence alignment reveals a high degree of conservation between the different morbillivirus C proteins at the C-terminus, nucleotides 100–167 (93–150 for DMV) (Mahapatra *et al.*, 2003). While the P protein is phosphorylated and found only in the cytoplasm in association with the nucleocapsids, the C is not phosphorylated and can be detected in both the nuclear and cytoplamic compartments of MV infected cells (Bellini *et al.*, 1985; Alkhatib *et al.*, 1988) but in RPV infections the C protein is uniformly distributed in the cytoplasm and is not found in the nucleus (Sweetman *et al.*, 2001).

Interactions of the morbillivirus C proteins with other virus proteins have been studied but the results are not consistent. The RPV C protein self inter-acts as well as binds to the L protein (Sweetman *et al.*, 2001), indicating a function in modulating RdRp activity. Other workers could not demonstrate an interaction either with itself or with any of the other viral proteins in MV infections (Liston *et al.*, 1995). As the C protein has an unusually high iso-electric point, creating a strong positive charge at physiological pH, a possible interaction with RNA has been suggested (Radecke and Billeter, 1996). The C-protein functions are very poorly understood in terms of their biological significance, although there is evidence that the C protein is a virulence fac-tor for MV (Patterson *et al.*, 2000). Using reverse genetics techniques it has been possible to produce viruses that do not express either or both of the non-structural proteins and MV C-minus mutants show no effect on viral multipli-cation or on the formation of progeny virus in some cells, for example in Vero cells, but produce reduced numbers of progeny virus in human peripheral blood mononuclear cells, a normal target cell for MV (Radecke and Billeter, 1996; Escoffier *et al.*, 1999). An RPV C knockout virus, however, showed impaired growth in Vero cells together with reduced viral RNA synthesis (Baron and Barrett, 2000). SeV C-minus mutants show impaired viral repli-cation *in vivo* (Tapparel *et al.*, 1997) and prevention of expression of all the four variants of the C protein in this virus results in severe attenuation of growth in tissue culture and the abrogation of pathogenicity in the natural host (Kurotani *et al.*, 1998). The non-structural proteins are also involved in over-coming the host's innate immunity to infection by blocking the IFN response to virus infection.

## The V protein

The edited mRNA produced from the P transcription unit is the template for the production of the V protein which is shorter than the P protein although the two share identical N-termini. The RPV V protein is phosphorylated and, like P, can bind to both N and L (Sweetman *et al.*, 2001), again indicating involvement of this protein in the regulation of viral RNA synthesis. The V protein has also been shown to bind unassembled N, but not encapsidated N in human parainfluenza virus 2 (Watanabe *et al.*, 1996), SeV (Horikami *et al.*, 1996) and simian virus 5 (SV5) (Randall and Bermingham, 1996), indicating that V may bind to N to keep it soluble prior to encapsidation (Precious *et al.*, 1995). Similar studies with MV using the yeast two-hybrid system, failed to show a V–N interaction (Liston *et al.*, 1995). These discrepancies may be due to the insensitivity of the systems used for detecting protein–protein interactions. The V-specific C-terminal region of the V protein is highly conserved among morbilliviruses and nine shared amino acids are found at the editing site in all, including seven highly conserved cysteine residues. These, along with a number of other residues, are conserved throughout the paramyxoviruses wherever V protein expression has been shown. This arrangement of cysteines at the C-terminus of V is similar to motifs found in metal ion-binding protein and, in fact, this domain of the SV5 and MV V proteins has been shown experimentally to bind to zinc ions (Liston and Briedis, 1994; Paterson *et al.*, 1995). It has also been reported that the cysteine-rich motif interacts with a host cell-derived protein, the 127 kD subunit of the damage-specific DNA binding protein (DDB1) (Lin *et al.*, 1998), although the significance of these interactions for the functioning of the V protein is not clear.

The presumed role of the V protein in regulating RNA synthesis has been studied by abolishing its expression by making alterations to the editing site of the virus which did not alter P protein coding. SeV lacking V grows to a comparable titre, and with a similar phenotype, to wild-type virus in tissue culture cells (Delenda *et al.*, 1997) but displays attenuated replication and pathogenesis in mice (Kato *et al.*, 1997). Mutant RPV and MV lacking V also are viable in tissue culture (Schneider *et al.*, 1997; Baron and Barrett, 2000). The absence of the V protein enhances viral replication in MV while overexpression attenuates RNA synthesis (Tober *et al.*, 1998), indicating a regulatory role of V protein in the transcription process. However, *in vivo* studies with the MV V-minus mutant showed reduced RNA synthesis and a reduced viral load in a mouse model with a consequent reduction in pathogenicity (Patterson *et al.*, 2000). Baron and Barrett (2000) also reported *in vitro* an enhanced synthesis of RPV genome and antigenome RNAs in a V-minus mutant of the vaccine virus but no studies have yet been carried out to establish the role of V in pathogenesis. The fact that these non-structural proteins are conserved in all morbilliviruses, and are present in many other paramyxoviruses, indicates that they have important functions with regard to growth and pathogenicity in the host species. Now that reverse genetics has been established as a tool to study site-specific mutations in these viruses it will be possible to carry out more detailed *in vitro* and *in vivo* studies to clearly define the functions of the non-structural virus proteins.

## The R protein

A third non-structural protein, the R protein, has been identified in MV-infected cells where its synthesis occurs as a result of ribosomal frameshifting during translation of the P protein mRNA. This frameshifting occurs 24 nucleotides upstream of the actual V protein stop codon and the new ORF terminates at the V protein stop, five codons downstream of the frameshift site and so only the last five amino acids at the C-terminal of R are shared with the V-specific region of the V protein. Both proteins have 299 amino acid residues of which 236 are identical; 231 of these are encoded by the sequence of the mRNA before the non-templated G insertion site, along with the last five amino acids at the C-terminus. It also has 294 residues in common with P. The fact that R has the same length as V, the two proteins migrating at the same position in one-dimensional polyacrylamide gels, means that it can only be differentiated from V by two-dimensional gel electrophoresis. The frameshift frequency has been estimated to be about 1.8%. This low frequency along with the fact that R and V co-migrate in one-dimensional protein gels and that there is no antibody specific to R (the first 294 amino acids are shared with P and the last five residues are in common with V), may have contributed to the R protein's existence being overlooked. Indeed MV is the only morbillivirus to date in which it has been described (Liston and Briedis, 1995).

# Molecular determinants of virulence

Reverse genetics now allows us to study the molecular basis underlying virus pathogenicity and host range in non-segmented negative strand viruses in much greater depth. Prior to its development basic molecular information on virus genomes gave some clues to the determinants of pathogenicity in some paramyxoviruses; for example changes at the $F_0$ cleavage site of NDV, which affects its susceptibility to cleavage by host cell proteases, were shown to correlate with virus virulence. Similarly, extensions at the C-terminus of the HN protein of NDV can attenuate the virus for chickens (Romer-Oberdorfer et al., 2003). This involvement of the sequence at the cleavage site of $F_0$ NDV in determining virus pathogenicity has now been confirmed using reverse genetics (Peeters et al., 1999; Panda et al., 2004).

The molecular changes that occurred during the passage of RPV in cells to attenuate the virus and make a safe vaccine (Plowright and Ferris, 1962) have also been investigated in an effort to relate specific changes to virus attenuation. The vaccine differs from the parent (Kabete 'O' strain) at only 87 nucleotide positions (approximately 0.054%) (Baron et al., 1996). These changes result in non-conservative amino substitutions in the N, P, F, H, and L proteins (Baron et al., 1996). Complete DNA copies (cDNA) of the RNA genomes were made for both the Kabete 'O' virus and the vaccine derived from it. These were rescued and have the expected pathogenic characteristics in cattle (Baron and Barrett, 1997; Baron *et al.*, 2005). Suitable restriction sites were introduced at the beginning and end of each protein ORF to facilitate swaps between these two viruses to try to identify which changes had an attenuating effect. The virulent virus then had each of its genes substituted one at a time by those from the vaccine, except for the M gene where no significant changes were found. Animals infected with chimeric viruses where the N, P, F or the first half of the L protein are replaced by the corresponding regions of the vaccine strain show reduced clinical disease, indicating that they each contribute to attenuation, however, no one gene is primarily responsible for attenuating the vaccine. Substitutions of the H gene, or the second half of L, do not affect virus virulence (Baron *et al.*, 2005). Mutations in the L protein of human respiratory syncytial (RS) and parainfluenza viruses are also associated with attenuation and cold sensitivity (Juhasz *et al.*, 1999; McAuliffe *et al.*, 2004).

The higher percentage of nucleotide differences seen within the UTRs, including the GP and AGP, compared to those found in the coding regions of the morbilliviruses, suggests that some of these untranslated promoters might also be involved in determining virus virulence. Studies *in vitro* using a minireplicon system for RPV identified several nucleotides in the GP whose conservation is essential for its function, while others, although not essential, greatly reduced its activity if changed (Mioulet *et al.*, 2001). Minor changes in promoters have been shown to have a significant effect on the pathogenicity of SeV in mice (Fujii *et al.*, 2002) and it was hypothesized that differences within these regions in RPV might profoundly affect its ability to replicate and cause disease in cattle. Recent studies carried out *in vivo* on viruses with chimeric GP and AGP regions confirmed their role in controlling virulence for cattle. For example when the GP and AGP from the highly virulent Saudi/81 strain of RPV were used to replace those of the virulent Kabete 'O' strain it does not affect virulence for cattle. In contrast, substitution of the same promoter regions with those of the vaccine strain greatly attenuates the virus (Banyard *et al.*, 2005). There are only 7 nucleotide changes in the vaccine compared to the wild-type virus in the GP and only 2 in the AGP. These results confirmed that minor changes in the promoter regions can significantly affect virus virulence and could be an explanation for the emergence of rinderpest virus strains varying greatly in their ability to cause disease in cattle and wild animals (Kock *et al.*, 1999). However, changes in the promoter regions are not the only ones that attenuate the RPV vaccine since replacing the vaccine promoters with those from the virulent strains did not make the vaccine pathogenic and so it is clear that the vaccine's attenuation is due to multiple mutations in several genes, as well as in the promoter regions. Taken together these data show that the Plowright vaccine has multiple mutations underlying its attenuation and these make for a highly safe and stable vaccine.

## Molecular determinants of host range

Each morbillivirus is generally only able to cause serious disease in one order of mammals and the basis for this host range variation probably lies both in the ability of the H protein to bind specific host cell receptors and also the interactions of host and virus proteins within the infected cell. For example, the Plowright vaccine strain is not able to replicate in rabbits but if the H gene of the lapinized strain is substituted it will replicate, albeit very poorly, in rabbits and generate an immune response (Yoneda *et al.*, 2002). However, the additional substitution of the P gene from the lapinized strain makes it highly pathogenic for rabbits. Since the non-structural proteins are also encoded in the P gene region, and they are known to be involved in overcoming the host's innate immune responses to virus infection, it could be that C and/or V, rather than the P protein itself, confer this virulence for rabbits but this remains to be confirmed experimentally (Yoneda *et al.*, 2004). Even a single amino acid change can alter the binding of this protein to receptors and affect tissue tropism (Hsu *et al.*, 1998; von Messling *et al.*, 2001). A stretch of amino acids (368–396) has been identified within the MV H protein that has been defined as a major antigenic determinant of the H protein and is assumed to play a role in neurotropism and virulence (Liebert *et al.*, 1994; Hummel and Bellini, 1995). Swapping the H gene from a brain-adapted neurovirulent strain of MV to a wild-type strain confers neurovirulence on the wild-type strain (Duprex *et al.*, 1999; Moeller *et al.*, 2002). Similar swaps between a wild-type strain of MV and the Edmonston vaccine strain enables growth of the vaccine strain in previously non-permissive cell lines since the vaccine has adapted to use CD46 rather than SLAM as a receptor molecule through passage in tissue culture (Johnston *et al.*, 1999; Takeuchi *et al.*, 2002).

## Conclusions

The contribution that reverse genetics has made to our knowledge of the molecular biology of Paramyxovirinae is difficult to overstate; however, there are still huge gaps in our understanding of the complexities of these viruses which current studies are attempting to fill. One of the most intriguing areas of research is to understand the complex interplay of virus and host cell proteins in infected cells. New post genomic technologies, such as microarray analysis to identify alterations in the transcription of mRNAs for different host proteins following infection, will further increase our knowledge of this aspect of virus replication and its relationship to virus virulence and cell tropism. No work has yet been carried out to investigate the molecular basis of the variations in virulence between wild-type morbillivirus strains, including rinderpest strains, for different hosts. In the 1990s there were three lineages of rinderpest virus in circulation; an Asian and two African (see Chapter 8). The only virus now in circulation is African lineage 2 in the Kenya-Somalia ecosystem and infections in cattle produce only a mild disease, however, infections in wildlife species such as buffalo and kudu result in severe disease (see Chapter 7). The basis for this variation is not known and it is not lineage related since historic strains of lineage 2 have been shown to be highly virulent in cattle. One question that remains uppermost is the likelihood of morbilliviruses crossing the species barrier, particularly now that rinderpest has been virtually eliminated from the world; will another morbillivirus, such as PPR, evolve to fill its niche?

# Acknowledgements

The contribution of many people has made this work possible and so we thank Professor Bert Rima and Drs Michael Baron, Paul Duprex and David Brown for their contribution to this work over many years. Mr Dalan Bailey provided invaluable help with the computer analyses of the sequence data.

# References

Alkahatib, G., Massie, B. and Briedis, D.J. (1988) Expression of bicistronic measles virus P/C mRNA by using hybrid adenoviruses: levels of C protein synthesised in vivo are unaffected by the presence or abscence of the upstream P initiator codon. *J. Virol.* **62**, 4059–69.

Alkhatib, G., Roder, J., Richardson, C., Briedis, D., Weinberg, R., Smith, D., Taylor, J., Paoletti, E. and Shen, S. H. (1994a). Characterization of a cleavage mutant of the measles virus fusion protein defective in syncytium formation. *J. Virol.* **68**, 6770–4.

Alkhatib, G., Shen, S.H., Briedis, D., Richardson, C., Massie, B., Weinberg, R., Smith, D., Taylor, J., Paoletti, E. and Roder, J. (1994b) Functional analysis of N-linked glycosylation mutants of the measles virus fusion protein synthesized by recombinant vaccinia virus vectors. *J. Virol.* **68**, 1522–31.

Bailey, D., Banyard, A., Dash, P., Ozkul, A. and Barrett, T. (2005) Full genome sequence of Peste des Petits Ruminants virus, a member of the Morbillivirus genus. *Virus Res.* **110**, 119–24.

Banerjee, A.K. (1987) Transcription and replication of rhabdoviruses. *Microbiol. Rev.* **51**, 66–87.

Bankamp, B., Horikami, S.M., Thompson, P.D., Huber, M., Billeter, M. and Moyer, S.A. (1996) Domains of the measles virus N-protein required for binding to P-protein and self-assembly. *Virology* **216**, 272–7.

Banyard, A.C., Baron, M.D. and Barrett, T. (2005) A role for virus promoters in determining the pathogenesis of Rinderpest virus in cattle. *J. Gen. Virol.* **86**, 1083–92.

Baron, M.D. and Barrett, T. (1995) Sequencing and analysis of the nucleocapsid (N) and polymerase (L) genes and the terminal extragenic domains of the vaccine strain of rinderpest. *J. Gen. Virol.* **76**, 593–602.

Baron, M.D. and Barrett, T. (1997) Rescue of rinderpest virus from cloned cDNA. *J. Virol.* **71**, 1265–71.

Baron, M.D. and Barrett, T. (2000) Rinderpest virus lacking the C and V proteins show specific defects in growth and transcription of viral RNAs. *J. Virol.* **74**, 2603–11.

Baron, M.D., Banyard, A.C., Parida, S. and Barrett, T. (2005) The Plowright vaccine strain of Rinderpest virus has attenuating mutations in most genes. *J. Gen. Virol.* **86**, 1093–101.

Baron, M.D., Kamata, Y., Barras, V., Goatley, L. and Barrett, T. (1996) The genome sequence of the virulent Kabete 'O' strain of rinderpest virus: comparison with the derived vaccine. *J. Gen. Virol.* **77**, 3041–6.

Barr, J.N., Whelan, S.P.J. and Wertz, G.W. (2002) Transcriptional control of the RNA-dependent RNA polymerase of vesicular stomatitis virus. *Biochim. Biophys. Acta-Gene Struct. Expr.* **1577**, 337–53.

Bellini, W.J., Englund, G., Rozenblatt, S., Arnheiter, H. and Richardson, C.D. (1985) Measles virus P gene codes for two proteins. *J. Virol.* **53**, 908–19.

Billeter, M.A., Baczko, K., Schmid, A. and ter Meulen, V. (1984) Cloning of DNA corresponding to four different measles virus genomic regions. *Virology* **132**, 147–59.

Billeter, M.A., Cattaneo, R., Spielhofer, P., Kaelin, K., Huber, M., Schmid, A., Baczko, K. and ter Meulen, V. (1994) Generation and properties of measles-virus mutations typically associated with subacute sclerosing panencephalitis. *Slow Infect. Centr. Nerv. Syst.* **724**, 367–77.

Blain, F., Liston, P. and Briedis, D.J. (1995) The carboxy-terminal 18 amino acids of the measles virus hemagglutinin are essential for its biological function. *Biochem. Biophys. Res. Commun.* **214**, 1232–8.

Blau, D.M. and Compans, R.W. (1995) Entry and release of measles virus are polarized in epithelial cells. *Virology* **210**, 91–9.

Blixenkrone-Møller, M., Sharma, B., Varsanyi, T.M., Hu, A., Norrby, E. and Kövamees, J. (1992) Sequence analysis of the genes encoding the nucleocapsid protein and phosphoprotein (P) of phocid distemper virus, and editing of the P gene transcript. *J. Gen. Virol.* **73**, 885–93.

Blumberg, B. and Kolakofsky, D. (1981) Intracellular vesicular stomatitis virus leader RNAs are found in nucleocapsid structures. *J. Virol.* **40**, 568–76.

Blumberg, B.M., Crowley, J.C., Silverman, J.I., Mennona, J., Cook, S.D. and Dowling, P.C. (1988) Measles virus L protein evidences elements of ancestral RNA polymerase. *Virology* **164**, 487–97.

Bolt, G. (2001) The measles virus (MV) glycoproteins interact with cellular chaperones in the endoplasmic reticulum and MV infection upregulates chaperone expression. *Arch. Virol.* **146**, 2055–68.

Bolt, G., Alexandersen, S. and Blixenkrone-Møller, M. (1995) The phosphoprotein gene of a dolphin morbillivirus isolate exhibits genomic variation at the editing site. *J. Gen. Virol.* **76**, 3051–8.

Bolt, G., Pedersen, I.R. and Blixenkrone-Møller, M. (1999) Processing of N-linked oligosaccharides on the measles virus glycoproteins: importance for the antigenicity and for production of infectious virus particles. *Virus Res.* **61**, 43–51.

Bourdin, P. and Laurent-Vautier, A. (1967) Note sur la structure du virus de la peste des petits ruminants. *Rev. Elev. Méd. Vét. Pays Trop.* **20**, 383–5.

Bourhis, J.M., Johansson, K., Receveur-Brechot, V., Oldfield, C.J., Dunker, K.A., Canard, B. and Longhi, S. (2004) The C-terminal domain of measles virus nucleoprotein belongs to the class of intrinsically disordered proteins that fold upon binding to their physiological partner. *Virus Res.* **99**, 157–67.

Brown, D.D., Rima, B.K., Allen, I.V., Baron, M.D., Barett, T. and Duprex, W.P. (2005a) Rational attenuation of a morbillivirus by modulating the activity of the RNA-dependent RNA polymerase. *J. Virol.*, in press.

Brown, D.D., Collins, F.M., Duprex, W.P., Baron, M.D., Barrett, T. and Rima, B.K. (2005b) 'Rescue' of mini-genomic constructs and viruses by combinations of morbillivirus N, P and L proteins. *J. Gen. Virol.* **86**, 1077–81.

Buckland, R., Malvoisin, E., Beauverger, P. and Wild, F. (1992) A leucine zipper structure present in the measles virus fusion protein is not required for its tetramerization but is essential for fusion. *J. Gen. Virol.* **73**, 1703–7.

Calain, P. and Roux, L. (1993) The rule of six, a basic feature for efficient replication of Sendai virus defective interfering RNA. *J. Virol.* **67**, 4822–30.

Cartee, T.L., Megaw, A.G., Oomens, A.G. and Wertz, G.W. (2003) Identification of a single amino acid change in the human respiratory syncytial virus L protein that affects transcriptional termination. *J. Virol.* **77**, 7352–60.

Castaneda, S.J. and Wong, T.C. (1989) Measles virus synthesises both leaderless and leader-containing polyadenylated RNA species *in-vivo*. *J. Virol.* **63**, 2977–86.

Castaneda, S. J. and Wong, T. C. (1990) Leader sequence distinguishes between translatable and encapsidated measles virus RNA. *J. Virol.* **64**, 222–30.

Cathomen, T., Buchholz, C.J., Spielhofer, P. and Cattaneo, R. (1995) Preferential initiation at the second AUG of the measles virus F mRNA: A role for the long untranslated region. *Virology* **214**, 628–32.

Cathomen, T., Mrkic, B., Spehener, D., Drillien, R., Naef, R., Pavlovic, J., Aguzzi, A., Billeter, M.A. and Cattaneo, R. (1998) A matrix-less measles virus is infectious and elicits extensive cell fusion: consequences for propagation in the brain. *EMBO J.* **17**, 3899.

Cattaneo, R., Kaelin, K., Baczko, K. and Billeter, M.A. (1989b) Measles virus editing provides an additional cysteine-rich protein. *Cell* **56**, 759–64.

Cattaneo, R., Schmid, A., Billeter, M.A., Sheppard, R.D. and Udem, S.A. (1988) Multiple viral mutations rather than host factors cause defective measles virus gene expression in a subacute sclerosing panencephalitis cell-line. *J. Virol.* **62**, 1388–97.

Cattaneo, R., Schmid, A., Spielhofer, P., Kaelin, K., Baczko, K., Meulen, V. ter, Pardowitz, J., Flanagan, S., Rima, B.K., Udem, S.A. and Billeter, M.A. (1989a) Mutated and hypermutated genes of persistent measles viruses which caused lethal human brain disease. *Virology* **173**, 415–25.

Chazal, N. and Gerlier, D. (2003) Virus entry, assembly, budding, and membrane rafts. *Microbiol. Mol. Biol. Rev.* **67**, 226–37, table of contents.

Chuang, J.L. and Perrault, J. (1997) Initiation of vesicular stomatitis virus mutant polR1 transcription internally at the N gene in vitro. *J. Virol.* **71**, 1466–75.

Collins, P.L., Mink, M.A. and Stec, D.S. (1991) Rescue of synthetic analogs or respiratory syncytial virus genomic RNA and effect of truncations and mutations on the expression of a foreign reporter gene. *Proc. Natl Acad. Sci. USA* **88**, 9663–7.

Coronel, E.C., Takimoto, T., Murti, K.G., Varich, N. and Portner, A. (2001) Nucleocapsid incorporation into parainfluenza virus is regulated by specific interaction with matrix protein. *J. Virol.* **75**, 1117–23.

Crowley, J.C., Dowling, P.C., Menonna, J., Silverman, J.I., Schuback, D., Cook, S.D. and Blumberg, B.M. (1988) Sequence variability and function of measles virus 3′ and 5′ ends and intercistronic regions. *Virology* **164**, 498–506.

Das, S.C., Baron, M.D. and Barrett, T. (2000) Recovery and characterization of a chimeric rinderpest virus with the glycoproteins of peste-des-petits-ruminants virus: Homologous F and H proteins are required for virus viability. *J. Virol.* **74**, 9039–47.

Delenda, C., Hausmann, S., Garcin, D. and Kolakofsky, D. (1997) Normal cellular replication of Sendai virus without the trans-frame, nonstructural V protein. *Virology* **228**, 55–62.

Diallo, A., Barrett, T., Barbron, M., Meyer, G. and Lefevre, P.C. (1994) Cloning of the nucleocapsid protein gene of peste-des-petits-ruminants virus: relationship to other morbilliviruses. *J. Gen. Virol.* **75** (Pt 1), 233–7.

Diallo, A., Barrett, T., Lefevre, P.C. and Taylor, W.P. (1987) Comparison of proteins induced in cells infected with rinderpest and peste des petits ruminants viruses. *J. Gen. Virol.* **68**, 2033–8.

Dimock, K. and Collins, P. (1993) Rescue of synthetic analogues of genomic RNA and replicative-intermediate RNA of human parainfluenza virus type 3. *J. Virol.* **67**, 2772–8.

Duprex, W.P., Collins, F.M. and Rima, B.K. (2002) Modulating the function of the measles virus RNA-dependent RNA polymerase by insertion of green fluorescent protein into the open reading frame. *J. Virol.* **76**, 7322–8.

Duprex, W.P., Duffy, I., McQuaid, S., Hamill, L., Cosby, S.L., Billeter, M.A., Schneider-Schaulies, J., Meulen, V. ter and Rima, B.K. (1999) The H gene of rodent brain-adapted measles virus confers neurovirulence to the Edmonston vaccine strain. *J. Virol.* **73**, 6916–22.

Durbin, A.P., Siew, J.W., Murphy, B.R. and Collins, P.L. (1997) Minimum protein requirements for transcription and RNA replication of a minigenome of human parainfluenza virus 3, and evaluation of the rule of six. *Virology* **234**, 74–83.

Ecker, A., Meulen, V. ter, Baczko, K. and Schneider-Schaulies, S. (1995) Measles virus-specific dsRNAs are targets for unwinding/modifying activity in neural cells in vitro. *J. Neurovirol.* **1**, 92–100.

Escoffier, C., Manie, S., Vincent, S., Muller, C. P., Billiter, M. and Gerlier, D. (1999) Nonstructural C protein is required for efficient measles virus replication in human peripheral blood cells. *J. Virol.* **73**, 1695–8.

Evans, S.A., Baron, M.D., Chamberlain, R.W., Goatley, L. and Barrett, T. (1994) Nucleotide sequence comparisons of the fusion protein gene from virulent and attenuated strains of rinderpest virus. *J. Gen. Virol.* **75**, 3611–17.

Evans, S.A., Belsham, G.J. and Barrett, T. (1990) The role of the 5′ nontranslated regions of the fusion protein mRNAs of canine distemper virus and rinderpest virus. *Virology* **177**, 317–23.

Fearns, R., Peeples, M.E. and Collins, P.L. (1997) Increased expression of the N protein of respiratory syncytial virus stimulates minigenome replication but does not alter the balance between the synthesis of mRNA antigenome. *Virology* **236**, 188–201.

Finke, S. and Conzelmann, K.K. (1997) Ambisense gene expression from recombinant rabies virus: random packaging of positive- and negative-strand ribonucleoprotein complexes into rabies virions. *J. Virol.* **71**, 7281–8.

Finke, S. and Conzelmann, K.K. (2003) Dissociation of rabies virus matrix protein functions in regulation of viral RNA synthesis and virus assembly. *J. Virol.* **77**, 12074–82.

Fujii, Y., Sakaguchi, T., Kiyotani, K., Huang, C., Fukuhara, N., Egi, Y. and Yoshida, T. (2002) Involvement of the leader sequence in Sendai virus pathogenesis revealed by recovery of a pathogenic field isolate from cDNA. *J. Virol.* **76**, 8540–7.

Gibbs, E.P., Taylor, W.P., Lawman, M.J. and Bryant, J. (1979) Classification of peste des petits ruminants virus as the fourth member of the genus Morbillivirus. *Intervirol.* **11**, 268–74.

Giraudon, P., Jacquier, M.F. and Wild, T.F. (1988) Antigenic analysis of African measles-virus field isolates – identification and localization of one conserved and 2 variable epitope sites on the Np protein. *Virus Res.* **10**, 137–52.

Gombart, A.F., Hirano, A. and Wong, T.C. (1993) Conformational maturation of measles virus nucleocapsid protein. *J. Virol.* **67**, 4133–41.

Gubbay, O., Curran, J. and Kolakofsky, D. (2001) Sendai virus genome synthesis and assembly are coupled: a possible mechanism to promote viral RNA polymerase processivity. *J. Gen. Virol.* **82**, 2895–903.

Gupta, A.K., Shaji, D. and Banerjee, A.K. (2003) Identification of a novel tripartite complex involved in replication of vesicular stomatitis virus genome RNA. *J. Virol.* **77**, 732–8.

Haffar, A., Libeau, G., Moussa, A., Cecile, M. and Diallo, A. (1999) The matrix protein gene sequence analysis reveals close relationship between peste des petits ruminants virus (PPRV) and dolphin morbillivirus. *Virus Res.* **64**, 69–75.

Harty, R.N. and Palese, P. (1995a) Measles virus phosphoprotein (P) requires the $NH_2$-terminal and COOH-terminal domains for interactions with the nucleoprotein (N) but only the COOH terminus for interactions with itself. *J. Gen. Virol.* **76**, 2863–7.

Harty, R.N. and Palese, P. (1995b) Mutations within noncoding terminal sequences of model RNAs of Sendai virus: influence on reporter gene expression. *J. Virol.* **69**, 5128–31.

Hausmann, S., Garcin, D., Delenda, C. and Kolakofsky, D. (1999) The versatility of paramyxovirus RNA polymerase stuttering. *J. Virol.* **73**, 5568–76.

Hinzman, E.E., Barr, J.N. and Wertz, G.W. (2002) Identification of an upstream sequence element required for vesicular stomatitis virus mRNA transcription. *J. Virol.* **76**, 7632–41.

Hoffman, M.A. and Banerjee, A.K. (2000) Precise mapping of the replication and transcription promoters of human parainfluenza virus type 3. *Virology* **269**, 201–11.

Horikami, S.M. and Moyer, S.A. (1995) Structure, transcription, and replication of measles virus. *Curr. Topics Microbiol. Immunol.* **191**, 35–50.

Horikami, S.M., Curran, J., Kolakofsky, D. and Moyer, S.A. (1992) Complexes of Sendai virus NP-P and P-L proteins are required for defective interfering particle genome replication *in vitro*. *J. Virol.* **66**, 4901–8.

Horikami, S.M., Smallwood, S., Bankamp, B. and Moyer, S.A. (1994) An amino-proximal domain of the L protein binds to the P protein in the measles virus RNA polymerase complex. *Virology* **205**, 540–5.

Horikami, S.M., Smallwood, S. and Moyer, S.A. (1996) The Sendai virus V protein interacts with the NP protein to regulate viral genome RNA replication. *Virology* **222** (2), 383–90.

Hsu, E.C., Sarangi, F., Iorio, C., Sidhu, M.S., Udem, S.A., Dillehay, D.L., Xu, W.B., Rota, P. A., Bellini, W.J. and Richardson, C.D. (1998) A single amino acid change in the hemagglutinin protein of measles virus determines its ability to bind CD46 and reveals another receptor on marmoset B cells. *J. Virol.* **72**, 2905–16.

Hu, A.H., Cattaneo, R., Schwartz, S. and Norrby, E. (1994) Role of N-linked oligosaccharide chains in the processing and antigenicity of measles virus hemagglutinin protein. *J. Gen. Virol.* **75**, 1043–52.

Huber, M., Cattaneo, R., Spielhofer, P., Örvell, C., Norrby, E., Messerli, M., Perriard, J.-C. and Billeter, M.A. (1991) Measles virus phosphoprotein retains the nucleocapsid protein in the cytoplasm. *Virology* **185**, 299–308.

Hummel, K.B. and Bellini, W.J. (1995) Localization of monoclonal antibody epitopes and functional domains in the hemagglutinin protein of measles virus. *J. Virol.* **69**, 1913–16.

Iakoucheva, L.M., Radivojac, P., Brown, C.J., O'Connor, T.R., Sikes, J.G., Obradovic, Z. and Dunker, A.K. (2004) The importance of intrinsic disorder for protein phosphorylation. *Nucleic Acids Res.* **32**, 1037–49.

Iseni, F., Baudin, F., Garcin, D., Marq, J., Ruigrok, R. and Kolakofsky, D. (2002) Chemical modification of nucleotide bases and mRNA editing depend on hexamer or nucleoprotein phase in Sendai virus nucleocapsids. *RNA* **8**, 1056–67.

Johansson, K., Bourhis, J.M., Campanacci, V., Cambillau, C., Canard, B. and Longhi, S. (2003) Crystal structure of the measles virus phosphoprotein domain responsible for the induced folding of the C-terminal domain of the nucleoprotein. *J. Biol. Chem.* **278**, 44567–73.

Johnston, I., ter Meulen, V., Schneider-Schaulies, J. and Schneider-Schaulies, S. (1999) A recombinant measles vaccine virus expressing wild-type glycoproteins: consequences for viral spread and cell tropism. *J. Virol.* **73**, 6903–15.

Juhasz, K., Murphy, B.R. and Collins, P.L. (1999) The major attenuating mutations of the respiratory syncytial virus vaccine candidate cpts530/1009 specify temperature-sensitive defects in transcription and replication and a non-temperature sensitive alteration in mRNA termination. *J. Virol.* **73**, 5176–80.

Karlin, D., Longhi, S. and Canard, B. (2002) Substitution of two residues in the measles virus nucleoprotein results in an impaired self-association. *Virology* **302**, 420–32.

Kato, A., Kiyotani, K., Sakai, Y., Yoshida, T. and Nagai, Y. (1997) The paramyxovirus, Sendai virus, V protein encodes a luxury function required for viral pathogenesis. *EMBO J.* **16**, 578–87.

Kaushik, R. and Shaila, M.S. (2004) Cellular casein kinase II-mediated phosphorylation of rinderpest virus P protein is a prerequisite for its role in replication/transcription of the genome. *J. Gen. Virol.* **85**, 687–91.

Kock, N.D., Kock, R.A., Wambua, J. and Mwanzia, J. (1999) Pathological changes in free-ranging African ungulates during a rinderpest epizootic in Kenya, 1993 to 1997. *Vet. Rec.* **145**, 527–8.

Kolakofsky, D., Le Mercier, P., Iseni, F. and Garcin, D. (2004) Viral DNA polymerase scanning and the gymnastics of Sendai virus RNA synthesis. *Virology* **318**, 463–73.

Kolakofsky, D., Pelet, T., Garcin, D., Hausmann, S., Curran, J. and Roux, L. (1998) Paramyxovirus RNA synthesis and the requirement for hexamer genome length: the rule of six revisited. *J. Virol.* **72**, 891–9.

Kozak, M. (1984) Compilation and analysis of sequences upstream from the translational start site in eukaryotic mRNAs. *Nucl. Acid Res.* **12**, 857–72.

Kurotani, A., Kiyotani, K., Kato, A., Shioda, T., Sakai, Y., Mizumoto, K., Yoshida, T. and Nagai, Y. (1998) Sendai virus C proteins are categorically nonessential gene products but silencing their expression severely impairs viral replication and pathogenesis. *Genes to Cells* **3**, 111–24.

Laine, D., Trescol-Biemont, M.C., Longhi, S., Libeau, G., Marie, J.C., Vidalain, P.O., Azocar, O., Diallo, A., Canard, B., Rabourdin-Combe, C. and Valentin, H. (2003) Measles virus (MV) nucleoprotein binds to a novel cell surface receptor distinct from FcgammaRII via its C-terminal domain: role in MV-induced immunosuppression. *J. Virol.* **77**, 11332–46.

Lamb, A. and Kolakofsky, D. (2001) Paramyxoviridae: the viruses and their replication. In: D. Knipe and P. Howley (eds), Fields *Virology*, 4th edn. Philadelphia: Lippincott Williams and Wilkins, pp. 1305–43.

Langedijk, J., Daus, F. and Oirschot, J. van (1997) Sequence and structure alignment of Paramyxoviridae attachment proteins and discovery of enzymatic activity for a morbillivirus hemagglutinin. *J. Virol.* **71**, 6155–67.

Lecouturier, V., Fayolle, J., Caballero, M., Carabaña, J., Celma, M. L., Fernandez-Muñoz, R., Wild, T. F. and Buckland, R. (1996) Identification of two amino acids in the hemagglutinin glycoprotein of measles virus (MV) that govern hemadsorption, HeLa cell fusion, and CD46 downregulation: phenotypic markers that differentiate vaccine and wild-type MV strains. *J. Virol.* **70**, 4200–4.

Li, T. and Pattnaik, A.K. (1997) Replication signals in the genome of vesicular stomatitis virus and its defective interfering particles: identification of a sequence element that enhances DI RNA replication. *Virology* **232**, 248–59.

Liebert, U.G., Flanagan, S.G., Loffler, S., Baczko, K., ter Meulen, V. and Rima, B.K. (1994) Antigenic determinants of measles virus hemagglutinin associated with neurovirulence. *J. Virol.* **68**, 1486–93.

Liermann, H., Harder,.T.C., Lochelt, M., von Messling, V., Baumgartner, W., Moennig, V. and Haas, L. (1998) Genetic analysis of the central untranslated genome region and the proximal coding part of the F gene of wild-type and vaccine canine distemper morbilliviruses. *Virus Genes* **17** (3), 259–70.

Lin, G.Y., Paterson, R.G., Richardson, C.D. and Lamb, R.A. (1998) The V protein of the paramyxovirus SV5 interacts with damage-specific DNA binding protein. *Virology* **249**, 189–200.

Liston, P. and Briedis, D.J. (1994) Measles virus V protein binds zinc. *Virology* **198**, 399–404.

Liston, P. and Briedis, D.J. (1995) Ribosomal frameshifting during translation of measles virus P protein mRNA is capable of directing synthesis of a unique protein. *J. Virol.* **69** (11), 6742–50.

Liston, P., Batal, R., DiFlumeri, C. and Briedis, D.J. (1997) Protein interaction domains of the measles virus nucleocapsid protein (NP). *Arch. Virol.* **142** (2), 305–21.

Liston, P., DiFlumeri, C. and Briedis, D.J. (1995) Protein interactions entered into by the measles virus P proteins, V proteins, and C proteins. *Virus Res.* **38**, 241–59.

Longhi, S., Receveur-Brechot, V., Karlin, D., Johansson, K., Darbon, H., Bhella, D., Yeo, R., Finet, S. and Canard, B. (2003) The C-terminal domain of the measles virus nucleoprotein is intrinsically disordered and folds upon binding to the C-terminal moiety of the phosphoprotein. *J. Biol. Chem.* **278**, 18638–48.

Mahapatra, M., Parida, S., Egziabher, B.G., Diallo, A. and Barrett, T. (2003) Sequence analysis of the phosphoprotein gene of peste des petits ruminants (PPR) virus: editing of the gene transcript. *Virus Res.* **96**, 85–98.

Maisner, A., Klenk, H.-D. and Herrler, G. (1998) Polarized budding of measles virus is not determined by viral surface glycoproteins. *J. Virol.* **72**, 5276–8.

Malur, A.G., Choudhary, S.K., De, B.P. and Banerjee, A.K. (2002) Role of a highly conserved NH(2)-terminal domain of the human parainfluenza virus type 3 RNA polymerase. *J. Virol.* **76**, 8101–9.

Manie, S.N., Debreyne, S., Vincent, S. and Gerlier, D. (2000) Measles virus structural components are enriched into lipid raft microdomains: a potential cellular location for virus assembly. *J. Virol.* **74**, 305–11.

McAuliffe, J.M., Surman, S.R., Newman, J.T., Riggs, J.M., Collins, P.L., Murphy, B.R. and Skiadopoulos, M.H. (2004) Codon substitution mutations at two positions in the L polymerase protein of human parainfluenza virus type 1 yield viruses with a spectrum of attenuation in vivo and increased phenotypic stability in vitro. *J. Virol.* **78**, 2029–36.

McIlhatton, M.A., Curran, M.D. and Rima, B.K. (1997) Nucleotide sequence analysis of the large (L) genes of phocine distemper virus and canine distemper virus (corrected sequence) *J. Gen. Virol.* **78**, 571–6.

Meyer, G. and Diallo, A. (1995) The nucleotide sequence of the fusion protein gene of the peste des petits ruminants virus – the long untranslated region in the 5′-end of the F-protein gene of morbilliviruses seems to be specific to each virus. *Virus Res.* **37**, 23–35.

Mioulet, V., Barrett, T. and Baron, M.D. (2001) Scanning mutagenesis identifies critical residues in the rinderpest virus genome promoter. *J. Gen. Virol.* **82**, 2905–11.

Mitra-Kaushik, S., Nayak, R. and Shaila, M.S. (2001) Identification of a cytotoxic T-cell epitope on the recombinant nucleocapsid proteins of Rinderpest and Peste des petits ruminants viruses presented as assembled nucleocapsids. *Virology* **279**, 210–20.

Moeller, K., Duffy, I., Duprex, P., Rima, B., Beschorner, R., Fauser, S., Meyermann, R., Niewiesk, S., ter Meulen, V. and Schneider-Schaulies, J. (2002) Recombinant measles viruses expressing altered hemagglutinin (H) genes: functional separation of mutations determining H antibody escape from neurovirulence. *J. Virol.* **75**, 7612–20.

Moll, M., Klenk, H.D., Herrler, G. and Maisner, A. (2001) A single amino acid change in the cytoplasmic domains of measles virus glycoproteins H and F alters targeting, endocytosis, and cell fusion in polarized Madin–Darby canine kidney cells. *J. Biol. Chem.* **276**, 17887–94.

Moll, M., Klenk, H.D. and Maisner, A. (2002) Importance of the cytoplasmic tails of the measles virus glycoproteins for fusogenic activity and the generation of recombinant measles viruses. *J. Virol.* **76**, 7174–86.

Moll, M., Pfeuffer, J., Klenk, H.D., Niewiesk, S. and Maisner, A. (2004) Polarized glycoprotein targeting affects the spread of measles virus in vitro and in vivo. *J. Gen. Virol.* **85**, 1019–27.

Moyer, S.A., Baker, S.C. and Horikami, S.M. (1990) Host cell proteins required for measles virus reproduction. *J. Gen. Virol.* **71**, 775–83.

Murphy, S.K. and Parks, G.D. (1999) RNA replication for the paramyxovirus simian virus 5 requires an internal repeated (CGNNNN) sequence motif. *J. Virol.* **73**, 805–9.

Naim, H.Y., Ehler, E. and Billeter, M.A. (2000) Measles virus matrix protein specifies apical virus release and glycoprotein sorting in epithelial cells. *EMBO. J.* **19**, 3576–85.

Nussbaum, O., Broder, C.C., Moss, B., Stern, L.B.L., Rozenblatt, S. and Berger, E.A. (1995) Functional and structural interactions between measles virus hemagglutinin and CD46. *J. Virol.* **69**, 3341–9.

Panda, A., Elankumaran, S., Krishnamurthy, S., Huang, Z. and Samal, S.K. (2004) Loss of N-linked glycosylation from the hemagglutinin-neuraminidase protein alters virulence of Newcastle disease virus. *J. Virol.* **78**, 4965–75.

Paterson, R.G., Leser, G.P., Shaughnessy, M.A. and Lamb, R.A. (1995) The paramyxovirus SV5 V protein binds two atoms of zinc and is a structural component of virions. *Virology* **208**, 121–31.

Patterson, J.B., Thomas, D., Lewicki, H., Billeter, M.A. and Oldstone, B.A. (2000) V and C proteins of measles virus function as virulence factors in vivo. *Virology* **267**, 80–9.

Peeples, M.E. (1991) Paramyxovirus M proteins: pulling it all together and taking it on the road. In: David W. Kingsbury (ed.), *The Paramyxoviruses*. New York: Plenum Press, pp. 427–56.

Peeters, B.P.H., de Leeuw, O.S., Koch, G. and Gielkens, A.L.J. (1999) Rescue of Newcastle disease virus from cloned cDNA: evidence that cleavability of the fusion protein is a major determinant for virulence. *J. Virol.* **73**, 5001–9.

Plemper, R.K., Hammond, A.L. and Cattaneo, R. (2000) Characterization of a region of the measles virus hemagglutinin sufficient for its dimerization. *J. Virol.* **74**, 6485–93.

Plemper, R.K., Hammond, A.L. and Cattaneo, R. (2001) Measles virus envelope glycoproteins hetero-oligomerize in the endoplasmic reticulum. *J. Biol. Chem.* **276**, 44239–46.

Plemper, R.K., Hammond, A.L., Gerlier, D., Fielding, A.K. and Cattaneo, R. (2002) Strength of envelope protein interaction modulates cytopathicity of measles virus. *J. Virol.* **76**, 5051–61.

Plowright, W. and Ferris, R.D. (1962) Studies with Rinderpest virus in tissue culture. The use of attenuated culture virus as a vaccine for cattle. *Res. Vet. Sci.* **3**, 172–82.

Precious, B., Young, D.F., Bermingham, A., Fearns, R., Ryan, M. and Randall, R.E. (1995) Inducible expression of the P, V, and Np genes of the paramyxovirus simian virus 5 in cell lines and an examination of NP-P and NP-V interactions. *J. Virol.* **69**, 8001–10.

Radecke, F. and Billeter, M.A. (1996) The nonstructural C protein is not essential for multiplication of Edmonston B strain measles virus in cultured cells. *Virology* **217**, 418–21.

Radecke, F., Spielhofer, P., Schneider, H., Kaelin, K., Huber, M., Ditsch, C., Christiansen, G. and Billeter, M.A. (1995) Rescue of measles virus from cloned DNA. *EMBO J.* **14**, 5773–84.

Rahaman, A., Srinivasan, N., Shamala, N. and Shaila, M.S. (2004) Phosphoprotein of the rinderpest virus forms a tetramer through a coiled coil region important for biological function: a structural insight. *J. Biol. Chem.* pp. 23606–14.

Randall, R.E. and Bermingham, A. (1996) NP-P and NP-V interactions of the paramyxovirus simian virus 5 examined using a novel protein-protein capture assay. *Virology* **224**, 121–9.

Rassa, J.C., Wilson, G.M., Brewer, G.A. and Parks, G.D. (2000) Spacing constraints on reinitiation of paramyxovirus transcription: The gene end U tract acts as a spacer to separate gene end from gene start sites. *Virology* **274**, 438–49.

Riedl, P., Moll, M., Klenk, H.D. and Maisner, A. (2002) Measles virus matrix protein is not cotransported with the viral glycoproteins but requires virus infection for efficient surface targeting. *Virus Res.* **83**, 1–12.

Rima, B.K., Baczko, K., Imagawa, D.T. and Termeulen, V. (1987) Humoral immune-response in dogs with old dog encephalitis and chronic distemper Meningoencephalitis. *J. Gen. Virol.* **68**, 1723–35.

Rodriguez-Boulan, E. and Nelson, W.J. (1989) Morphogenesis of the polarized epithelial cell phenotype. *Science* **245**, 718–25.

Romer-Oberdorfer, A., Werner, O., Veits, J., Mebatsion, T. and Mettenleiter, T.C. (2003) Contribution of the length of the HN protein and the sequence of the F protein cleavage site to Newcastle disease virus pathogenicity. *J. Gen. Virol.* **84**, 3121–9.

Ryan, K.W. and Portner, A. (1990) Separate domains of Sendai virus P protein are required for binding to viral nucleocapsids. *Virology* **174**, 515–21.

Samal, S.K. and Collins, P.L. (1996) RNA replication by a respiratory sycytial virus analog does not obey the rule of six and retains a nonviral trinucleotide extension at the leader end. *J. Virol.* **70**, 5075–82.

Schneider, H., Kaelin, K. and Billeter, M.A. (1997) Recombinant measles viruses defective for RNA editing and V protein synthesis are viable in cultured cells. *Virology* **227**, 314–22.

Schneider-Schaulies, S., Kreth, H.W., Hofmann, G., Billeter, M.A. and ter Meulen, V. (1991) Expression of measles virus RNA in peripheral blood mononuclear cells of patients with measles SSPE and autoimmune diseases. *Virology* **182**, 703–11.

Seki, F., Ono, N., Yamaguchi, R. and Yanagi, Y. (2003) Efficient isolation of wild strains of canine distemper virus in Vero cells expressing canine SLAM (CD150) and their adaptability to marmoset B95a cells. *J. Virol.* **77**, 9943–50.

Seth, S. and Shaila, M.S. (2001) The hemagglutinin-neuraminidase protein of peste des petits ruminants virus is biologically active when transiently expressed in mammalian cells. *Virus Res.* **75**, 169–77.

Shaji, D. and Shaila, M.S. (1999) Domains of rinderpest virus phosphoprotein involved in interaction with itself and the nucleocapsid protein. *Virology* **258**, 415–24.

Sidhu, M.S., Chan, J., Kaelin, K., Spielhofer, P., Radecke, F., Schneider, H., Masurekar, M., Dowling, P.C., Billeter, M.A. and Udem, S.A. (1995) Rescue of synthetic measles virus minireplicons: measles genomic termini direct efficient expression and propagation of a reporter gene. *Virology* **208**, 800–7.

Simons, K. and Garoff, H. (1980) The budding mechanisms of enveloped animal viruses. *J. Gen. Virol.* **50**, 1–21.

Skiadopoulos, M.H., Vogel, L., Riggs, J.M., Surman, S.R., Collins, P.L. and Murphy, B.R. (2003) The genome length of human parainfluenza virus type 2 follows the rule of six, and recombinant viruses recovered from non- polyhexameric-length antigenomic cDNAs contain a biased distribution of correcting mutations. *J. Virol.* **77**, 270–9.

Smallwood, S., Ryan, K.W. and Moyer, S.A. (1994) Deletion analysis defines a carboxyl-proximal region of Sendai virus P protein that binds to the polymerase L protein. *Virology* **202**, 154–63.

Spehner, D., Drillien, R. and Howley, P.M. (1997) The assembly of the measles virus nucleoprotein into nucleocapsid- like particles is modulated by the phosphoprotein. *Virology* **232**, 260–8.

Spielhofer, P., Bächi, T., Fehr, T., Christiansen, G., Cattaneo, R., Kaelin, K., Billeter, M.A. and Naim, H.Y. (1998) Chimeric measles viruses with a foreign envelope. *J. Virol.* **72**, 2150–9.

Stallcup, K.C., Raine, C.S. and Fields, B.N. (1983) Cytochalasin B inhibits the maturation of measles virus. *Virology* **124**, 59–74.

Stillman, E.A. and Whitt, M.A. (1998) The length and sequence composition of vesicular stomatitis virus intergenic regions affect mRNA levels and the site of transcript initiation. *J. Virol.* **72**, 5565–72.

Stillman, E.A. and Whitt, M.A. (1999) Transcript initiation and 5'-end modifications are separable events during vesicular stomatitis virus transcription. *J. Virol.* **73**, 7199–209.

Sugiyama, M., Ito, N., Minamoto, N. and Tanaka, S. (2002) Identification of immunodominant neutralizing epitopes on the hemagglutinin protein of rinderpest virus. *J. Virol.* **76**, 1691–6.

Suryanarayana, K., Baczko, K., ter Meulen, V. and Wagner, R.R. (1994) Transcription inhibition and other properties of matrix proteins expressed by M genes cloned from measles viruses and diseased human brain tissue. *J. Virol.* **68**, 1532–43.

Sweetman, D.A., Miskin, J. and Baron, M.D. (2001) Rinderpest virus C and V proteins interact with the major (L) component of the viral polymerase. *Virology* **281**, 193–204.

Takeuchi, K., Takeda, M., Miyajima, N., Kobune, F., Tanabayashi, K. and Tashiro, M. (2002) Recombinant wild-type and edmonston strain measles viruses bearing heterologous H proteins: role of H protein in cell fusion and host cell specificity. *J. Virol.* **76**, 4891–900.

Tapparel, C. and Roux, L. (1996) The efficiency of Sendai virus genome replication: the importance of the RNA primary sequence independent of terminal complementarity. *Virology* **225**, 163–71.

Tapparel, C., Hausmann, S., Pelet, T., Curran, J., Kolakofsky, D. and Roux, L. (1997) Inhibition of Sendai virus genome replication due to promoter-increased selectivity: a possible role for the accessory C proteins. *J. Virol.* **71**, 9588–99.

Tapparel, C., Maurice, D. and Roux, L. (1998) The activity of Sendai virus genomic and antigenomic promoters requires a second element past the leader template regions: a motif $(GNNNNN)_3$ is essential for replication. *J. Virol.* **72**, 3117–28.

Tatsuo, H., Okuma, K., Tanaka, K., Ono, N., Minagawa, H., Matsuura, Y. and Yanagi, Y. (2000) Virus entry is a major determinant of cell tropism of Edmonston and wild-type strains of measles virus as revealed by vesicular stomatitis virus pseudotypes bearing their envelope proteins. *J. Virol.* **74**, 4139–45.

tenOever, B.R., Servant, M.J., Grandvaux, N., Lin, R. and Hiscott, J. (2002) Recognition of the measles virus nucleocapsid as a mechanism of IRF-3 activation. *J. Virol.* **76**, 3659–69.

ter Meulen, V. and Martin, S.J. (1976) Genesis and maintenance of a persistent infection by canine distemper virus. *J. Gen. Virol.* **32**, 431–40.

Tober, C., Seufert, M., Schneider, H., Billeter, M.A., Johnston, I.C.., Niewiesk, S., ter Meulen, V. and Schneider-Schaulies, S. (1998) Expression of measles virus V protein is associated with pathogenicity and control of viral RNA synthesis. *J. Virol.* **72**, 8124–32.

Tuckis, J., Smallwood, S., Feller, J.A. and Moyer, S.A. (2002) The C-terminal 88 amino acids of the Sendai virus P protein have multiple functions separable by mutation. *J. Virol.* **76**, 68–77.

Udem, S.A. and Cook, K.A. (1984) Isolation and characterization of measles virus intracellular nucleocapsid RNA. *J. Virol.* **63**, 57–65.

Valsamakis, A., Schneider, H., Auwaerter, P.G., Kaneshima, H., Billeter, M.A. and Griffin, D.E. (1998) Recombinant measles viruses with mutations in the C, V, or F gene have altered growth phenotypes in vivo. *J. Virol.* **72**, 7754–61.

Vincent, S., Gerlier, D. and Manie, S.N. (2000) Measles virus assembly within membrane rafts. *J. Virol.* **74**, 9911–15.

von Heijne, G. (1998) Life and death of a signal peptide. *Nature* **396** (111), 113.

von Messling, V., Zimmer, G., Herrler, G., Haas, L. and Cattaneo, R. (2001) The hemagglutinin of canine distemper virus determines tropism and cytopathogenicity. *J. Virol.* **75**, 6418–27.

Vongpunsawad, S., Oezgun, N., Braun, W. and Cattaneo, R. (2004) Selectively receptor-blind measles viruses: Identification of residues necessary for SLAM- or CD46-induced fusion and their localization on a new hemagglutinin structural model. *J. Virol.* **78**, 302–13.

Vulliémoz, D. and Roux, L. (2001) 'Rule of six': how does the Sendai virus RNA polymerase keep count? *J. Virol.* **75**, 4506–18.

Watanabe, M., Hirano, A., Stenglein, S., Nelson, J., Thomas, G. and Wong, T.C. (1995a) Engineered serine protease inhibitor prevents furin-catalyzed activation of the fusion glycoprotein and production of infectious measles virus. *J. Virol.* **69**, 3206–10.

Watanabe, M., Wang, A., Sheng, J., Gombart, A. F., Ayata, M., Ueda, S., Hirano, A. and Wong, T.C. (1995b) Delayed activation of altered fusion glycoprotein in a chronic measles virus variant that causes subacute sclerosing panencephalitis. *J. Neurovirol.* **1**, 177–88.

Watanabe, N., Kawano, M., Tsurudome, M., Kusagawa, S., Nishio, M., Komada H., Shima, T., Ito, Y. (1996) Identification of the sequences responsible for nuclear targeting of the V protein of human parainfluenza virus type 2. *J. Gen. Virol.* **77** (Pt 2 ), 327–38.

Wertz, G.M.R. and Ball L.A. (2002) Adding genes to the RNA genome of VSV: positional effects on stability of expression. *J. Virol.* **76**, 7642–50.

Wertz, G.W., Perepelitsa, V.P. and Ball, L.A. (1998) Gene rearrangement attenuates expression and lethality of a nonsegmented negative strand RNA virus. *Proc. Natl Acad. Sci. USA* **95**, 3501–6.

Whelan, S.P.J. and Wertz, G.W. (1999a) The 5′ terminal trailer region of vesicular stomatitis virus contains a position-dependent cis-acting signal for assembly of RNA into infectious particles. *J. Virol.* **73**, 307–15.

Whelan, S.P.J. and Wertz, G.W. (1999b) Regulation of RNA synthesis by the genomic termini of vesicular stomatitis virus: identification of distinct sequences essential for transcription but not replication. *J. Virol.* **73**, 297–306.

Whelan, S.P.J. and Wertz, G.W. (2002) Transcription and replication initiate at separate sites on the vesicular stomatitis virus genome. *Proc. Natl Acad. Sci. USA* **99**, 9178–83.

Wong, T.C. and Hirano, A. (1987) Structure and function of bicistronic RNA encoding the phosphoprotein and matrix protein of measles virus. *J. Virol.* **61**, 584–9.

Wright, P.E. and Dyson, H.J. (1999) Intrinsically unstructured proteins: re-assessing the protein structure-function paradigm. *J. Mol. Biol.* **293**, 321–31.

Wu, X., Gong, X., Foley, H.D., Schnell, M.J. and Fu, Z.F. (2002) Both viral transcription and replication are reduced when the rabies virus nucleoprotein is not phosphorylated. *J. Virol.* **76**, 4153–61.

Yang, J., Koprowsgi, H., Dietzschold, B. and Fu, Z.F. (1999) Phosphorylation of rabies virus nucleoprotein regulates viral RNA transcription and replication by modulating leader encapsidation. *J. Virol.* **73**, 1661–4.

Yoneda, M., Bandyopadhyay, S.K., Shiotani, M., Fujita, K., Nuntaprasert, A., Miura, R., Baron, M.D., Barrett, T. and Kai, C. (2002) Rinderpest virus H protein: role in determining host range in rabbits. *J. Gen. Virol.* **83**, 1457–63.

Yoneda, M., Miura, R., Barrett, T., Tsukiyama-Kohara, K. and Kai, C. (2004) Rinderpest virus phosphoprotein gene is a major determinant of species-specific pathogenicity. *J. Virol.* **78**, 6676–81.

Yoshida, E., Shin, Y.S., Iwatsuki, K., Gemma, T., Miyashita, N., Tomonaga, K., Hirayama, N., Mikami, T. and Kai, C. (1999) Epitopes and nuclear localization analyses of canine distemper virus nucleocapsid protein by expression of its deletion mutants. *Vet. Microbiol.* **66**, 313–20.

Zhang, X., Glendening, C., Linke, H., Parks, C.L., Brooks, C., Udem, S.A. and Oglesbee, M. (2002) Identification and characterization of a regulatory domain on the carboxyl terminus of the measles virus nucleocapsid protein. *J. Virol.* **76**, 8737–46.

# Rinderpest and peste des petits ruminants – the diseases: clinical signs and pathology

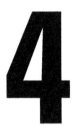

**4**

## PETER WOHLSEIN* AND JEREMIAH SALIKI[†]

*Tierärztliche Hochschule Hannover, Institut für Pathologie, Hannover, Germany
[†]Oklahoma Animal Disease Diagnostic Laboratory, College of Veterinary Medicine, Stillwater, Oklahoma, USA

## Introduction

Rinderpest and peste des petits ruminants (PPR) are contagious morbilliviral infections in cloven hoofed animals, both domestic and wild, which share common clinical and morphological features. The classical course of rinderpest and PPR is characterized by profuse diarrhoea and inflammation of various mucous membranes. Morphologically, erosive lesions of the mucous membranes of the digestive tract are the main changes seen in both rinderpest and PPR but respiratory signs are a distinguishing feature typical for PPR where an interstitial and suppurative pneumonia may occur. In highly susceptible animals each virus causes similar severe clinical signs and high mortality rates. Today, however, as a result of the successful rinderpest eradication campaign, virtually all countries have stopped vaccinating against rinderpest and the virus remaining in the last endemic focus is a mild strain for cattle with low numbers of fatalities but it causes severe and mostly fatal infections in wildlife species (see Chapter 7). As yet no strains of PPR have been characterized as mild, although they probably do exist. Due to the clinical and morphologic similarities of both diseases, there was considerable confusion regarding which of these viruses was most prevalent

ISBN-13: 978-0-12-88385-1
ISBN-10: 0-12-88385-6

in small ruminants in Asia until molecular tests were available to rapidly and unequivocally distinguish the two viruses in clinical specimens (Nanda *et al.*, 1996).

## Rinderpest clinical disease

The clinical disease of rinderpest has been extensively described over the past eight decades (Curasson, 1932; Scott, 1964, 1981a, 1981b, 1990a). The severity of clinical signs and lesions in affected animals varies greatly according to the virulence of the strain of rinderpest virus (RPV) involved and the infected host's innate resistance (Wohlsein *et al.*, 1995; Anderson *et al.*, 1996). In cattle, host resistance to RPV infection varies considerably among the different breeds. The severe acute clinical disease may occur in fully susceptible breeds like unhumped cattle (*Bos taurus*), water buffalo (*Bubalus bubalis*) and yaks (*Bos grunniens*). In humped (zebu) cattle (*Bos indicus*), clinical disease may be less severe. In naive cattle populations, RPV affects animals of all ages and mortality rates exceeding 90% may occur. Today, this severe form of the disease would only arise if a less virulent endemic strain entered and enjoyed an uncontrolled period of spread in a population of (susceptible) bovines large enough to allow for the selection of a highly virulent strain. The last outbreak of this nature was documented in Pakistan in the 1990s (Rossiter *et al.*, 1998). This outbreak was not reported for 6 months so the virus may have increased in virulence in the course of the outbreak, although this was never proven.

In areas where rinderpest is endemic, natural infection increasingly results in mild disease with greatly reduced or inapparent clinical signs. Therefore, wide variations in intensity and frequency of disease occur in these areas. The incidence of the disease typically varies with age and immune status: yearlings are the most susceptible, while adults are immune either through vaccination or recovery from infection and suckling animals are passively protected. Together, these factors account for the great variations in morbidity and mortality rates observed, both of which typically range from 0 to 10%. It is important to note that in recent years many strains have been isolated in East Africa that cause only mild disease (mortality rates of 20% or less) even in highly susceptible animals (Robson *et al.*, 1959; Plowright, 1963; Wamwayi *et al.*, 1995). This mild form of the disease, which is often characterized by lack of one or more of the typical clinical and epidemiological features, appears to typify the disease still present in what increasingly appears to be the last remaining focus of rinderpest in the world (see Chapter 15). In the classic, acute form of the disease, not all clinical signs may be present in an individual animal, but among the members of an affected herd, the totality of the signs may be observed. Typical clinical signs include: a sudden onset of fever; muco-purulent oculo-nasal discharges; mucosal necrosis, erosions and ulcerations in the upper digestive and respiratory tracts; abomaso-enteritis followed by diarrhoea, dehydration and death. The clinical course of the disease can be divided into five stages (Plowright, 1965):

- Incubation period
- Prodromal phase
- Mucosal phase
- Diarrhoeic phase
- Convalescent phase in non-fatal cases.

The *incubation period* varies from 3 to 9 days in acute natural infections and experimental parenteral inoculation, depending on the route of infection and the dose and strain of virus. The incubation period following experimental contact infection or with mild strains may require up to 15 days until sudden onset of fever, the first sign of the prodromal phase.

The *prodromal phase* lasts about 3 days on average, with a range of 2–5 days. The temperature rises steadily and peaks between the third and fifth days, reaching 40.0 to 41.5 °C. In addition to pyrexia, affected animals exhibit non-specific signs of illness comprising restlessness, depression, anorexia, and dryness of the muzzle. The respiration is shallow and rapid, the milk yield drops, and the hair coat is rough. The visible mucous membranes become congested and copious serous nasal and lachrymal secretions are present. The water intake is increased and rumination is retarded.

The *mucosal or erosive phase* starts 2–5 days after the onset of pyrexia as pinhead-sized greyish-white foci of necrotic epithelium in the mucous membranes lining the mouth (see Figure 4.1; Plate 3), nares maybe (but never on the turbinates) and vagina. The oral lesions on the gums and on the inside of the lower lip extend rapidly with accompanying involvement of large areas of the buccal mucosa and the ventral and lateral aspects of the tongue. Subsequently, necrotic epithelial lesions are found on the posterior dorsum of the tongue, in the pharynx and in the nares and vagina. The necrotic surface is readily abraded and the hyperaemic submucosa is visible through the basal layer of the sharply eroded epithelium. The erosions enlarge, coalesce and are covered with yellow, caseous patches of cellular debris, encrusted inflammatory exudates, and secretions, producing a fetid necro-purulent discharge. The mucosa of the muzzle may crack. The animals salivate profusely, probably due to oropharyngeal discomfort when swallowing. They drink excessively, stop eating and produce controlled soft faeces frequently. Usually there are no signs of constipation, but an absence of defecation may be observed before diarrhoea starts.

The *diarrhoeic phase* starts 4–5 days after the onset of pyrexia and 1–3 days after the first appearance of erosions. It is accompanied by a drop in temperature to subnormal values. This phase is characterized by uncontrolled profuse diarrhoea. The stool is liquid, dark green, occasionally yellowish or grey, malodourous, and contains huge amounts of mucus, epithelial debris and blood. The hair coat of the hind quarters is soiled by faeces and tenesmus while prolapse of the rectal mucosa may be observed. The muzzle dries out and may display large areas of epithelial loss. Necrosis of the mucus membranes of the nasal vestibulum, vulva, vagina and prepuce may occur.

Cutaneous lesions in the form of maculo-papular rashes are rarely observed on areas of soft skin such as the udder, scrotum, axillae or groin. Lymphadenopathy is usually not detectable by palpation. The oculo-nasal discharges become muco-purulent and the animals display photophobia due to conjunctivitis. The breathing becomes accelerated, laboured, painful and often abdominal with grunting exhalation and occasional coughing. Affected animals are reluctant to move, and exhibit depression, severe loss of condition, rapid and progressive dehydration with sunken eyes, emaciation, and prostration. They grind their teeth and stand with arched backs and stooped heads. Animals in recumbency face their flanks in a typical 'milk fever' posture. The rapid loss of fluid and salts and the profound weakness result in death 5–14 days after the onset of illness in most animals, while a few survive until the end of the third week.

The *convalescent phase* is prolonged and the return to full health can take several weeks. The mucosal lesions heal within a week after their first appearance in cases without secondary bacterial infections and the diarrhoea slowly stops afterwards. Pregnant animals abort during the convalescent phase, but there is no evidence of viral teratogenicity or the development of persistently infected offspring. Latent or chronic infections, especially those caused by haemoparasites such as *Anaplasma marginale*, may be activated and, if untreated, may increase the mortality rate.

Haematologically, a mild lymphocytosis is present during the incubation period followed by a marked leukopenia, particularly lymphopenia, starting the day before or on the day of initial temperature rise and persisting until death or for several weeks during convalescence if the animal survives. Immunosuppression resulting from the destruction of lymphocytes predisposes the affected animal to the activation of latent infections, allowing the establishment of concomitant infections. In the diarrhoeic phase, haemoconcentration with elevated numbers of erythrocytes and a rise in the packed cell volume are both observed, while the total serum protein and electrolytes decline. In particular, serum chloride levels decline during terminal illness. Blood clotting may be impaired in severely affected animals (Thiéry, 1956; Anderson *et al.*, 1996).

Besides the typical acute form of rinderpest in susceptible cattle, peracute and mild forms of the disease have been described. The *peracute form* occurs exceptionally and causes death during the prodromal phase within 1 or 2 days after the onset of fever in highly susceptible animals infected with a highly virulent strain of RPV. The affected animals exhibit anorexia, depression, high body temperature and sudden death. The *mild form* is caused by strains of low virulence in susceptible animals. This form of the disease is characterized by a prolonged clinical course with an incubation period up to 15 days, variable morbidity and low mortality rates. Affected animals show variable clinical features, ranging from an inapparent infection in some cattle to disease indistinguishable from that caused by highly virulent strains in others, but generally with only occasional mortality. Typically, mild strains give rise to cases in which all, some, or none of the following signs may be observed: a slight rise in temperature of 3–7 days' duration, serous nasal and ocular discharges, salivation, scant oral erosions and diarrhoea. Recovery is rapid.

For differential diagnosis, all diseases that cause oral lesions should be considered. These include bovine viral diarrhoea–mucosal disease (BVD–MD), malignant catarrhal fever (MCF), foot-and-mouth disease (FMD), and infectious bovine rhinotracheitis (IBR).

Small ruminants that become infected with African strains of RPV may show transient fever, sometimes accompanied by slight nasal and ocular discharges, but usually they are infected subclinically. In India, small ruminants infected with Indian strains of RPV develop clinical signs similarly to cattle (Anderson et al., 1990). Fever, diarrhoea and oculo-nasal discharges are associated with erosive mouth lesions, which are less obvious than in cattle. Pneumonia is encountered more frequently, probably due to secondary bacterial infections.

The clinical disease in pigs depends on the breed of pigs involved. European breeds are more resistant to RPV than the Asian breeds. The former often, but not always, exhibit a subclinical course (Govindarajan et al., 1996) while the latter show clinical signs consisting of pyrexia, anorexia, depression, nasal and ocular discharges, congestion of oral mucous membranes, erosions and gastroenteritis with diarrhoea. The diarrhoea lasts 5–10 days and severely affected animals die from dehydration (Ramani et al., 1974). Pregnant sows may abort and erythematous skin lesions may occur. The lymphatic tissues display degeneration and necrosis of lymphocytes with subsequent regeneration. However, both groups of pigs shed virus and have to be considered as a potential source of RPV infection.

RPV may infect a broad range of susceptible wild ungulates resulting in clinically variable disease depending on the innate resistance of the species infected and the strain of virus involved (Scott, 1964; see also Chapter 7). Clinical disease is seen most frequently in African buffaloes (*Syncerus caffer*), lesser kudu (*Tragelaphus imberbis*), impala (*Aepyceros melampus*), eland (*Taurotragus oryx*), and giraffe (*Giraffa camelopardalis*). Warthogs (*Phacochoerus* spp.) and wildebeest (*Connochaetes taurus*) are sometimes involved. In Asia, the disease has been recorded in Indian axis deer (*Axis axis*), and numerous species of wild pigs and ruminants including mithun (*Bos frontalis*), gaur (*Bos gaurus*) and banteng (*Bos javanicus*). In the African buffalo morbidity and mortality rates exceeding 90% may be seen. Virus causing mild disease in cattle may result in about 80% mortality in buffaloes. Clinical signs in buffalo comprise fever, malaise, diarrhoea and dehydration. Affected animals may become approachable or even aggressive. In the lesser kudu, clinical signs of RPV infection are characterized by fever, blindness and keratoconjunctivitis with severe ocular discharge. The animals segregate themselves from others and become disorientated. In some cases swelling of the knee and hock joints is observed. Diarrhoea is observed rarely. Affected eland are depressed and anorectic. The animals display marked ocular discharge with crusting, and occasionally diarrhoea, dehydration, and emaciation (Kock *et al.*, 1999).

# Rinderpest pathology

The morphological alterations of RPV infection in naturally infected animals have been extensively described (Khera, 1958a,b,c; Maurer *et al.*, 1956). For the most part, the lesions observed in rinderpest are a direct result of the viral cytopathogenicity and the severity and frequency of lesions is directly related to the virulence of the virus strain involved. The carcass is emaciated and dehydrated with sunken eyes and reduced skin turgor. The hair coat is rough and soiled by muco-purulent discharges and watery faeces.

The most prominent gross lesions are found in the mucous membranes of the digestive tract. They are located on the lingual side of the lower lips, the lower gum, the papillae of the buccal mucosa close to the commissures, the dental plate and the adjacent gum, the ventral surface of the rostral part of the tongue, and in advanced cases, on the caudal hard and soft palate, pharynx, and upper part of the oesophagus. The fore stomachs are rarely affected, with lesions occurring preferentially on the pillars of the rumen or leaves of the omasum.

The alterations to the oral stratified squamous epithelium consist of circumscribed, pinpoint, raised (Figure 4.1a), partially coalescing, greyish-white necroses, which, after shedding of the debris, exhibit shallow erosions with hyperaemic submucosa (Figure 4.1b). The mucosal defect may be covered with a yellowish exudate. Occasionally, ulcerations occur due to mechanical alterations and/or secondary bacterial infections.

The abomasum is one of the most common sites for lesions in rinderpest. The abomasal folds are oedematous and haemorrhagic. Ulcerations which are covered with black-coloured clotted blood are found mostly along the mucosal folds of the pyloric region. During the acute phase, the intestinal contents consist of necrotic mucosal shreds, blood, inflammatory exudate and mucus. In the small intestine, lesions occur less frequently than in the oral cavity, abomasum, and large intestine. Erosions are also observed in the duodenum and ileum. The Peyer's patches of the small intestine are particularly affected. They appear initially swollen and haemorrhagic and, after lymphocyte depletion and sloughing of the necrotic surface, exhibit deep ulcerative craters. The ileo-caecal valve is congested, haemorrhagic, and displays large necrotic areas and erosions. The mucosa of the large intestine is oedematous and congested and exhibits petechial haemorrhages. The congested submucosal capillaries along the crests of the mucosal folds of the caecum, colon and rectum give a characteristic appearance, termed 'zebra-stripes' or 'tiger-stripes' (Figure 4.2). The lymphoglandular complexes of the large intestine are depleted and closure of the orifice at the

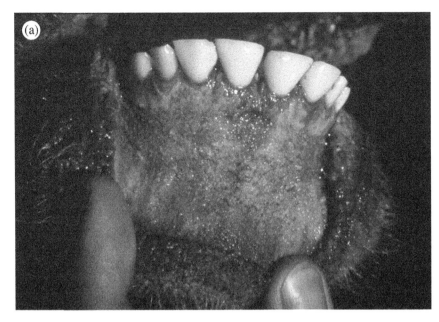

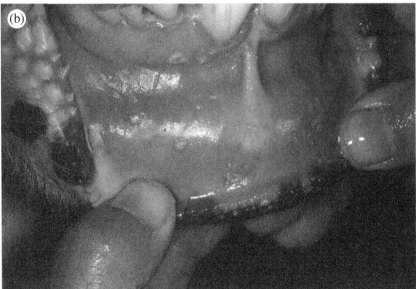

**Figure 4.1** Rinderpest in cattle: Panels (a) and (b): Erosive stomatitis.

neck of the infundibulum results in accumulation of cellular debris and exudate. Lesions in the gall bladder vary from petechial to extensive haemorrhages; erosions seldom occur.

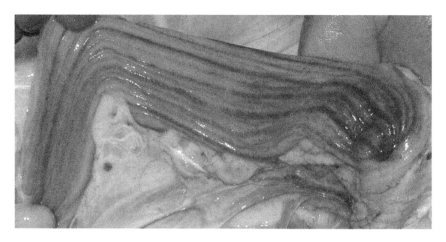

**Figure 4.2**   Zebra striping in the large intestine in an animal infected with the virulent Kabete 'O' strain of rinderpest virus.

Lymph nodes are swollen due to oedema and congestion. The spleen is slightly enlarged and subserosal petechiae and ecchymoses are present. The bone marrow may show local congestion. In animals that die after a prolonged course, lymph nodes are shrunken. Erosive lesions occur in the nares associated with petechiae on the nasal mucosa. Pinpoint haemorrhages and erosions are found on the larynx. In the trachea streaks of haemorrhages are observed, and alveolar and interstitial pulmonary emphysema may be prominent in animals that die late in the disease. Bronchopneumonia is observed in cases with secondary bacterial infections. In the heart, subendocardial haemorrhages are found in the left ventricle and subendocardial petechiae and ecchymoses are present on the base of the heart and along the coronary grooves. Haemorrhages and occasional erosions are encountered in the uro-genital tract, especially in the urinary bladder and vagina. The conjunctiva is affected by a muco-purulent inflammation and occasionally corneal ulcers are observed. The skin exhibits occasionally erosive changes on medial thighs, udder and scrotum. The gross lesions in mild cases of rinderpest are similar to those described for severely affected animals but are less extensive and appear less frequently.

Histologically, mild and highly virulent strains of RPV display both epithelio- and lympho-tropism. The microscopic changes observed in the stratified squamous epithelium of the mouth are characterized by syncytial cell formation, occurrence of cytoplasmic eosinophilic inclusions and, less frequently, similar nuclear inclusions. Circumscribed ballooning degeneration of epithelial cells of the spinous cell layer without formation of vesicles extends upwards (Figure 4.3) and is followed by sloughing of the necrotic cellular debris leaving clearly demarcated erosions. Adjacent infiltrations of mononuclear cells and granulocytes are present. In the lymphoid tissues, syncytial cell formations

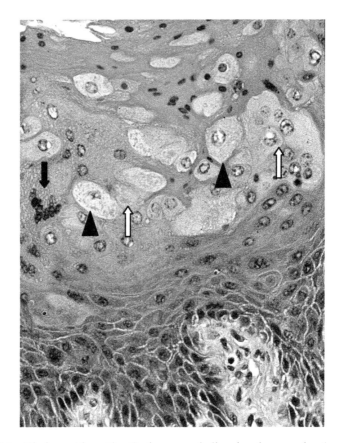

**Figure 4.3** Rinderpest in cattle: Oral mucosa: ballooning degeneration (arrowheads) and syncytia of epithelial cells (black arrow); cytoplasmic inclusions (white arrows); H&E; magnification ×400.

with cytoplasmic and nuclear inclusions are observed. Subsequently and depending on the virulence of the virus involved, lymphoid tissues display progressive lymphocytic destruction and depletion, first seen in the germinal centres and later in the T cell areas (Figure 4.4a). RPV destroys both B and T lymphocytes. In addition to necrosis, apoptosis is involved in the depletion of lymphoid cells. In lymphoid follicles of tonsils, lymph nodes, spleen and mucosa-associated lymphoid tissues, lytic destruction of lymphocytes leaves a residual network of branching reticular cells (Stolte *et al.*, 2002; Wohlsein *et al.*, 1995). In animals with a prolonged clinical course, fibrosis with focal lymphoid regeneration has been observed (Khera, 1958c). In animals with mild clinical disease, tissue samples show unremarkable histopathological changes in the gastrointestinal tract and the lymphoid tissues. Erosive lesions are limited in number and extent.

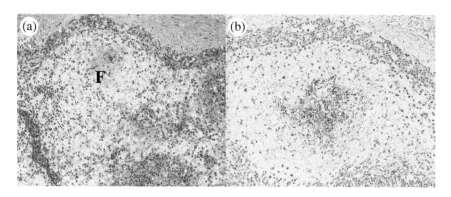

**Figure 4.4**    Rinderpest in cattle: mesenteric lymph node
(a) Severe depletion of lymphocytes in a follicle (F); H&E; magnification ×200
(b) Immunohistochemical labelling of RP virus antigen; magnification ×200.

Immunohistochemical studies have been performed on tissues from experimentally and naturally infected animals (Gathumbi *et al.*, 1989, 1990; Wohlsein *et al.*, 1993, 1995; Brown, 1997). The immunohistochemical results show the presence of viral antigen in areas with microscopic lesions. Cattle infected with highly virulent RPV strains reveal widespread infection with presence of viral antigen in numerous tissues and organs. In infected cells, antigen is located in the nucleus or the cytoplasm or both. The distribution of RPV antigen in tissues displays a lympho- and epithelio-tropism. In contrast to other morbilliviruses, neurotropism has not been confirmed under natural conditions. In lymphoid tissues (tonsil, lymph nodes, spleen, Peyer's patches), viral antigen is identified in reticular cells of the lymphoid follicles, macrophages, single lymphoid cells and endothelial cells lining the sinuses (Figure 4.4b). Immunolabelling in the thymus is located in epithelial reticular cells and occasionally in Hassal's corpuscles.

Epithelial cells of the upper and lower digestive tract and of the respiratory and urogenital tracts have been found to harbour viral antigen. Additionally, viral antigen is detectable in multinucleated syncytial cells, mononuclear cells of the intestinal lamina propria, epithelial cells of the conjunctiva, bronchiolar epithelial cells, sebaceous epithelial cells, salivary epithelial cells, bile duct epithelial cells, epithelial cells of the exocrine pancreas, hepatocytes, thyroid epithelial cells, and cells of the adrenal cortex. Viral antigen of low virulent strains is detected only in low quantities in both epithelial and lymphoid tissues (Brown and Torres, 1994).

Ultrastructurally, RPV and PPRV share common findings. Infected cells contain arrays of tubular nucleocapsid material probably corresponding to the inclusions observed by light microscopy. Nucleocapsids of PPRV are slightly bigger in size than those of RPV (Durojaiye *et al.*, 1985; see also Chapter 3).

The diameter of intact particles varies between 130 and 390 nm. Virus release occurs by budding through the cell membrane.

Lesions in small domestic ruminants are similar to those observed in cattle but tend to be less intense. Pulmonary involvement is more prominent. In Asian pigs morphological changes resemble those in cattle but there is a wide individual variation.

In wildlife, gross lesions comprise dehydration, emaciation and erosions of the nares, lips, tongue and buccal mucosa. In advanced cases, there may be more confluent necroses with extensive epithelial loss resulting in a fetid odour. The abomasum displays congestion, oedema and petechial haemorrhages. Catarrhal enteritis with liquid intestinal contents is accompanied by depletion and collapse of the gut-associated lymphoid tissue. The mucosa of the large intestine may show zebra striping. Additional gross findings in the lesser kudu include ulcerative keratoconjunctivitis with corneal oedema, most often in both eyes, and synovitis and tenosynovitis around the radial and tarsal joints. Liver and kidneys are congested (Kock *et al.*, 1999).

# PPR clinical disease

PPR (peste des petits ruminants) is an acute to subacute viral disease of goats and sheep caused by PPR virus (PPRV). It is similar to rinderpest in its clinical signs, morphological lesions and immunological response. The clinical disease in naturally and experimentally infected small ruminants has been described extensively (Braide, 1981; Obi *et al.*, 1983; Furley *et al.*, 1987; Bundza *et al.*, 1988; Shaila *et al.*, 1989; Scott 1990b; Brown *et al.*, 1991; Kulkarni *et al.*, 1996). Goats are reported to be more susceptible than sheep (Nanda *et al.*, 1996), but outbreaks have occurred with both species being equally affected or with sheep being more affected than goats. The mortality rate in susceptible goats ranges from 10 to 90% and varies with degree of innate resistance, body condition, age, virulence of the virus involved, and occurrence of complications resulting from secondary bacterial and parasitic infections. West African goats are commonly more severely affected than European breeds. The recovery rate in sheep is significantly higher than in goats in most instances. Cattle and pigs are susceptible to PPRV infection but exhibit no clinical disease and are incapable of transmitting the virus; however, they seroconvert and cattle become protected against RPV infection following subclinical PPRV infection. However, PPRV infection of cattle may impair the immune response to rinderpest vaccination (Anderson and McKay, 1994).

Depending on the clinical outcome, peracute, acute, subacute and subclinical forms can be distinguished. The *peracute* form of the disease starts often after a short incubation period of 2 days with a sudden high rise in body temperature up to 40–42 °C accompanied by serous oculo-nasal discharges, depression, dyspnoea, anorexia and constipation. The oral mucous membranes become congested and occasionally eroded. Affected animals develop profuse watery diarrhoea and die within 4–6 days after the onset of fever.

The *acute* form represents the most common course of the disease. It is characterized by an incubation period of 3–4 days followed by a sudden rise in temperature, serous ocular and nasal discharges (Figure 4.5), depression, anorexia, restlessness, dry muzzle and dull coat. Diarrhoea starts 2–3 days after the onset of pyrexia and is accompanied by severe dehydration, emaciation and prostration. The epithelium of the oral and nasal mucous membranes displays numerous, partially coalescing pin-point greyish necrotic foci, which leave sharply demarcated, hyperaemic, but non-haemorrhagic erosions after sloughing off the necrotic debris. The predilection sites of epithelial lesions are lips, gums, dental plate, tongue, buccal papillae adjacent to the commissures of the mouth, and in female animals the labial surface of the vulva. The oral lesions may be accompanied by profuse salivation. The initial serous nasal and ocular discharges become progressively more profuse and muco-purulent followed by crusting and the animal develops a fetid odour. The nares are covered by prominent crusty scales that cause sneezing and coughing. Additional clinical signs include tachypnoea, dyspnoea, and moist and productive cough with catarrhal discharges from the eyes. Most goats die within 10–12 days after the onset of pyrexia, but some survive for three weeks.

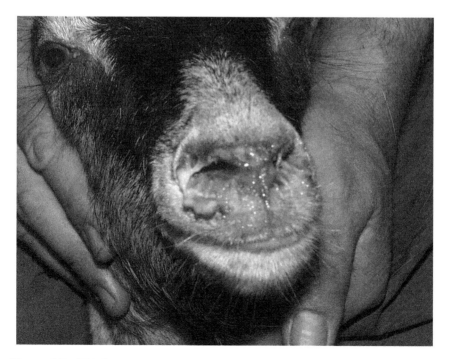

**Figure 4.5**   PPR in goats: muco-purulent oculo-nasal discharges.

In pregnant animals abortion may occur. Laboratory findings include a severe leukopenia, which correlates with the severity of the clinical disease.

In *subacute* forms less severe illness is observed after an incubation period of 6 days and low-grade fever. Affected animals do not display all the clinical signs described above and the mortality rate is much lower. Many animals will recover after an illness of 10–14 days. *Subclinical* infections are characterized by seroconversion alone.

The clinical disease may be complex due to the involvement of many different secondary pathogens. The most frequent complications arise from secondary bacterial infections caused by *Pasteurella* spp. or *Mycoplasma* spp. resulting in severe pneumonia. Additionally, infections with *E. coli* produce a heat-labile enterotoxin which will increase the severity of the clinical signs and the mortality rate. Cutaneous lesions may be complicated by recrudescence of infection with *Dermatophilus congolensis*. PPRV may activate latent intestinal or blood parasites, increasing the number of fatalities.

For clinical differential diagnosis, the following diseases and conditions have to be considered: contagious caprine pleuropneumonia, bluetongue, contagious ecthyma, caprine or ovine pox virus infections, foot-and-mouth disease, Nairobi sheep disease, various respiratory and enteric bacterial infections, intestinal and blood endoparasitoses, and plant and mineral poisoning. In Asia there are some strains of RPV adapted to sheep and goats which may cause lesions similar to those caused by PPRV.

Cattle and pigs can be infected with PPRV experimentally, but do not display clinical signs. PPRV infection in wildlife has been reported in a zoological collection of Dorcas gazelle (*Gazella dorcas*) and gemsbok (*Oryx tragocamelus*) and in gazelle (*Gazella thompsonii*) in Saudi Arabia.

# PPR pathology

Morphological alterations have been described in detail by several authors (Braide, 1981; Taylor, 1984). Animals that die from the *peracute* form do not exhibit gross lesions other than congestion of the oral mucosa and the ileo-caecal valve occasionally accompanied by erosions of the oral mucosa. In the *acute* form, the carcass is dehydrated, emaciated and soiled with green to greyish faeces. The eyelids, nostrils and lips are encrusted with a purulent discharge. The lips are hyperaemic and oral lesions may vary from a single erosion to a severe, extensive, ulcerative to necrotizing stomatitis involving the dental plate, hard palate, buccal mucosa and papillae, and the dorsum of the rostral part of the tongue (Figure 4.6). The mucosal alterations may extend to the pharynx. Occasionally, erosions are found on the ruminal pillars and the leaves of the omasum. The mucosa of the abomasum exhibits severe congestion and multiple erosions. Occasionally, a diffuse congestion is found throughout the intestinal tract, but in most cases it is restricted to the duodenum, ileum, caecum and upper colon.

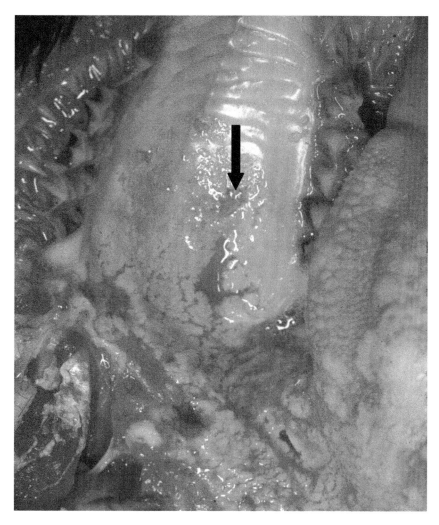

**Figure 4.6**    PPR in goats: erosive to ulcerative stomatitis (arrow) [Courtesy of C. Brown].

Haemorrhages are observed most commonly in the ileo-caecal valve. The crests of the longitudinal folds of the large intestine occasionally display severe congestion giving a zebra-stripe appearance. The gut-associated lymphoid tissue is necrotic and collapsed. Mesenteric lymph nodes are slightly enlarged and oedematous, and the spleen may be swollen. The conjunctiva displays mucopurulent conjunctivitis. The mucosa of the upper respiratory tract may exhibit severe hyperaemia accompanied by erosions in the nares and trachea. In the lungs, diffuse or patchy congestion is found (Figure 4.7a). The apical and cardiac lobes most commonly display a fibrinous or suppurative pneumonia obscuring the underlying primary viral pneumonia. The lungs are firm in consistency and display a purulent or muco-purulent exudate in the deeper airways caused by secondary bacterial infections. The pulmonary lymph nodes are swollen and oedematous. In the kidney and urinary bladder congestion may be present. In females, erosions may occur in the vulvo-vaginal mucosa. Heart, liver and skin do not present significant gross findings.

Histological changes in the oral mucosa consist of hydropic to ballooning degeneration of epithelial cells in the stratum granulosum followed by coalescing necrosis of epithelial cells, occasionally accompanied by multinucleated syncytial cells (see Figure 4.3). Nuclear and cytoplasmic eosinophilic inclusion bodies are found in epithelial cells and syncytia. These changes resemble those of other mucous membranes. The mucosal alterations are surrounded by a mild inflammatory infiltration of macrophages and lymphocytes at the borders of the lesions. The deep abomasal glands are necrotic and in the intestinal mucosal crypts are dilated with accumulation of cellular debris. The lamina propria is infiltrated with lymphocytes, macrophages and eosinophilic granulocytes. The nasal or oral crusts, which have been reported by some authors as 'proliferative changes', display neither hyperplasia nor proliferation of tissue structures, but rather consist of cellular debris, encrusted inflammatory exudate, neutrophilic granulocytes and macrophages. Spleen, lymph nodes, tonsil and the gut-associated lymphatic tissues exhibit extensive necrosis and depletion of lymphocytes. Reticulo-endothelial cells appear hyperplastic and occasionally contain nuclear inclusion bodies. In the lung, interstitial pneumonia

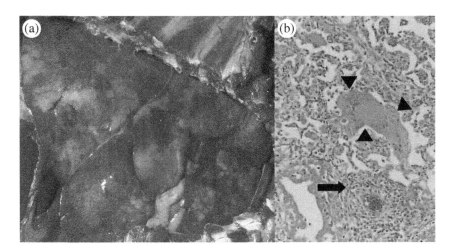

**Figure 4.7** PPR in goats:
(a) Severe, diffuse, interstitial pneumonia [Courtesy of C. Brown]
(b) Syncytial cell (arrowheads) and non-purulent interstitial pneumonia (arrow); H&E; magnification ×400 [Courtesy of C. Brown].

with hyperaemia together with infiltration of mononuclear cells and granulocytes is observed. Epithelial necrosis is present in the mucosa of the deeper airways. There is marked proliferation of type II pneumocytes and infiltration of numerous alveolar macrophages. Multinucleated giant cells are observed scattered throughout the lung (Figure 4.7b), a feature which is not characteristic of rinderpest. Cytoplasmic and nuclear inclusion bodies are found in epithelial and multinucleated cells. Fibrinous or suppurative bronchopneumonia with lobular infiltration of neutrophils is found due to secondary bacterial infections. In some animals, small foci of hepatocellular necrosis are present.

Immunohistochemistry of tissues from animals infected experimentally or naturally with PPRV reveals viral antigen in conjunctival, tracheal, bronchial, bronchiolar, and ileal epithelial cells, type II pneumocytes, syncytial cells and alveolar macrophages (Eligulashvili *et al.*, 1999; Saliki *et al.*, 1994).

# References

Anderson, J., Barrett, T. and Scott, G.R. (1996) *Manual on the Diagnosis of Rinderpest.* Rome: FAO.

Anderson, E.C., Hassan, A. *et al.* (1990) Observations on the pathogenicity for sheep and goats and the transmissibility of the strain of virus isolated during the rinderpest outbreak in Sri Lanka in 1987. *Vet. Microbiol.* **21** (4), 309–18.

Anderson, J. and McKay, J.A. (1994) The detection of antibodies against peste des petits ruminants virus in cattle, sheep and goats and the possible implications to rinderpest control programmes. *Epidemiol. Infect.* **112** (1), 225–31.

Braide, V.B. (1981) PPR – a review. *World Anim. Rev.* **39**, 25–8.

Brown, C.C. (1997) A review of three pathology-based techniques for retrospective diagnosis of rinderpest, with comparison to virus isolation. *Res. Vet. Sci.* **63** (2), 103–6.

Brown, C.C. and Torres, A. (1994) Distribution of antigen in cattle infected with rinderpest virus. *Vet. Pathol.* **31**, 194–200.

Brown, C.C., Mariner, J.C. *et al.* (1991) An immunohistochemical study of the pneumonia caused by peste des petits ruminants. *Vet. Pathol.* **28**, 166–70.

Bundza, A., Afshar, A. *et al.* (1988) Experimental peste des petits ruminants (goat plague) in goats and sheep. *Can. J. Vet. Res.* **52** (1), 46–52.

Curasson, G. (1932) *La Peste bovine.* Paris: Vigot Frères.

Durojaiye, O.A., Taylor, W.P. *et al.* (1985) The ultrastructure of peste des petits ruminants virus. *Zentralbl. Veterinarmed.* B **32** (6), 460–5.

Eligulashvili, R., Perl, S. *et al.* (1999) Immunohistochemical detection of peste des petits ruminants viral antigen in formalin-fixed, paraffin-embedded tissues from cases of naturally occurring infection. *J. Vet. Diagn. Invest.* **11** (3), 286–8.

Furley, C.W., Taylor, W.P. *et al.* (1987) An outbreak of peste des petits ruminants in a zoological collection. *Vet. Rec.* **121** (19), 443–7.

Gathumbi, P., Jonsson, L. *et al.* (1989) Immunohistological localization of rinderpest virus in formalin-fixed, paraffin-embedded tissues from experimentally infected cattle. *J. Vet. Med. Series B Infect. Dis. Immunol. Food Hyg. Vet. Publ. Hlth (Zentralbl Veterin. Reihe B)* **36**, 261–70.

Gathumbi, P.K., Wafula, J.S., Wamwayi, H.M. and Mbuthia, P.G. (1990). Immunohistological confirmation of a diagnosis of rinderpest from a recent natural outbreak. *Bull. Anim. Hlth Prod. Afr.* **38**, 375–7.

Govindarajan, R., Muralimanohar, B., Koteeswaran, A., Venugopalan, A.T., Varalakshmi, P., Shaila, M.S. and Ramachandran, S. (1996) Occurrence of rinderpest in European pigs in India. *Vet. Rec.* **139**, 473.

Khera, K.S. (1958a) Histological study on rinderpest. I. Pathogenesis of rinderpest virus in lymphatic glands; II. Histological lesions of the digestive tract; III. Lesions in various organs. *Rev. Elev. Méd. Vét. Pays Trop.* **11**, 399–405.

Khera, K.S. (1958b) Histological study on rinderpest. I. Pathogenesis of rinderpest virus in lymphatic glands; II. Histological lesions of the digestive tract; III. Lesions in various organs. *Rev. Elev. Méd. Vét. Pays Trop.* **11**, 406–15.

Khera, K.S. (1958c) Histological study on rinderpest. I. Pathogenesis of rinderpest virus in lymphatic glands; II. Histological lesions of the digestive tract; III. Lesions in various organs. *Rev. Elev. Méd. Vét. Pays Trop.* **11**, 416–20.

Kock, R.A., Wambua, J.M. *et al.* (1999) Rinderpest epidemic in wild ruminants in Kenya 1993–97. *Vet. Rec.* **145** (10), 275–83.

Kulkarni, D.D., Bhikane, A.U. *et al.* (1996) Peste des petits ruminants in goats in India. *Vet. Rec.* **138** (8), 187–8.

Maurer, F.D., Jones, T.C. and DeTray, D. (1956). The pathology of rinderpest. Proceedings Book of the 92nd Annual Meeting of the American Veterinary Medical Asssociation, Minneapolis.

Nanda, Y.P., Chatterjee, A. *et al.* (1996) The isolation of peste des petits ruminants virus from northern India. *Vet. Microbiol.* **51** (3–4), 207–16.

Obi, T.U., Ojo, M.O. *et al.* (1983) Peste des petits ruminants (PPR) in goats in Nigeria: clinical, microbiological and pathological features. *Zentralbl. Veterinarmed. B* **30** (10), 751–61.

Plowright, W. (1963) Some properties of strains of rinderpest virus recently isolated in East Africa. *Res. Vet. Sci.* **4**, 96–108.

Plowright, W. (1965) Symposium: the smallest stowaways. 3. Rinderpest. *Vet. Rec.* **77** (48), 1431–7.

Ramani, K., Charles, Y.S., Srinivas, R.P., Narayanaswamy, M. and Ramachandran, S. (1974) Isolation of rinderpest virus from an outbreak in domestic pigs in Karnataka. *Ind. Vet. J.* **51**, 36–41.

Robson, J., Arnold, R.M., Plowright, W. and Scott, G.R. (1959) The isolation from an eland of a strain of rinderpest virus attenuated for cattle. *Bull. Epizoot. Dis. Afr.* **7**, 97–102.

Rossiter, P.B., Hussain, M. *et al.* (1998) Cattle plague in Shangri-La: observations on a severe outbreak of rinderpest in northern Pakistan 1994–1995. *Vet. Rec.* **143** (2), 39–42.

Saliki, J.T., Brown, C.C. *et al.* (1994) Differential immunohistochemical staining of peste des petits ruminants and rinderpest antigens in formalin-fixed, paraffin-embedded tissues using monoclonal and polyclonal antibodies. *J. Vet. Diagn. Invest.* **6** (1), 96–8.

Scott, G.R. (1964) Rinderpest. *Adv. Vet. Sci.* **9**, 113–224.

Scott, G.R. (1981a) Rinderpest and peste des petits ruminants. In: E.P.J. Gibbs (ed.), *Virus Disease of Food Animals.* London: Academic Press, vol. 2, pp. 401–32.

Scott, G.R. (1981b) Rinderpest. In: J.W. Davis, L.H. Karstad and D.O. Trainer (eds), *Infectious Diseases of Wild Animals.* Ames, IO: Iowa State University Press, vol. 2, pp. 18–30.

Scott, G.R. (1990a) Rinderpest virus. In: Z. Dinter, and B. Morein (eds), *Virus Infections in Vertebrates.* Amsterdam: Elsevier, pp. 341–54.

Scott, G.R. (1990b) Peste-des-petits-ruminants (goat plague) virus. In: Z. Dinter and B. Morein (eds), *Virus Infections of Vertebrates*. Amsterdam: Elsevier, pp. 355–61.

Shaila, M.S., Purushothaman, V., Bhavasar, D., Venugopal, K. and Venkatesan, R.A. (1989) PPR of sheep in India. *Vet. Rec.* **125**, 602.

Stolte, M., Haas, L. *et al.* (2002) Induction of apoptotic cellular death in lymphatic tissues of cattle experimentally infected with different strains of rinderpest virus. *J. Comp. Pathol.* **127** (1), 14–21.

Taylor, W.P. (1984) The distribution and epidemiology of peste des petits ruminants. *Prev. Vet. Med.* **2**, 157–66.

Thiéry, G. (1956) Haematology, histopathology and histochemistry of rinderpest. *Rev. Elev. Méd. Vét. Pays Trop.* **9**, 117–40.

Wamwayi, H., Fleming, M. *et al.* (1995) Characterization of African isolates of rinderpest virus. *Vet. Microbiol.* **44**, 151–63.

Wohlsein, P., Trautwein, G. *et al.* (1993) Viral antigen distribution in organs of cattle experimentally infected with rinderpest virus. *Vet. Pathol.* **30**, 544–54.

Wohlsein, P., Wamwayi, H.M. *et al.* (1995) Pathomorphological and immunohistological findings in cattle experimentally infected with rinderpest virus isolates of different pathogenicity. *Vet. Microbiol.* **44** (2–4), 141–9.

# Rinderpest – an old and worldwide story: history to c.1902

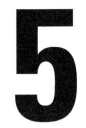

**PAUL-PIERRE PASTORET,[¶] KAZUYA YAMANOUCHI,[†]
UWE MUELLER-DOBLIES,[*] MARK M. RWEYEMAMU,[‡]
MARIAN HORZINEK,[§] AND THOMAS BARRETT[*]**
[¶]*Biotechnology and Biological Science Research Council, UK*
[*]*Institute for Animal Health, Pirbright Laboratory, Surrey, UK*
[†]*Nippon Institute for Biological Sciences, Tokyo, Japan*
[‡]*Woking, Surrey, UK*
[§]*Veterinary Faculty, Department of Infectious Diseases and Immunology,
Utrecht University, The Netherlands*

## Introduction

The history of rinderpest is one of the best documented of all animal diseases. Originating in Asia it frequently spread into Europe and at the end of the nineteenth century Africa was stricken with rinderpest. Early in the twentieth century Australia and the Americas faced accidental incursions: Brazil in 1920 and Australia in 1923, with each outbreak originating with importation of cattle from Asia. The outbreaks in Australia and Brazil were quickly contained and so descriptions of outbreaks and epizootics in this chapter will be limited to Asia, Europe and Africa. Two major publications provide detailed accounts of the many outbreaks or epizootics of the disease around the world. In 1890 W. Dieckerhoff wrote a book in German entitled *Geschichte der Rinderpest und Ihrer Literatur* (History of Rinderpest and its Literature), which is still a valuable and well-documented source of information. More recently, C.A. Spinage published in 2003 *Cattle Plague: A History*, which is a remarkable historical recollection. These two major works are invaluable sources of historical information and give access to relevant published papers. The purpose of this chapter is therefore not to duplicate those works, but rather to give a brief overview of the concepts prevailing about rinderpest until the discovery of the virus by Nicolle and Adil-Bey in 1902.

ISBN-13: 978-0-12-88385-1
ISBN-10: 0-12-88385-6

# Rinderpest: a terrible disease

Rinderpest has been described as the most dreaded of all animal diseases. In its classical, virulent form, infection can result in 80–90% mortality in cattle, buffalo, yaks and many wildlife ungulate species (Scott, 1964; Rossiter et al., 1998). Wherever it has occurred, rinderpest has caused terrible destruction of cattle, adversely affecting livestock, agriculture and rural livelihoods bringing famine and starvation (Barrett and Rossiter, 1999). In all languages the name given to this disease reflects its devastating nature in cattle. It is a classical plague, hence the name – cattle plague; the German, English, Latin, French, Spanish and other Latin-based languages refer to this disease as the terrible pest of cattle, i.e. *rinder-pest, peste bovine, pesta bovina*. In Kiswahili, it is called *sotoka*, meaning a debilitating killer disease of cattle.

Rinderpest in England was originally known as the 'Steppe murrain'. According to Scott (2000) and Scott and Provost (1992), this term reflected the European belief that:

> its homeland was the Steppe country around the Caspian Basin between Europe and Asia from where century after century it swept west over and around Europe and east over and around Asia with every marauding army, causing disaster, death and devastation that preceded the fall of the Roman Empire, the conquest of Christian Europe by Charlemagne, the French Revolution, the impoverishment of Russia and the colonization of Africa.

Invasion by Huns into Europe in 370 resulted in an outbreak of a highly contagious disease suspected of being rinderpest. Pandemics of rinderpest were brought by Mongol invasions of Western Europe, the first led by Genghis Khan in 1222. Although Genghis Khan died five years later, his commanders continued their operations, causing two further pandemics in 1233 and 1238, these latter being introduced into England with trade cattle imported from mainland Europe (Scott, 1996). Rinderpest was probably the first agro-biological weapon ever to be employed. Scott (2000) recounts that:

> the secret weapons of the invaders were Grey Steppe oxen. Their value was a strong innate resistance manifested by slow spread of virus and by the absence of clinical signs. A troop of Grey Steppe cattle could shed rinderpest virus for months provoking epidemics that devastated buffalo and cattle populations of invaded countries. The sequelae were no transport, untilled fields, starving peasants, and overthrown governments.

While outbreaks in virgin territory were dramatic, its endemic effects were just as serious. Edwards (1930) observed that in India:

> in the absence of artificial obstacles towards its spread, the virus showed a cyclical pattern. Three-year periods of recrudescence of the disease, when outbreaks

would be high and the spread of the disease most difficult to check, alternated with three-year periods of abatement, when outbreaks were few, mortality low, and the disease tending to become extinguished spontaneously, smouldering on without any tendency to spread.

In East Africa endemicity saw the emergence of a virus of reduced virulence. For example, Lowe and others (1947) described the occurrence of mild rinderpest in Tabora (western Tanzania) which they had encountered in 1942 and demonstrated experimentally that the virus caused only a mild clinical disease in cattle, and that the case mortality rate was very low. Later, Robson *et al.* (1959) described the isolation of a strain of rinderpest virus from an eland in northern Tanzania which was naturally attenuated for cattle although still virulent for certain wildlife species. The interplay of mild and virulent forms of rinderpest is described in greater detail in other chapters in this monograph (see Chapters 6 and 7).

# The early recognition of the disease

There is still controversy regarding interpretation of descriptions of the disease in ancient times. According to Leclainche (1936) and Mammerickx (1967, 2003), it was on the occasion of the epizootics of 376–386 that rinderpest was clearly identified for the first time by the Latin writer Severus Sanctus Endeleichus, who described a contagious disease occurring as a major epizootic in cattle. Nevertheless, according to Aristotle (384–322 BC), in *Stagiritae de Historia Animalium*, cattle suffer from two major diseases: the *Podagra* and the *Struma*. The *Podagra* (disease of the feet) was most probably foot-and-mouth disease and, according to the description given, the *Struma* (fever) would be typical of rinderpest. We have also evocations of rinderpest in the writings of Columella and later those of Flavius Vegetius Renatus. Since the sixth century rinderpest has been seen on a regular basis in Western Europe, but it was not until the eighteenth century that we had a clear description of the disease and the first scientific enlightenments; the epizootics from 1709 to 1714 were the first to be scientifically described. The disease originated in Tartary from where it invaded the greater part of Europe, eventually burning itself out in the region of Liège in Belgium.

# The first scientific descriptions of the disease and the first control measures

Bernardino Ramazzini (1633–1714), the principal professor of medicine at the University of Padua, seems to be the first to clearly describe rinderpest, in 1712. He saw similarities between rinderpest and smallpox and his views were widely accepted. It is also during this period that the first breakthrough was made in the control of rinderpest by Giovanni Maria Lancisi (1654–1720) and that the contagious nature of the disease was acknowledged by Johann Kanold (1679–1729) in Prussia, who recognized in 1711 that rinderpest was a specific '*contagio*', rejecting origins other than transmission as scientifically unfounded and observed that recovered cattle were no longer susceptible. He also defined a 'plague' by three cardinal criteria, analogous to those of Galen (AD 129–200): dissemination by contagion, high morbidity and mortality along with severe clinical findings. During the Italian outbreak, Pope Clement XI (1649–1721) ordered his physician, Dr Lancisi, to investigate the cause and prescribe measures for the control of the plague that had killed so many cattle in the papal herds (Wilkinson, 1992). A detailed account of the historical epidemiological status of rinderpest is given by Lancisi (1715); Scott (2000); Blancou (2003); and Spinage (2003). Lancisi's recommendations and their success were underpinned by two thrusts (see also Chapter 9):

- zoo-sanitary measures, including stamping-out
- strong legal enforcement of control measures.

Thus Lancisi's technical recommendations included: slaughter to reduce spread, restricted movement of cattle, burial of whole animals in lime, and inspection of meat. Their implementation was enforced rigorously by the papal edicts by which Draconian penalties, including even hanging of guilty laymen and condemning of clergy to the galleys, were enforced. This led to the first effective control of rinderpest within a country, the state then known as Romagna. The same measures were successfully applied to control an epidemic of rinderpest that invaded England in 1714 with cattle shipped from the Netherlands. Their rigorous application was recommended and advocated by Thomas Bates, surgeon to King George I of England (Bates, 1718). Bates, having been stationed as a naval surgeon in Sicily, was familiar with the edicts of Lancisi. In addition to following Lancisi's recommendations Bates also recommended the segregation of animals into small groups. Similarly enforced measures were successful in containing rinderpest in France and Germany through orders of the French Royal Council in 1714 and by Friedrich Wilhelm I in 1716, both of which included movement control measures. In other parts of Europe where these control measures were not applied with the same rigour, rinderpest elimination was not possible. Blancou in Chapter 9 of this monograph, describes in more detail the evolution and impact of rinderpest control strategies.

It quickly became necessary to train a cadre of specialists to control rinderpest and other animal diseases through the application of Lancisi's methods as all attempts to find a cure for rinderpest had proved fruitless. Thus the first veterinary school was founded in 1761 in Lyon under an order of the French Controller-General of Finances. Over the next few years other European countries opened veterinary schools. In effect, the necessity to control rinderpest led to the founding of the veterinary profession. This was followed by the establishment of State Veterinary Services in European countries to regulate and enforce its control. During the nineteenth century several scholars established that the spread of rinderpest was primarily due to the movement of infected animals. This led to the enacting of preventive measures. It also led to strong debates on the risk of communication of the disease. Thus, for example, in 1857, Professor Simmond of London, argued that:

> Rinderpest is a disease which specially belongs to the Steppe of Russia. … In general terms rinderpest had not visited Central and Western Europe for a period of 40 years … No fear need be entertained that this destructive pest will reach our shores.

However, four years later, alarmed by a relaxation in the strict prohibition of cattle importation, the removal of import duties and permission for uncontrolled entrance of each kind of animal used for food, Professor Simmond declared his conviction that 'nothing could save the country from a visitation of rinderpest unless the authorities realized the probability of such an event arising and adopted vigorous measures to prevent it'.

Although Simmond vacillated, Professor John Gamgee of the Royal Dick Veterinary School in Edinburgh, Scotland, was a persistent advocate of strict import restrictions and slaughter of infected cattle with compensation. In 1863, he wrote to warn Professor Simmond and others that rinderpest would enter the country with cargo from a Baltic port. Two years later Gamgee's prediction was vindicated and Britain was invaded by just that route (Spinage, 2003). During the second half of the eighteenth century and early nineteenth century incursions of rinderpest were less efficiently eradicated in England than in continental Europe. Each episode was costing a lot and taking longer to eradicate than in France. This was attributed partly to an inadequate number of trained veterinarians and less vigour in the implementation of stamping-out and zoo-sanitary measures. Thus for example, Edwards, writing in 1928 (Edwards, 1930) observed that:

> this great expenditure was attributable most largely to the authorities paying heed to medical opinion and delaying with the disease initially by attempted treatment, instead of placing confidence at once in the methods recommended by the experienced veterinarians of the country. In France, where there already existed an organized veterinary service, the disease was exterminated at this time at relatively negligible cost.

Accordingly, when in 1865 the State Veterinary Service was established in England by Order of the Privy Council to deal with cattle plague, the epidemic was eliminated within two years (Pearce *et al.*, 1965).

The control measures adopted in the eighteenth and nineteenth centuries comprised:

- Quarantine measures to segregate infected from unaffected herds
- Import restrictions
- Movement restrictions for animals and people

- Slaughter of all diseased and in contact animals
- Safe carcass disposal – usually deep burial in lime
- Prohibition of the sale of meat and milk from sick animals
- Compulsory notification of disease to the authorities
- Enabling legislation, enforcement and heavy penalties for offenders.

These measures remain valid today and now form the core of the stamping-out policy for the control of highly contagious animal diseases, also referred to as transboundary animal diseases, i.e. those that are of significant economic, trade and/or food security importance for a considerable number of countries; which can easily spread to other countries and reach epidemic proportions; and where control/management, including exclusion, requires cooperation between several countries (FAO, 1996).

This zoo-sanitary policy was undoubtedly the most logical approach to combat the rinderpest epizootics but it met with much resistance and was therefore applied only sparingly, especially at the beginning. In some countries, the measures were seen as too drastic and costly, as is still the case today in most African and Asian countries. In addition, their strict application required a strong central authority, which was often lacking.

Against this background it was not surprising that attempts were made to apply the inoculation principle applied to smallpox (variolation) by analogy to rinderpest. It was also extrapolated to measles by Francis Homes (1719–1813) a few years later (Homes, 1759). Both rinderpest and measles were seen as closely related to smallpox since one attack was known to provide lifelong protection. Several of the most fervent and experienced smallpox inoculators, such as Pieter Camper (1722–1789) in the Netherlands, became the most enthusiastic promoters of applying a similar procedure to rinderpest, especially because all attempts to cure the disease had failed; the whole range of the then known drugs used in human medicine had been tried without success to treat rinderpest (Theves, 1994; see also Chapter 9).

# The first inoculations in England and The Netherlands

The first written report of rinderpest inoculation was published as a letter signed 'T.S.' in the November 1754 issue of the *Gentleman's Magazine*, a journal then widely read by educated people in Britain and also on the Continent. This magazine also supported the practice of smallpox inoculation (Huygelen, 1997). After some initial experiments in England, the focus of activity shifted to The Netherlands where in early 1755 funds were raised to purchase cattle for an inoculation experiment to be carried out in Beverwijk by Corneel Nozeman, a teacher in Haarlem, along with Agge Roskamkool, and Jan Tak, two physicians in Leiden. In the preface to their publication (1755), they stated that neither before nor during their experiment had they had any knowledge of the report published in the *Gentleman's Magazine*. They described their trials in great details using in most cases a seton, a thread or a wick soaked in the nasal or conjunctival secretions of infected animals; with a needle they pierced the skin between two incisions in the buttock and left the thread under the skin.

Of the seventeen inoculated animals, only three survived, one of these having had the disease previously. The authors concluded that inoculation could not be recommended and tried to find an explanation for their failure and wondered whether it would be possible to make the operation less lethal by using a 'weaker' inoculum. They referred to smallpox in which inoculators always tried to take material from patients with a mild form of the disease. They also wondered whether the disease could be made milder by adequate treatment of the inoculated animals (Nozeman *et al.*, 1755). A few further trials were also performed in England. Daniel Peter Layard (1721–1802), Fellow of the Royal Society and medical practitioner in Huntingdon, published his results in a letter read to the Royal Society on 2 February 1759. Layard advocated inoculation, except for young calves and pregnant cows, and made detailed recommendations on how to proceed. In his book on rinderpest published previously he had stressed the analogy between rinderpest and smallpox. Due to the subsequent receding of rinderpest in England, the interest in inoculation declined and almost all further experimentations were done in The Netherlands, Northern Germany and Denmark. At that time the question of smallpox inoculation in man was also vividly debated. The main arguments against inoculation were either medical (inoculation maintaining the disease in a given area because of transmission between inoculated persons to others in their neighbourhood), ethical (nobody having the right to intentionally inflict a disease on somebody else), or even theological (disease being a divine punishment, trying to prevent it by inoculation was acting against God's will).

Among all the inoculation trials against rinderpest carried out during that period, it is worth mentioning the work of Geert Reinders (1737–1815) in The Netherlands (Reinders, 1776) (Figure 5.1). He was a farmer in the Province of Groningen and a self-taught man. He contacted Pieter Camper and, in collaboration with Munniks (1744–1806), carried out several trials with variable success in the 1769–1770 period. Similar experiments were done by Stolte in Germany (Stolte, 1793). These authors tried different inoculation procedures and a variety of treatments to alleviate the clinical signs, all of them without measurable effect. During his experiments Reinders noticed that calves from recovered cows were resistant, representing most probably the first recognition of the phenomenon of maternally derived immunity, since, according to him, this resistance was not of hereditary origin, depending solely on the immunity of the dam. He also noticed that the transferred immunity gradually disappeared, leaving the calves just as susceptible as those from dams who had not had the disease. He also took advantage of this temporary resistance to inoculate calves with minimal risk and realized that he increased his chances of

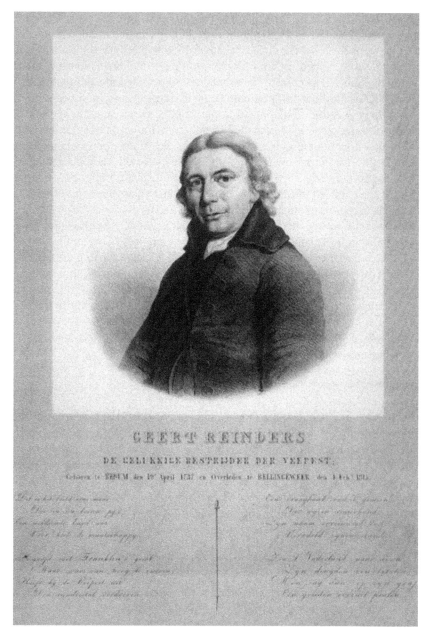

**Figure 5.1**   Geert Reinders (1737–1815) who worked on rinderpest control in The Netherlands.

successful inoculation by repeating the procedure at different ages because in some of the calves the first inoculation would not produce a 'take' (Huygelen, 1997). Nevertheless, in the end it became obvious that inoculation was not a valid solution for rinderpest control. Not only were the losses after inoculation too high but, more importantly, the procedure perpetuated the circulation of the causative agent in the cattle population. At least all these experiments proved that smallpox was not unique in being preventable by inoculation and that the procedure, when successful, provided lifelong protection. It also reinforced the concept that infectious diseases are caused by specific aetiological agents and that rinderpest was a transmissible, reproducible disease. It should also be mentioned that in the early 1760s Jan Engelman published a paper on rinderpest and was the first to observe the close similarity between rinderpest and measles, as opposed to smallpox (Engelman, 1763).

After the discovery of vaccination against smallpox by Edward Jenner (1749–1823) in 1796, and due to the suspected analogy between the two diseases, there were trials to vaccinate cattle against rinderpest using the smallpox vaccine. This practice created a real passion in England during the epizootics of 1865–1867 (Dele, 1870); finally one of the main advocates of this practice, a Dr Murchison (1830–1879), wrote to *The Times* (30 January 1866) that:

> the analogies between smallpox and rinderpest were so obvious that it was logical to try to vaccinate cattle against rinderpest; but it is becoming also obvious that, despite all the trials, there are nowadays sufficient evidence that vaccination does not confer a continuous protection against rinderpest.

As mentioned in Chapter 1, Henri Bouley (1814–1885) in fact demonstrated the total lack of cross-protection between rinderpest, smallpox and vaccinia in 1865. For this purpose he sent eight cows to England, where the rinderpest epizootics were raging. These cows, which had already been used in France to produce the anti-smallpox vaccine, all contracted rinderpest. This proved conclusively the contention of Joseph Reynal (1873) of 'the utter futility of the doctrine propounding the similarity between these two afflictions'.

# The 1865–1867 epizootics in England

One of the best documented epizootics in Europe occurred in England from 1865 to 1867 (see Plate 4) (Third Report of the Commissioners, 1866; Dele, 1870). At that time there were vigorous debates about the origin of this epizootic after such a long absence. The most prominent popular opinion was that the disease emerged spontaneously on the island, even though at that time England imported huge numbers of cattle from the Continent. It must be noted here that the controversy about spontaneous generation was still ongoing, despite the scientific evidence already presented by Lazzaro Spalanzani

(1729–1799) and later by Louis Pasteur (1822–1895) in the early 1860s (Spalanzani, 1769; Pasteur, 1922). The plague was also seen as a sign from God and interpreted as part of a continuing dialogue between the Almighty and His fallen children. It was necessary to lose more than one hundred thousand head of cattle due to trials of all preventive treatments (see Chapter 9) before, thanks to the veterinarians, the outbreak was arrested using the zoo-sanitary measures of Lancisi.

# History of rinderpest in Asia

From ancient times, numerous outbreaks of rinderpest must have occurred in Asia. Based on the fragmented information available, the historical aspects of rinderpest in three Asian countries, India, Korea and Japan are described.

## Rinderpest in India

There is almost no extant literature on cattle diseases and veterinary work, although much of India's ancient literature indicates that cattle were considered essential and valuable to society and were for centuries the basic unit of currency in trading (Dunlop and Williams, 1996). In 1893 James Mills, former director of the Bombay Veterinary College, discovered an old treatise written on palm leaves which showed that in ancient times bovine diseases were classified and treated, and that rinderpest, anthrax, staggers, dysentery, piroplasmosis, meningoencephalitis and ague must have been known. These diseases were characterized by their cardinal signs and treated accordingly. Among them, rinderpest can be confidently recognized (Leclainche, 1936).

In 1890, the Government of India appointed Alfred Lingard, a Welsh medical doctor, as Imperial Bacteriologist charged with investigating animal diseases all over India, the main task being the prevention and cure of epizootic diseases. Laboratory accommodation was provided for him at the Science College, Poona, where a commemorative plaque still testifies to its earlier existence. In 1893 the laboratory was moved to its present situation at Mukteswar in the foothills of the Himalayas at 7500 feet elevation above sea level. It was then named the Imperial Bacteriological Laboratory (Datta, 1948), later becoming the Indian Veterinary Research Institute after independence (Figure 5.2). Rinderpest was the major target for its research efforts. At the invitation of the Government of India, Robert Koch (1843–1910) came to India, directly following his visit to South Africa to deal with the rinderpest pandemic there (Figure 5.3). He arrived at Mukteswar via Bombay in May 1897 with his colleagues, bacteriologists George Gaffky (1850–1918) and Richard Pfeiffer (1858–1926). There they carried out autopsies on diseased animals and subsequently expressed it as Koch's opinion that 'the pathological changes found in the intestines were identical with those found by him in

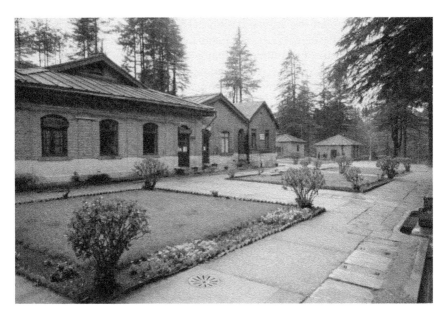

**Figure 5.2** Indian (formerly Imperial) Veterinary Laboratory (IVRI) at Mukteshwar.

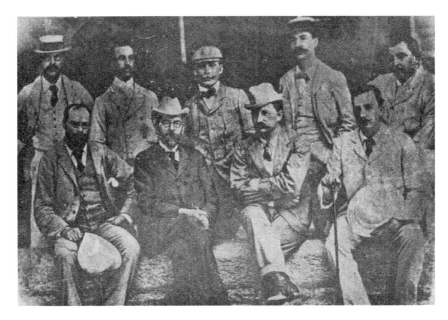

**Figure 5.3** Robert Koch and others at the IVRI in 1897.

animals dead of rinderpest in South Africa, and therefore the Indian and the South African diseases are identical'.

During his two week stay at Mukteswar Koch conducted experiments similar to those he had just recently carried out in South Africa on the immunizing effects of bile taken from the gall bladder of an animal which had succumbed to a virulent attack of rinderpest. However, the results were again inconclusive (Lingard, 1897). It was not until the 1920s that an effective vaccine for rinderpest was developed in India (see Chapter 11).

## Rinderpest in Korea

In the Koryo period (AD 918–1392) an official post of 'Doctor of Veterinary Medicine' existed and several cattle diseases are mentioned in documents from those times. Outbreaks of highly contagious cattle disease suspected of being rinderpest were described in 1142 and 1278. However, some of them appear to have been due to anthrax, as human infection was also noticed. Sakae Miki, a Japanese medical doctor, comprehensively investigated the old medical history of Korea. By taking a high contagion rate and an 80% mortality in cattle as a rinderpest case description, he identified six outbreaks of disease that could have been rinderpest, in 1541–42, 1577–78, 1636–37, 1644–45, 1668–72 and 1680–84 (Miki, 1962). Sporadic outbreaks of suspected rinderpest continued to occur in 1690, 1693, 1701, 1718, 1738, 1748–49 and 1763. In 1871 a rinderpest outbreak in Siberia spread to Korea and there are several records of rinderpest in Korea every two to three years after that.

## Rinderpest in Japan

### The Edo period (1603–1867)

Rinderpest was first mentioned in a Japanese–Portuguese dictionary published in 1603. In this dictionary a disease known as 'Tachi' in Japanese was described, which resembled rinderpest. Later, in 1720, a Japanese handbook entitled *Gyuka Satsuyo* (compendium of bovine diseases) was published, and it mentioned a highly contagious disease with high mortality also called 'Tachi' (Figure 5.4). The disease was characterized by fever, conjunctivitis, nasal or ocular discharge with a staring coat and is considered to have been rinderpest. Shigeru Kishi, a veterinary officer in Yamaguchi Prefecture in the western part of the Main Island of Japan, conducted a comprehensive historical survey of rinderpest using the Yamaguchi prefecture archives (Kishi, 1974, 1976). Until this study, the first outbreak of rinderpest in Japan was considered in most of the veterinary textbooks to be the one that occurred in 1872. However, Kishi's study revealed that records from the Edo period mentioned acute deaths of over 500 000 cattle in the period 1637–1642 and he concluded that this was the first record of rinderpest in Japan. The disease first occurred in Nagato region in the

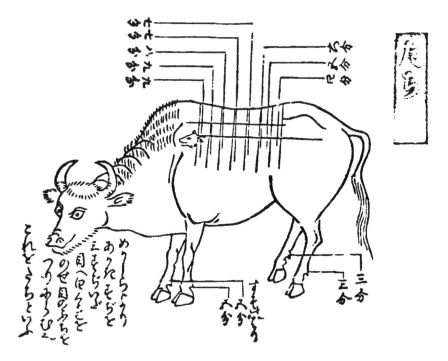

**Figure 5.4** Japanese veterinary illustration of rinderpest, 'Tachi'.

current Yamaguchi prefecture, located on the western coast of the Sea of Japan very close to Korea. Another outbreak, also in Nagato, occurred in 1672–1673. The rate of spread was estimated at 400 km in six months. Chronological examination suggested that the source of the outbreak in 1637 was an introduction from a Korean outbreak that occurred between 1636 and 1637, and the one in 1672 from a Korean outbreak that occurred between 1668 and 1672. The number of cattle deaths in the western part of mainland Japan during these two outbreaks was estimated at over 400 000. In those days dead cattle were usually discarded at a designated cattle disposal area and, as the only preventive measure taken was praying to god, rinderpest spread widely (Plate 5). In 1958, large numbers of cattle bones were found in the sand on the coast of the Sea of Japan where more than 50 000 cattle were suspected to have died in 1672. As the bones are now kept in Tokyo University of Agriculture and Technology, it would be interesting if traces of rinderpest virus could be found in them if in future a sufficiently powerful molecular biological technique for RNA analysis becomes available.

Illegal imports of cattle were considered to be one possible source of rinderpest; however, as Japan had a strict policy of seclusion in those days this is considered unlikely and cattle owners were mostly peasants with low income. By analysing old records for Korean ship wrecks on the coast of the Sea of

Japan in the seventeenth century, Kishi suggested this as a possible alternative explanation for the introduction of the disease (Kishi, 1976).

## The Meiji period (1868–1912)

The newly established Japanese government under the Emperor Meiji (1852–1912) abrogated the policy of seclusion of the country and introduced western science and technology, including veterinary medicine. In 1869 a rinderpest outbreak occurred in the Shanghai district of China and continued until 1871. An American stationed in Japan (C.E. DeLong), received a letter warning of rinderpest from Daniel Jerome McGowan, an American medical doctor in Shanghai and consultant physician to the Ministry of Foreign Affairs of Japan, in June 1871. The Japanese government recognized the importance of rinderpest for the first time and immediately banned the import of livestock from Shanghai, Siberia and the whole area of Korea. However, importation was resumed in October, only 4 months after the import ban (possibly to protect the hide industry in the Osaka region) and consequently a rinderpest outbreak occurred in 1872, probably due to the importation of either live cattle or hides. The outbreak continued until 1873 and caused the deaths of a total of 42 297 cattle in 22 prefectures throughout Japan. At the time, according to the statistical records published in 1878, most cattle in Japan were used for cultivation and these made up 92% of the livestock population and so the outbreak must have caused severe damage to agriculture.

The autopsies on early cases from the outbreak were conducted by Thomas Antisell, an American doctor, who diagnosed typhus fever. Another American, Edward Selton, considered it to be due to an incurable infectious disease and ordered the immediate incineration of the affected cattle. Apparently he had knowledge of rinderpest. Subsequently two Japanese medical doctors dealt with the diagnosis, with advice from Antisell and two Dutch doctors (Ermerins and Beukema). The experience of Dr Beukema, who had served as a Red Cross surgeon in the Franco-Prussian war of 1870, may have made the most substantial contribution to the diagnosis of rinderpest (Kishi, 1977). Most of the diseased cattle were of Japanese domestic breeds. The first symptom was a high fever, followed by swelling of the abdomen and vomiting followed by wasting. It was reported that a strong fetid smell filled the cattle barns. Acute cases died at 3–4 days and others at 7–8 days. On Shikoku island, the mortality was over 98%. Diseased cattle were treated by bleeding from the tail vein as it was believed that cattle enduring a profuse blood loss would survive, while those with less bleeding died consistently. This outbreak accelerated the establishment of nationwide preventive measures against infectious diseases of domestic animals. In 1878 the first agricultural school consisting of a division of veterinary medicine and a division of agriculture was founded. Later, this became the Faculty of Agriculture, University of Tokyo. In 1891 the Laboratory of Veterinary Diseases was established in the Agriculture Station of the Ministry of Agriculture in Tokyo. This became the current Institute of Animal Health. In 1896 the 'Law of

Prevention of Domestic Animal Diseases' was enacted and a quarantine system, with special emphasis on rinderpest, was introduced.

## The great African rinderpest epizootic

Rinderpest was probably introduced into Egypt in the early 1800s but it did not spread across the continent as did the great rinderpest pandemic of the late 1880s. This pandemic started in Eritrea early in 1887 and the disease was thought to have been introduced by Italian imports of infected zebu cattle from Aden or Bombay to Massowah (Eritrea) and was apparently the first incursion of the virus into sub-Saharan Africa. The progress of the African rinderpest pandemic is well documented by Mack (1970). Over a ten-year period the plague swept over a whole continent of susceptible animals from Abyssinia through Eastern Africa and finally on into southern Africa at a time when veterinary services, with the exception of South Africa, were virtually non-existent (Figure 5.5). Eighty to ninety per cent of cattle, buffalo (*Syncerus caffer*), eland (*Taurotragus* spp.), giraffe (*Giraffa camelopardalis*), wildebeest (*Connochaetes* spp.), kudu (*Tragelaphus* spp.) and various species of antelope succumbed (Edington, 1899).

The pandemic may have been aided by a secondary introduction of rinderpest into Tanzania. According to Littlewood (1905), a certain Major von Wiessmann living in German East Africa (modern day Tanzania) may have imported cattle from either the ports of Aden or Bombay for a German expedition that was being organized to the interior in 1888–89. Apparently he had done this despite prior warnings by Littlewood of the risk of introducing cattle plague, as had happened with the recent Italian importations of Asian cattle. In any case, the resulting rinderpest pandemic caused widespread destruction of the livestock and wildlife and led to starvation among the pastoral communities. In Kenya, the Masai people suffered starvation and, together with a smallpox epidemic that followed the cattle plague, were severely reduced in numbers so facilitating the subsequent colonization of Kenya's great tracts of empty land, probably formerly populated by the Masai. Lugard (1893), describing the impact of rinderpest in Masailand, wrote that 'never before in the memory of man, or by the voice of tradition, have the cattle died in such numbers; never before has the wild game suffered'.

Branagan and Hammond (1965) reported that a Masai young man at the time described how the Engaruka Basin in Ngorongoro, northern Tanzania, was littered with the remains of cattle and people: 'so many and so close that the vultures had forgotten to fly'. And Ranger (1992), in 'Plagues of beasts and men', describes this same rinderpest pandemic in sub-Saharan Africa as though it:

> seemed to threaten a levelling of society to a uniform impoverishment. Its threat was all the more felt because rinderpest did not strike alone but combined with smallpox and drought to create a general ecological crisis in eastern Africa in the late 1880s and 1890s and in southern Africa after 1896.

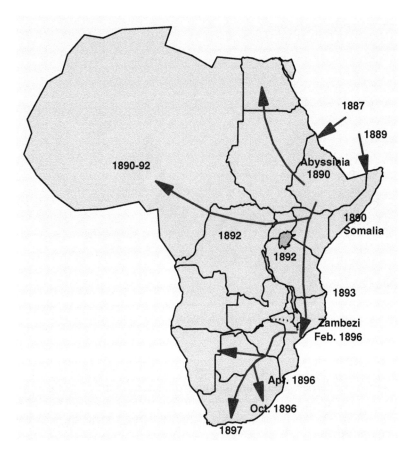

**Figure 5.5**    Spread of rinderpest in Africa 1887–1897 (after Mack, 1970).

In South Africa oxen, which were cheap and readily available, were then the main means of transport as horses were expensive and had to be imported. The disease caused enormous economic losses and dramatically increased the cost of transportation. It struck rapidly and dramatically; cattle that were healthy at the start of a journey would collapse and die before it had ended (Figure 5.6). Some were left in wild country facing hunger and thirst many days away from the nearest human habitation. Mule carts had to be used to rescue some and it was suggested that camels be employed for transport. There was also a shortage of meat, which had to be imported at a huge cost from Australia. Governments of the Cape Colony and the Transvaal called on European expertise to help fight the disease, most notably that of Robert Koch, the foremost microbiologist of the day. He and his assistant Paul Kohlstock arrived at the beginning of December 1896 and immediately set up a laboratory some distance from Kimberley, near the frontier with Transvaal. The history of their

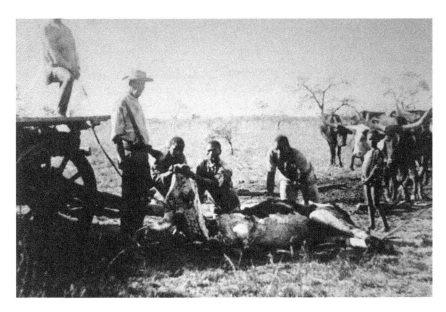

**Figure 5.6** Rinderpest in South Africa. An ox stricken by the disease in 1897.

efforts to isolate the disease-causing agent and their attempts to vaccinate cattle against rinderpest are outlined in more detail in Chapter 11. The opportunities presented at the end of the nineteenth century with new scientific breakthroughs finally led to the discovery of the rinderpest virus by Nicolle and Adil-Bey in 1902.

# References

Barrett, T. and Rossiter, P. (1999) Rinderpest: the disease and its impact on humans and animals. *Adv. Virus Res.* **53**, 89–110.

Bates, T. (1718) A brief account of the contagious disease which raged among the milch cows near London, in the year 1714 and of the methods that were taken for suppressing it. *Phil Trans. R. Soc.*, 30.

Blancou, J. (2003) *History of the Surveillance and Control of Transmissible Animal Diseases*. Paris: Office International des Épizooties.

Branagan, D. and Hammond, J.A. (1965) Rinderpest in Tanganyika: a review. *Bull. Epizoot. Dis. Afr.* **13** (3), 225–46.

Datta, S. (1948) The nature and significance of veterinary problems in ancient and modern India. *Ind. Vet. J.* **25**, 115–21.

Dele, E. (1870) La peste bovine ou thypus contagieux épizootique en Angleterre (1865–1867). Brussels: Combe et Van de Weghe.

Dieckerhoff, W. (1890) *Gesichte der Rinderpest und ihrer Literatur*. Berlin: Verlag von Th. chr. Fr. Enslin.

Dunlop, R.H. and Williams, D.J. (1996) *Veterinary Medicine. An Illustrated History*. St Louis: Mosby, p. 130.

Edington, A. (1899) A retrospect of the rinderpest campaign in South Africa *Lancet*, **i**, 357–9.

Edwards, J.T. (1930) The problem of rinderpest in India. *Bull. Imp. Inst. Agr. Res. Pusa* **199**, 1–16.

Engelman, J. (1763) Nader verhandeling over de rundveesterfte betre klijk tot de waarneemingen vervat in't VIde deel, II° stuk. *Verhand. Holl. Maatsch. Wetenschap*, **7**, 247–318.

FAO (1996) Prevention and control of transboundary animal diseases. Report of the FAO Expert Consultation on the Emergency Prevention System (EMPRES) for Transboundary Animal and Plant Pests and Diseases (Livestock Diseases Programme) including the Blueprint for Global Rinderpest Eradication. Rome, Italy, 24–26 July 1996. FAO Animal Production and Health Paper 133, FAO, Rome.

Homes, F. (1759) *Medical Facts and Experiments*. London: A. Miller.

Huygelen, C. (1997) The immunisation of cattle against rinderpest in eighteenth-century Europe. *Med. Hist.* **41**, 182–96.

Kishi, H. (1974) The study on the history of rinderpest that broke out during the Edo era in Japan. Jui Chikusan Shimpo, No. 625, 1099–1104 and 1146–1154. (In Japanese with English abstract.)

Kishi, H. (1976) A historical study on outbreaks of rinderpest during the Edo era in Japan. *Yamaguchi J. Vet. Med.*, **3**, 33–40.

Kishi, H. (1977) A historical study on the diagnosis of rinderpest at the beginning of Meiji period. *Jpn. J. Vet. Hist.* **11**, 1–14. (In Japanese.)

Lancisi, G.M. (1715) *Dissertatio historica de bovilla peste, ex campaniae finibus anno MDCCXlll Latio importata*. Rome: Ex Typographia Joannis Mariae Salvioni.

Layard, D.P. (1759) A discourse on the usefulness of inoculation of the horned cattle to prevent the contagious distemper among them. *Phil. Trans. R. Soc.*, **50**, 11.

Leclainche, E. (1936) *Histoire de la médecine vétérinaire*. Toulouse: Office du Livre.

Lingard, A. (1897) Preliminary note on rinderpest at Imperial Bacteriological Laboratory, by Prof. R. Koch, 4th to 15th June, 1897.

Littlewood, W. (1905) Cattle Plague in Egypt in 1903–04–05. *J. Comp. Pathol.* **18**, 312–21.

Lowe, H.J., Wilde, J.K.H., Lee, R.P., Stuchbery, H.M. (1947) An outbreak of an aberrant type of rinderpest in Tanganyika territory. *J. Comp. Pathol. Ther.* **57** (3), 175–83.

Lugard, F.J.D. (1893) *The Rise of Our East African Empire, 1893: Early Efforts in Nyasaland and Uganda* (Cass Library of African Studies). International Specialized Book Services; New Impression (May, 1968).

Mack, R. (1970) The great African cattle plague epidemic of the 1890s. *Trop. Anim. Hlth Prod.*, **2**, 210–19.

Mammerickx, M. (1967) Histoire de la médecine vétérinaire belge: suivie d'un répertoire bio-bibliographique des médecins vétérinaires belges et de leurs écrits. Brussels: Académie Royale de Médecine de Belgique.

Mammerickx, M. (2003) La peste bovine, Jules Bordet et le centre sérumigène de Cureghem. *Ann. Méd. Vét.* **147**, 197–205.

Miki, S. (1962) *History of Korean Medicine and of Diseases in Korea*. Ishiyaku Shuppan. (In Japanese.)

Nicolle, M. and Adil-Bey, M. (1902) Études sur la peste bovine (3ᵉ mémoire). *Ann. Institut Pasteur* **16**, 50–67.

Nozeman, C., Roskamkool, A. and Tak, J. (1755) *Eerste proefneeming over de uitwerkingen van de inentinge der besmettende ziekte in het rundvee gedaan in de Beverwijk.* Amsterdam: K van der Sys and K de Veer.

Pasteur, L. (1922) *Oeuvres.* Paris: Masson.

Pearce, J.W.R., Pugh, L.P. and Ritchie J. (1965) *Animal Health: A Centenary, 1865–1965.* London: HMSO.

Ranger, T. (1992) Plagues of beasts and men: prophetic responses to epidemic in eastern and southern Africa. In: T. Ranger and P. Slack (eds), *Epidemics and Ideas: Essays on the Historical Perception of Pestilence.* Cambridge: Cambridge University Press, pp. 241–68.

Reinders, G. (1776) *Waarneemingen en proeven meest door inёntinge op het rundvee gedaan, dienende ten bewijse, dat wij onze kalvers van gebeterde koejen geboren, door inёntinge tegen de veepest kunnen beveiligen.* Groningen: L. Huisingh.

Reynal, J. (1873) *Traité de police sanitaire des animaux domestiques.* Paris: P. Asselin.

Robson, J., Arnold, R.M., Plowright, W. and Scott, G.R. (1959) The isolation from an eland of a strain of rinderpest virus attenuated for cattle. *Bull. Epizoot. Dis. Afr.* **7**, 97–102.

Rossiter, P.B., Hussain, M., Raja, R.H., Moghul. W., Khan, Z. and Broadbent D.W. (1998) Cattle plague in Shangri-La: observations on a severe outbreak of rinderpest in northern Pakistan 1994–1995. *Vet. Rec.* **143** (2), 39–42.

Scott, G.R. (1964) Rinderpest. *Adv. Vet. Sci.* **9**, 113–224.

Scott, G. (1996) The history of rinderpest in Britain. *State Vet. J.* **6**, 8–10.

Scott, G. (2000) The Murrain now known as Rinderpest. *Newsl. Trop. Agr. Assoc. U.K.* **20**, 14–16.

Scott, G. and Provost, A. (1992). Global eradication of rinderpest. Background paper prepared for the FAO expert consultation on the strategy for Global Rinderpest Eradication. Rome, October 1992, p. 109.

Spalanzani, L. (1769) *Nouvelles recherches sur les êtres microscopiques, et sur la génération des corps organisés.* London and Paris: Lacombe.

Spinage, C.A. (2003) *Cattle Plague: A History.* New York, Boston, Dordrecht: Kluwer Academic/Plenum.

Stolte, J.H. (1793) Schreiben wegen Einimpfung des jungen Rindviehes, 1 November 1777. In: W. Schumacher, *Die sichersten Mittel wider die Gefahr beym Eintritte der Rindvieseuche aus Erfahrungen und Urkunden bestätiget 1777,* 2nd edn. Berlin: Oemigke.

Theves, G. (1994) De la maladie des bêtes à cornes au Duché de Luxembourg, pendant le XVIIIᵉᵐᵉ siècle: traitement et prophylaxie. *Ann. Méd. Vét.* **138**, 81–8.

*Third report of the Commissioners appointed to inquire into the origin and nature, etc. of the Cattle Plague,* London: Eyre and Spottiswoode, 1866.

Wilkinson L. (1992) *Animals and Disease: An Introduction to the History of Comparative Medicine.* Cambridge: Cambridge University Press.

# Rinderpest in the twentieth and twenty-first centuries

# 6

## PETER L. ROEDER,* WILLIAM P. TAYLOR,† AND MARK M. RWEYEMAMU‡

*Food and Agriculture Organization, Animal Health Service, Animal Production and Health Division, Rome, Italy
†Littlehampton, Sussex, UK
‡Woking, Surrey, UK

## Introduction

Whilst the early years of the twentieth century were marked by widespread experience of cattle plague throughout Asia, parts of Europe and Africa, the written record is meagre and generally only exceptional events are described. Sadly few sought to record rinderpest events as diligently as Nawathe and co-workers in Nigeria (see, for example, Nawathe and Lamorde, 1982, 1985; Nawathe et al., 1983). Because of this it can be difficult to discern any epidemiological pattern within the overall picture of viral persistence which is obscured by long-lived epizootic, even panzootic, waves of infection interspersed with times of apparent disease absence. Yet, as recognized in recent years, these epizootics must have had their origin in areas of enzootic persistence and indeed the epidemiological situation can be glimpsed by examination of such 'grey literature' as does exist. Few formal publications on rinderpest occurrence in the field are available to consult after about 1970 because few chose to publish their observations. Recording rinderpest occurrence came to be seen as 'sensitive' because of the potential impact on international trade in livestock and their products. In fact this is probably the single most important factor that has bedevilled rinderpest investigation and control leading to an under-recording of enzootic disease situations and even epizootics.

ISBN-13: 978-0-12-88385-1
ISBN-10: 0-12-88385-6

During this period, the disease was confined essentially to Asia and Africa, although its potential to invade other continents was clearly demonstrated by the movement of virus in trade cattle to Belgium and then on to Brazil from India in 1920 and via cattle infected by pigs in Singapore to Australia in 1923 (Throssel, 1980), where it infected 28 herds within seven weeks. Fortunately, even though the virus did start to become established, all three of these long-distance rinderpest movements were eliminated rapidly by stamping-out combined with livestock movement controls.

Although progress was frequently disrupted by global and regional conflicts which favoured resurgence of rinderpest, overall the twentieth century saw a progressive increase in control and reduction of the impact of the disease particularly once vaccines became widely available in mid-century. In the post-colonial era collapse in effectiveness of official veterinary services allowed resurgence of rinderpest in Africa from reservoirs of infection not eliminated by institutionalized annual mass vaccination.

A brief history of rinderpest occurrence and its determinants since 1900 follows. In it an attempt is made to provide an epidemiological overview rather than a precise catalogue of outbreaks in order to understand why and how rinderpest has been brought to the brink of extinction. It owes much to a retrospective analysis of events using information from many official meetings and informal discussions combined with the evidence provided by molecular epidemiology. On a phylogenetic basis field strains of rinderpest virus can be placed in one of three lineages (Wamwayi *et al.*, 1995). Even though few viruses have survived to be preserved in the archive the information provided by genetic characterization has been valuable in determining the source of outbreaks in recent years.

# Progressive control and eradication

No one reading an account of veterinary services during the early years of the twentieth century can fail to be struck by the preoccupation of veterinary services with rinderpest control, for indeed this was the prime reason in most countries for their foundation. However, as the twentieth century entered its last decade we could be reasonably confident that rinderpest viruses were restricted primarily to a small number of persisting reservoirs of infection. Now, half-way through the first decade of the twenty-first century, only one of the rinderpest virus lineages is possibly extant and in a relatively small area of the Greater Horn of Africa at that. This is significant progress, suggesting that eradication could be achieved in the near future if lessons are learnt from the past and commitment to eradication is sustained for the five years or less required.

Vaccines were initially used year-round to combat outbreaks but once they became routinely available many countries implemented annual, pulsed vaccination campaigns throughout their territory or in border areas considered to be particularly vulnerable to invasion. However, little progress was made towards eradication in Africa until the advent of international coordination with the inception of Joint Project 15 (JP15; Lepissier, 1971), the first of the three internationally supported and internationally coordinated rinderpest eradication campaigns that dominate the history of African rinderpest during the second half of the twentieth century. It had earlier been demonstrated in Asia by FAO that intensified vaccination and international coordination of vaccination across international borders could be a successful technique in freeing large areas from rinderpest (Hambridge, 1955; Hudson, 1960). JP15 demonstrated this again in Africa but it neglected to develop the capacity to stamp out residual reservoirs of infection and in the early 1980s a second rinderpest epizootic swept across sub-Saharan Africa undoing most of what had been achieved. The resulting Pan African Rinderpest Campaign (PARC) succeeded in reclaiming much of the situation (Taylor, 1990), yet it too ended in 1999 without eradicating the virus from Africa. At the present time the Pan African Control of Epizootics (PACE) programme is mandated to take the credit for the eradication of rinderpest from Africa (Plate 6).

Coordinated mass vaccination undoubtedly suppressed the disease considerably and even cleared large areas completely. It did not, however, prevent periodic resurgences in panzootic form or eliminate the reservoirs of infection which were not clearly defined until the advent of the Global Rinderpest Eradication Programme (GREP) in the 1990s. In the mid-1990s it became clear that ultimately eradication of rinderpest would depend on assured elimination of the remaining persisting reservoirs of infection. A series of FAO Technical and Expert Consultation meetings held in Rome (FAO, 1996, 1998, 1999) identified six areas of prime concern because of known or suspected existence of reservoirs of rinderpest virus. These comprised four in Asia (Pakistan with Afghanistan; Asiatic Russia with Mongolia and China; Yemen with Saudi Arabia; and Turkey with Iraq and Iran – 'The Kurdish Triangle'), and two in Africa (southern Sudan with contiguous areas of Kenya, Ethiopia and Uganda, and southern Somalia with eastern Kenya and southern Ethiopia – the 'Somali pastoral ecosystem') with periodic involvement of southern Kenya and northern Tanzania. This proved to be an accurate assessment and there has been no cause to suspect the presence of rinderpest outside the areas defined for special attention. These areas will be given emphasis in the following account together with an explanation of the development of control/eradication precepts. The 'Intensified GREP', which was implemented from 1999 to 2004, focused primarily on containment of infection within reservoirs, raising community and professional awareness of rinderpest and the factors facilitating its persistence, epidemiological clarification to guide strategy, intensive, focused immunization to eliminate epidemiologically defined foci with seromonitoring of vaccination efficacy where possible and timely withdrawal of vaccination to allow verification of freedom. Accompanying the eradication effort was a drive to enlist countries in the process of accreditation of rinderpest freedom by means of the 'OIE Pathway' (OIE, 2004).

As a result, progress in assured rinderpest eradication has been rapid in the past ten years. All but one of the 'areas of concern' identified above, in five of which rinderpest was endemic into the second half of the last decade of the twentieth century, yielded to the eradication effort and have been cleared of infection. At the time of writing (end of 2004), there can be little doubt that the whole of Asia has been free from rinderpest virus infection since 2000 and the same can be assuredly stated for most of Africa except for a small part of eastern Africa. Remarkably there has been no re-appearance of rinderpest in any of the former endemic foci or any resurgence of rinderpest elsewhere which could have indicated the presence of cryptic foci of infection. Its absence even from the warfare and its aftermath in Afghanistan and Iraq is quite remarkable and in sharp contrast to the situation that pertained in the previous decade when, for example, a resurgence of rinderpest in Turkey, Iraq and Iran resulted from the Gulf War of 1991 and rinderpest spread in Afghanistan in 1995 was facilitated by civil disturbance.

## The freeing of Europe from rinderpest

Strict enforcement of zoo-sanitary procedures in Europe saw the disease defeated early in the twentieth century, including European Russia west of the Ural mountains by 1908. It has stayed free apart from upsurges after the First World War, most notably in Poland, and rapidly dealt with introductions into Belgium in 1920 with cattle from South Asia, Rome zoological gardens in 1950 by importation of antelopes from Somalia, Georgia in 1989 (which will be discussed later) and, possibly as reported in local newspapers at the time, Turkish Thrace in 1996. Interestingly, in 1954 Italy, and Europe, narrowly escaped a rinderpest outbreak when the disease was detected in two buffaloes (presumably African *Syncerus caffer*) on board a ship docked at Trieste harbour (Boldrini, 1954). The buffaloes had been embarked at Mombasa and were destined to move by train from Trieste to Yugoslavia. Subsequent investigations disclosed that the ship had taken on board at Mogadishu, Somalia, 300 cattle which had been unloaded at Suez.

## The demise of the Asian lineage of rinderpest virus

The twentieth century opened with rinderpest widespread across Asia. Writing in 1918, Kakizaki stated 'It exists permanently in Siberia and Mongolia, whence it spread over Chosen (Korea), Taiwan, The Philippines, British India, Egypt, Siam, China etc.', but indicated that Nippon (Japan) had been free since 1909.

The middle of the twentieth century witnessed a dramatic upsurge of rinderpest in Asia as a result of the Second World War; its control took many years and was a prime reason for the founding of FAO. In 1948 the great cattle plague was killing millions of cattle, buffaloes and yaks in China and Mao Zedong decreed that its eradication was to be a priority for the new nation for it was seen that there was little or no prospect of the agricultural development needed to feed the masses unless the disease was removed from the equation. As recently as 1957 Thailand had to appeal to the international community for food aid because so many buffaloes had died that paddies could not be prepared for rice planting and famine loomed.

## The China, Russia and Mongolia focus

Lenin attached great importance to the eradication of rinderpest, personally signing several decrees on the subject of the elimination of rinderpest (Laktionov, 1967) and, as a result, the European part of the USSR was freed when the last disease was eliminated from the Transcaucasian countries of Armenia, Azerbaijan and Georgia in 1928. Essentially these countries have remained free until today apart from an incident in Georgia in 1989 (Kurchenko *et al.*, 1993).

The far east of Russia was repeatedly invaded by rinderpest from China and Mongolia until the 1930s and 1940s, the last invasion being from the Manchurian region of China in 1945 and 1946. Further west, after the 1940s the Central Asian Republics were maintained essentially free from rinderpest apart from serious incursions into Turkmenistan in 1950 and Tajikistan in 1944 and 1951 from Afghanistan/Iran. This understanding of long-term freedom made it difficult to explain how outbreaks could have occurred in Russia close to the border with Mongolia in 1991 and in 1998 in Amur Region in the Far East of the Russian Federation in a single village near the border with China. These enigmatic events in Georgia and the Russian Far East will be dealt with later.

During the war period of 1938 to 1941 more than one million cattle died from rinderpest in western China (including Sichuan, Qinghai, Gansu and Tibet provinces), and rinderpest occurred widely in China in 1948/49 (Prof. Zhang Nianzu, personal communication). An intensive vaccination programme was at first constrained in China because early live vaccines retained unacceptable virulence for some breeds of Chinese cattle and yaks. However, passage of the Japanese lapinized vaccine virus in goats and sheep produced a safe attenuated vaccine made from lymphoid organs and blood of affected animals.

In May 1951 a meeting in Beijing launched a five-year eradication plan prepared by Dr. Cheng Shaojiong. Rooting out pockets of infection in the Himalayas at a time when there was little or no motorized transport and no cold chain involved heroic feats to transport vaccine virus in live, infected goats on the back of horses and yaks to the sites where vaccine was produced for immediate use. According to Academician Shen Rong-Xian, who led the final eradication effort, success came rapidly and no outbreak has occurred since 1955, when vaccination ceased. Only once since then has vaccination been resorted to and that was briefly in 1994 in a small area of Xinjiang in response to the perceived risk of spread from cattle plague in the Northern Areas of Pakistan.

Rinderpest was first officially recorded in Mongolia in 1910, at which time annual losses approximated 120 000 cattle and yaks per year. Repeated re-invasions, controlled by movement restrictions and immunization, were noted in the 1930s and 1940s. Kurchenko (1995) referred to the conclusion from studies conducted in the 1950s that rinderpest had most frequently been introduced into the country by infected *dzeren* gazelles (*Procapra gutturosa*) during their migrations across the border with China, just as occurs today with foot-and-mouth disease. From the 1950s the country remained free until 1991 to 1993, when outbreaks of rinderpest occurred on both sides of the Mongolia/Russia border.

This area was selected for special attention by GREP because, despite the lack of any evidence of persisting rinderpest, the disease had occurred in Mongolia and Russia in the 1990s. Lack of clarification of this event led to a situation where each of the three countries knew themselves to be free from rinderpest whilst believing the other two to be harbouring infection. A similar situation continues to exist today in the case of Kazakhstan, which suspects China and Mongolia of harbouring rinderpest.

## The Georgia–Mongolia–Russia rinderpest enigma

As mentioned earlier, the restricted outbreaks of rinderpest occurring between 1989 and 1998 in countries of the former USSR were difficult to explain. The first localized outbreak on three farms in Georgia in October/November 1989 was assumed to have been caused by introduction from Turkey, which was not unreasonable at that time. In the Russian/Mongolian incidents of 1991 to 1993 there appear to have been two separate elements. The first in June/July 1991 involved rinderpest on one farm in the Russian province of Chita; a group of cattle was vaccinated there, as was customary, with rinderpest vaccine and then moved to grazing in Mongolia. The second occurred in October of the same year, further west, when rinderpest was discovered in yaks on farms in Tuva province (Semenikhin *et al.*, 1995). These yaks had earlier been at grazing in Mongolia where rinderpest was also seen in feral/wild yaks. A salient feature of the epizootic is that recognition of the disease in Russia as rinderpest was delayed until 1992 by the earlier vaccination of cattle masking the epizootic appearance. As a result infection spread widely and persisted into 1993. The last of the three outbreaks involved a single village in the Amur region of the Russian Far East close to the border with China, but separated from it by the broad Amur River, fortifications and severely enforced movement restrictions.

In order to explain the enigmatic events, scientists have hypothesized about the roles that deer and gazelles could play in maintaining rinderpest in the region. Russian scientists have also proposed s*uroks* and *susliks* (rodents of the genera *Marmuta* and *Citellus* respectively) as potential hosts and a means of introduction across a heavily guarded border with China, their susceptibility to laboratory infection having been established. However, it is unlikely that any of the wild fauna could have sustained rinderpest virus for 50 years without its presence being shown in local cattle and wild ungulates.

All three incidents were associated with the vaccination buffer zone which had been maintained in border areas of the USSR, and subsequent to its dissolution by many of its former member countries, from the Pacific Ocean to the Caspian Sea, since the time of the rinderpest incidents in Tajikistan and the Russian Far East in the1940s. The vaccine in use during the period in question was derived by attenuation of the Kabul 1961 virulent strain of rinderpest virus which is designated K37/70 (Dr Sergei Starov, personal communication). Molecular characterization of the K37/70 virus and that isolated from the Amur Region outbreak demonstrated a very close relationship between them (Roeder and Reichard, 1999, relating the work of Drs Sergei Starov and Pavil Ayanot of the All Russia Research Institute for Animal Health, Vladimir, Russia). Within a 321 nucleotide section of the F gene examined, the viruses are identical except for one substitution. Both these viruses also share a single substitution of another nucleotide with the progenitor Kabul 1961 virus. Conclusively, perhaps, sequencing or partial sequencing of viruses derived from Tuva and Georgia outbreaks also demonstrate a very close relationship with the K37/70 vaccine virus (Barrett *et al.*, 1993; Prof. Tom Barrett personal communication). Molecular characterization of rinderpest viruses derived from Turkish outbreaks also suggests this to be an unlikely candidate for the origin of the Georgia outbreak. Therefore it is suggested that the outbreaks occurring in the vaccination buffer zone of the USSR/Russian Federation between 1989 and 1998 resulted from reversion to virulence of the vaccine virus. In contrast it must be stated that extensive *in vivo* testing had never disclosed such a tendency to regain virulence yet the origin of the outbreaks in this manner remains a plausible hypothesis. The Russian Federation no longer continues to try to maintain border vaccination, which is only practised now in Tajikistan and Kazakhstan.

## South-East Asia

Rinderpest was well known in South-East Asia in the first half of the twentieth century. Myanmar (then Burma) reported a serious epizootic comprising 743 outbreaks as early as 1925–26. Indo-China (now referred to generally as South-East Asia) and the archipelagic area of East Asia suffered severely after the Second World War but slowly control was regained. The War provoked a dramatic increase in incidence of outbreaks signalled by a grave epizootic in Laos in 1944–45, which is reckoned to have killed 75% of cattle and buffaloes. Thailand had become free by 1949 and Laos had been free for several years by 1956 but rinderpest persisted in neighbouring countries and Thailand again experienced outbreaks from 1956 to 1958 on the border with Cambodia. Looming famine in Thailand, and epizootics in neighbouring countries, sparked intensive control efforts in that year, spearheaded by FAO. The last cases of rinderpest in Myanmar occurred on the border with Bangladesh in 1958; Burma, Laos and Thailand were considered free in 1958 as was Malaysia. Yet further east rinderpest persisted without attracting much attention. An epizootic of rinderpest occurred from 1957 to 1961 in Cambodia and in 1964 the country was still infected. How and when rinderpest was finally eliminated from this focus is unclear but the Vietnamese official veterinary service has stated that an outbreak was experienced in the southern highlands of Vietnam in 1974 and that the virus persisted throughout the Vietnam war until as late as 1977 (Dr Le Min Chi, personal communication).

The USA colonized Indonesia and the Philippines in the 1870s and 1880s and in the process introduced rinderpest from mainland Asia. The epidemics were savage, causing up to 90% losses (Scott, 2000). Both invading administrations quickly established veterinary departments yet both took 30 years to eliminate the disease. Rinderpest was again a major problem in the Philippines during the 1940s and into the 1950s but had been eliminated by 1956 only to be re-introduced in 1965 by riverine buffaloes imported from India. Having escaped from quarantine the disease started to spread locally and was eliminated only with some difficulty. In 1960 'the disease continued to have a stronghold in Indonesia' (FAO, 1984) but was eliminated soon after, freeing the archipelagic area of East Asia from endemic rinderpest.

## South Asia

India mounted a valiant effort to eliminate rinderpest for almost the whole of the twentieth century. Repeatedly the disease was pushed out of the northern part of the subcontinent only to resurge periodically, as it did in the 1950s and 1980s. The fortunes of the other countries comprising the Indian sub-continent mirrored the evolution of the disease and its control in India. In the 1990s it became abundantly evident that India's problem with rinderpest emanated from a reservoir of enzootic persistence in the southern states of Tamil Nadu, Karnataka and Kerala, where the virus was persisting enzootically (see Chapter 13), with frequent involvement of Andhra Pradesh. This realization led to a final effort coordinated by the National Programme for Rinderpest Eradication with EU support which achieved the remarkable result of eliminating the last infection in 1995. There had been much confusion earlier over the role that small ruminants played in the maintenance and transmission of rinderpest in the southern peninsula of India. Taylor *et al.* (2002a) however, showed that much (but not all) of what had been thought to be rinderpest was in fact peste des petits ruminants (PPR), which had been recognized as present only in 1987 (Shaila *et al.*, 1987). Yet, goats were incriminated in the inadvertent transfer in 1978 by the Indian Peacekeeping Force of rinderpest to Sri Lanka, which had been free of the disease for 30 years. It spread widely and persisted in the troubled north-east and east of the island where civil disturbance largely but not completely reduced access to the affected villages. However, extensions of rinderpest from the affected area were few and there is good evidence that rinderpest failed to persist there after 1994.

Bangladesh appears to have been free from rinderpest as early as 1958, in which year approximately three million cattle and buffaloes had died in the north-east of the country. Prior to that, the history of rinderpest had been one of occasional introduction from neighbouring countries with epidemic spread within the country, but not of persistence. Like Bangladesh, as disease was eliminated from northern India so did it depart from Bhutan and Nepal. Nepal was invaded by rinderpest from India on 13 occasions between 1952 and 1989, which was the last year it was so affected. After losing 25% of its cattle and yak herds in 1969, Bhutan remained free.

History records few outbreaks in Afghanistan since 1950: 1955, 1960, 1982, 1988 and the last in 1995 (Dr Azizullah Osmani, personal communication). Although certainly an incomplete record, this does suggest that rinderpest might be a relatively rare event in that country. However, rinderpest in Afghanistan was of major regional significance, for it moved on from there into Iran on several occasions and in 1950 and 1951 breached the defences of the USSR to enter Turkmenistan and Tajikistan (as it had previously in 1944) respectively. In terms of rinderpest ecology Afghanistan can be considered as an extension of the western Pakistan ecosystem because the two are linked by contiguous livestock populations, by transhumance, and by two-way trade in livestock. An outbreak, the last encountered in Afghanistan, in Khost province of eastern Afghanistan in 1995 was traced back to Sarghoda market in Punjab province of Pakistan, which itself received buffaloes from Sindh province. Assessing the situation and exerting appropriate control was difficult at that time but fortunately the European Union and the United Nations Development Programme supported FAO in this effort. Despite this the disease lingered on until 1997, fortunately without extensive spread, when the disease was also detected for the last time in the contiguous North-West Frontier province and adjacent tribal areas of Pakistan. Combined with the absence of overt disease, serological investigations in 1998 (Majok et al., 2000) and 2000/1 (Table 6.1) conducted by FAO start to provide confidence that Afghanistan does not present a risk of harbouring rinderpest.

The area of the Indian sub-continent which became Pakistan, like India per se, was severely affected by rinderpest throughout most of the twentieth century, with enzootic persistence interspersed with periods of epizootic resurgence in 1947 to 1951 and again from 1959 to 1962, suppressed by vaccination. The last such dramatic epizootic occurred in 1994, when rinderpest was introduced into

**Table 6.1**  The serological results obtained from a risk-focused random survey conducted in 2001–02 in Afghanistan using the OIE-prescribed rinderpest competitive ELISA

| Region | Tested | Positive |
|---|---|---|
| North | 7212 | 12 |
| South-west | 6194 | 1 |
| South-east | 5963 | 35 |
| **Total** | **19 369** | **48** |

Source: Drs Daad Mohammed and Aggrey Majok

the Northern Areas by buffaloes from Punjab Province where an upsurge of rinderpest had been recorded in 1993. Classical cattle plague resulted, with more than 40 000 cattle, yaks, cattle/yak hybrids and buffaloes dying during the first year of the epizootic in the Gilgit and Hunza valleys (Rossiter *et al.*, 1998). The epizootic spread slowly but progressively until 1996 when it was eliminated by intensive vaccination campaigns conducted by the government of Pakistan aided by FAO and assisted by the EU. From 1999 FAO mounted a strong programme of assistance to the Pakistan authorities in their desire to eradicate rinderpest and from 2002 the EU added additional valuable financial support for strengthening surveillance. Studies rapidly revealed that far from being ubiquitous rinderpest had in fact generally been restricted in the preceding decade to the Indus River buffalo tract of Sindh province where the disease was suppressed by vaccination focused on outbreaks. However, starting in the early 1990s it appears that problems related to the quality of rinderpest vaccine led to both an upsurge of rinderpest along the Indus River in Sindh province and the seeding of virus into other areas of Pakistan to generate epizootics, such as that in the Northern Areas in 1994 and more restricted outbreaks in the North-West Frontier region (1995–96), Punjab (1994–95; 1997) and Balochistan province (1990; 1995), as shown in Figure 6.1.

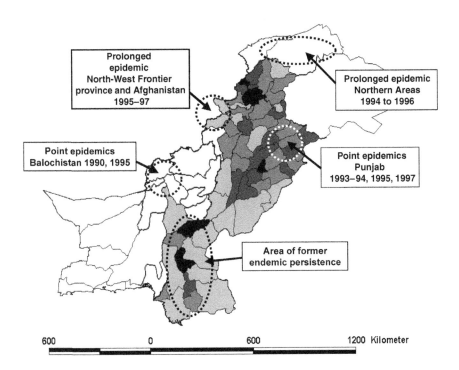

**Figure 6.1**   Pakistan: epidemiological situation outlined in 2001. The depth of shading indicates density of combined cattle and buffalo population.

The Landhi Dairy Colony near Karachi, founded in the 1950s to house 28 000 cattle and buffaloes, developed to become a home for hundreds of thousands of buffaloes and cattle and became notorious for being continuously infected with rinderpest during the 50 years since its establishment. The colony was clearly harbouring infection in 1997 (Brüning *et al.*, 1999), as were other dairy colonies serving Karachi. Some investigators even considered the Landhi Dairy Colony to have been the prime source of rinderpest virus for the outbreaks experienced in the 1980s and 1990s in Pakistan. With the use of quality-assured potent vaccine after 1995 faith in rinderpest vaccination was restored and the incidence of rinderpest decreased. However, studies conducted between 1999 and 2003 indicated clearly that although rinderpest had been eliminated from the large dairy colonies such as Landhi, rinderpest continued to circulate in the small herds of buffaloes in the more remote areas of Sindh until late 2000 and possibly early 2001. The last cases of rinderpest were detected in October 2000 in small farms near to Karachi (Hussain *et al.*, 2001). In addition to routine and emergency disease reporting systems, active village searches using participatory disease searching methodology (Catley, 1997; Mariner *et al.*, 2003) for evidence of rinderpest were put in place throughout the country but concentrating on Sindh and Punjab provinces. The initial findings in 2002 provided strong confirmation that rinderpest ceased to circulate after 2000 (Table 6.2) and a greatly expanded and continuing nationwide programme of searching in 2003 to 2004 adds further confidence.

Vaccination was withdrawn in 2000 and serological studies are now also in progress. Risk-focused randomized surveys of buffaloes and cattle gave a clear

**Table 6.2**  Findings of the first participatory disease search exercise conducted in Sindh province, Pakistan in 2002

| Name of colony/village | Cattle/buffalo population | Year of last reported rinderpest case |
|---|---|---|
| *Dairy colonies* | | |
| Landhi | 190 000 | 1997 |
| Bilal | 12 000 | 1995 |
| Surjani | 85 000 | 1996 |
| Al-Momin | 10 000 | 1994 |
| Nagori | 12 500 | 1994 |
| Baldia with Lyari | 300 000 | 2000 |
| Hyderabad | 10 000 | 2000 |
| *Scattered farms near Karachi* | | |
| Keyamari, Marnipur | | |
| Baba Bhit, | | |
| Malir,* Korangi,* Memon Ghot* | 25 000 | 2000 |

*Villages in which the last reported cases were detected by the pen-side test and confirmed by laboratory testing.

**Table 6.3**  Findings of the first randomized serosurveillance exercise conducted in Pakistan in 2003 using the OIE-prescribed rinderpest competitive ELISA

| Province or Area | Cattle/buffaloes sampled | Positive (percentage) |
| --- | --- | --- |
| Sindh | 2000 | 13 (0.65) |
| Punjab | 2222 | 4 (0.20) |
| North-West Frontier | 1000 | 4 (0.40) |
| Balochistan | 1000 | 7 (0.70) |
| Azad Jammu and Kashmir | 750 | 0 |
| Northern Areas | 580 | 1 (0.20) |
| Islamabad Capital Territory | 509 | 2 (0.40) |
| **Total** | **8061** | **31 (0.38)** |

indication of rinderpest absence even in a population in which vaccination was used so recently (Table 6.3). These studies are also continuing to demonstrate rinderpest freedom as are all other elements of the national animal disease surveillance system.

## West Asia and the Middle East

For decades from the early years of the twentieth century, epizootics of rinderpest swept into Iran from its neighbours causing great losses. The source could not always be identified, as in 1916 and 1932, but in 1924 it came from the Caucasus and Turkey to the north-west. In 1949 and 1969 the disease entered from the north-east establishing a trend of epizootics originating from the eastern borders with Afghanistan and Pakistan separated by extended periods of apparent freedom. It is conceivable that even then the epizootics had their origin in the Indus Valley. These epizootics extended through the country along cattle trading routes, on into Turkey and Iraq and on occasion on to other countries in the Arabian Peninsula and the Levant. Typical of these panzootics, and most reported, is that often referred to as the Near East Panzootic of 1969–73, which swept from Afghanistan through Iran to the Mediterranean littoral and into the Arabian Peninsula invading virtually all countries (FAO, 1993). The virus spread widely in the region, with Israel, Lebanon, Syria, Jordan (Anon, 1971), Kuwait and Yemen known to have become affected between 1970 and 1972. Another wave of rinderpest engulfed Iraq from 1985, resulting from 600 Indian dairy buffaloes being introduced into Iraq through the port of Basrah (or possibly via Kuwait). The buffaloes were distributed widely in Iraq and caused a country-wide virgin epizootic which in Baghdad's Al-Fedeliya Dairy Village alone killed half the 30 000 buffaloes resident at that time. Rinderpest appears to have been endemically established in Saudi Arabia during the 1970s and 1980s (Hafez *et al.*, 1985) persisting until the mid-1990s in feedlots in Al Qassim and Al Hoffuf which were stocked with traditional indigenous and Friesian calves from dairy farms.

The last of the introductions into Iran from South Asia took place in the mid-1980s at which time there was a distinct change in the pattern of rinderpest incursions. Incursions in 1987 and 1989 entered from the north of its western neighbour, Iraq, as happened also in Turkey. Rinderpest invasion of Turkey in 1991 caused alarm in Europe and was met by action for control from FAO. However, another upsurge of rinderpest in the 'Kurdish Triangle' in 1993/4 elicited a strong FAO response to initiate coordinated activities between the three countries to resolve the rinderpest problem.

The Near East Panzootic of 1963–73 and the subsequent pandemic resulting from the 1985 introduction into Iraq, appeared to leave in their wake pockets of infection in Lebanon, from where the disease re-emerged in 1982/3 to re-infect Syria and Israel before being eliminated, as well as in Iraq and Saudi Arabia where pockets persisted until the mid-1990s. However, it seems also that these reservoirs were augmented by repeated re-introductions of rinderpest from South Asia (especially Pakistan and India) in traded cattle and buffaloes into northern Iraq, Saudi Arabia and the United Arab Emirates (UAE). Certainly this is indicated by the pattern from 1979 to 1996 of repeated rinderpest epizootics in Oman which occurred at regular short intervals (for example 1979, 1982, 1984, 1986, 1988 and 1991–93). Many of these appear to have originated by introduction of cattle from Al Ain market on the border with the UAE, which received animals from both the Horn of Africa and South Asia. Another source of rinderpest was the 'illegal' importation of fighting bulls, of which the best and most sought-after came from Pakistan, being transported to Oman by truck through UAE from the port of Khasab on the Musamdan Peninsula. The last of the rinderpest introductions into Oman occurred in 1996 at the same time as the last known outbreaks in Saudi Arabia and Qatar. As was the case in earlier outbreaks, after introduction rinderpest spread steadily along the Batinah coast from market to market before elimination by vaccination campaigns.

Rinderpest persisted in the Central and Southern Governorates of Iraq until September 1994 when it was eliminated by intensive, repeated vaccination of buffaloes, targeting especially the dairy villages close to Baghdad and the areas adjacent to the marshes near Basrah in the south. The latter was a long-standing reservoir of rinderpest from which invasions of western Iran occurred in 1987 and 1994 by the movement of buffaloes across the Shatt al-Arab waterway. Infection was also detected in wild boar (*Sus scrofa*) at the time of the latter incursion (Dr Gholam Ali Kiani, personal communication). Rinderpest lingered on in the Northern Governorates of Dohuk, Erbil and Sulimaniya until 1996, when it was last detected near Dohuk in feedlots causing a very mild disease syndrome with a mortality rate less than 5%. It was eliminated by the intensive vaccination campaigns organized by FAO in 1994–96.

Rinderpest introduced into Yemen in 1971, not for the first time, generated an epizootic which persisted for many years with fluctuating incidence. Outbreaks with high incidence were generally experienced in the coastal Tihama region, from where the traditional movement of milking cattle to highland markets and villages led to a slowly evolving epizootic throughout highland areas with occasional years of exceptional incidence, such as 1987–89 when there were more than 200 outbreaks recorded. The pattern continued into the 1990s, although it is not clear whether this represented continuous endemic persistence or was the result of repeated introductions by trade in cattle from Asia and Africa. The last recorded outbreaks occurred at the turn of 1994/5 in widely separated villages in the extreme north and south of the country.

From 1999 to 2003 intensive efforts by the Directorate of Animal Resources of Yemen to strengthen the national animal disease surveillance system and establish the country's rinderpest status were supported by FAO. The risk-focused randomized village searches conducted in 2001–03 provided no evidence for the persistence of rinderpest after 1992 in the 468 villages searched in areas selected as high risk for enzootic persistence of rinderpest virus (Table 6.4). Elsewhere, outbreaks had been detected in 1994 and separate village search studies indicated that the final occurrence of rinderpest could be dated to 1996. Rinderpest was ruled out after thorough investigation of two disease outbreaks which raised suspicions of rinderpest in 2001 and 2002. In the first serosurveillance studies conducted, antibodies to rinderpest were found in approximately 10% of the cattle sampled throughout the country. When different age categories were compared, the prevalence values were 7% in calves less than one year old, 6% in animals 1–2 years old,

**Table 6.4**    Villages in Yemen reporting the last time they experienced outbreaks of rinderpest and had received rinderpest vaccination

| Village | District | Governorate | Last year of suspected rinderpest | Last vaccination |
|---|---|---|---|---|
| Hagal | Alrogom | Al Mahwit | 1984 | 1996 |
| Bani Alsala | Alrogom | Al Mahwit | 1985 | 1997 |
| Hagarah | Al Sod | Sana'a | 1985 | 1986 |
| Al Ashraf | Al Luhaya | Al Hodeidah | 1985 | 1996 |
| Biot Al Bota | Al Soknah | Al Hodeidah | 1986 | 1995 |
| Bit Soreh | Maswar | Sana'a | 1986 | 1988 |
| Dhi Addirm | Assaddah | Ibb | 1986/7 | Never |
| Khalaqah | Annadirah | Ibb | 1986/7 | Never |
| Al Maidan | Otomah | Dhamar | 1987 | Never |
| Al Lakamah | Otomah | Dhamar | 1987 | Never |
| Al Mibhaya | Otomah | Dhamar | 1987 | Never |
| Al Hajar | Otomah | Sana'a | 1992 | 1997 |
| Assalah | Otomah | Sana'a | 1992 | 1997 |
| Al Arkah | Al Tial | Sana'a | 1990 | 1995 |
| Al Qihadi | Maghrib | Sana'a | 1990 | 1996 |
| Abr Simak | Maghrib | Sana'a | 1991 | 1995 |
| Al Ahyas | Maghrib | Sana'a | 1992 | 1995 |

16% in 2–3-year-olds, and 21% in animals over 3 years. These results suggest that rinderpest has not been widespread for ten years or more and constitute a useful study against which further serosurveillance studies can be assessed. As Yemen follows the process of verification of rinderpest freedom, surveillance continues to fail to disclose any evidence of rinderpest.

The virus derived from the north of Yemen in 1994 was characterized as belonging to the Asian lineage as were all the other four viruses available from the Arabian Peninsula, including one from each of Iraq, Yemen, Kuwait and Oman; all were obtained between 1979 and 1985. The archive of viruses preserved for identification is meagre yet the fact that only Asian lineage viruses were found has been taken as evidence that the Horn of Africa has not been a source of rinderpest for the Middle East. However, even though it might have been only an infrequent event, there does exist evidence for outbreaks in Muscat, Oman, in 1983 (OIE, 1983a, b), around Al-Hodeidah port in north Yemen in 1988 and inland from Aden in south Yemen in 1991 which were associated with eastern African cattle imports. It is also relevant to note that the GCC (Gulf Cooperation Council) states were notified in April 1998 through their animal health information system that rinderpest had been detected in a consignment of cattle on board a ship off Dubai in the Gulf after jettisoned carcasses were washed ashore at Dubai; these cattle were reported to have been loaded in southern Somalia. The ship attempted to dock at Kuwait but entry to all GCC states was blocked and the fate of what was left of the cattle consignment is not recorded.

It is clear that elimination of rinderpest from India in 1995 and progressive reduction of the weight of infection in Pakistan from 1995 onwards was an important factor in reducing the risk of rinderpest virus transmission by livestock trade to the Middle East and that eradication of the Iraqi reservoirs between 1994 and 1996 eliminated the risk of rinderpest resurgence within the 'Kurdish Triangle' of Iraq, Turkey and Iran.

# The control of rinderpest in Africa

## North Africa

Egypt appears to have entered the twentieth century free from rinderpest as the three recorded introductions of rinderpest in the previous century (1827, 1841–43 and 1865–66) had all died out. The source of these outbreaks was taken to be Turkey, although bizarrely, Edwards (1949) mentions Nubia (Sudan) as another early source of infection. He also referred to the risk of importation of disease along with cattle entering Upper Egypt from (the then) Anglo-Egyptian Sudan. Although the only contemporary trade between the Sudan and Upper Egypt is of live camels, at an earlier time there was a flourishing trade in cattle. It is accepted however, that an outbreak that started in 1903, had its origins in cattle imported from Asia Minor (the Baghdad region).

Although its entry was anticipated, the mildness of the virus allowed it to elude the sanitary precautions put in place in Alexandria (Littlewood, 1905). On entering the then wholly susceptible Egyptian cattle population the virus apparently reverted to virulence and spread all over the country and was still causing problems in 1912. From that time onwards Egypt was subject to alternating epizootics and periods of apparent freedom from the disease. Surviving Edward's attempt to eradicate it in 1946 by introducing the Vom sub-strain of goat attenuated virus in place of inactivated virus, the last and among the most severe of these epizootics was recorded between 1982 and 1986 (Dr Mustafa Osman Ramadan, personal communication), when over 11 000 cattle died. The origins of this outbreak could not be back-traced to an external source although various authors have attributed its occurrence to spread of the virus from Sudan at the time of the early 1980s panzootic. If we assume that the highly virulent Nigerian lineage 1 isolate of 1983 was typical of the virus which was circulating in eastern Africa at that time, in comparison with a virus isolated in Egypt in 1984, the two have radically different virulence profiles suggesting that the Egyptian and Nigerian strains had possibly been separated for a number of years. Equally, there is no contemporary account of the spread of rinderpest from Sudan into Egypt. On this occasion, phylogenetic analysis does not help to resolve the issue as the Egypt 1984 virus, identified as belonging to African lineage 1, is closely related to other representatives of this clade such as the Nigeria 1983 virus and an isolate obtained from Sudan in 1993. Actually, the Egyptian isolate appears to contain sub-populations of virus capable of causing either mild or severe clinical disease in cattle, and as such to offer both a connection with, and explanation of, the alternating waves of rinderpest afflicting Egypt after 1903. In fact the presence of such a long-standing cryptic-to-virulent-to-cryptic endemic focus of rinderpest in Egypt might not have been detected had the virus not been introduced into feedlot cattle under conditions of stress which lowered their innate resistance. Fortunately, once detected, Egypt was freed of infection by comprehensive vaccination.

The rest of North Africa has never recorded the presence of rinderpest except for Libya, which suffered an outbreak in 1966; the circumstances are unclear but a virus was isolated as referred to by Singh and Ata (1967).

## Sub-Saharan Africa

After its introduction into eastern Africa in the late nineteenth century, rinderpest moved down the eastern seaboard of Africa in the form of a disease of grazing animals both domestic and wild, reaching the Transvaal before the end of the nineteenth century but never penetrated the dense forests on the western side. Madagascar stayed free but rinderpest raged in Reunion between 1900 and 1902 and the disease even gained entry to one of the Comoros Islands in 1901.

When the first Great Rinderpest Panzootic died down it left behind pockets of infection from which background arose periodic epizootics and panzootics, a pattern which continued until the last years of the century. Curasson (1936) gives an interesting account of the behaviour of rinderpest in Africa in the early years of the century, describing the occurrence of repeated epizootics and alarms. For example, he indicates that only sporadic foci existed up to 1912 in West Africa but in the following year 'French Equatorial Africa' (modern-day Chad, Central African Republic, Congo Republic and Gabon) was invaded from 'Soudan' (Curasson was probably referring to the area then known as French Soudan centred on Mali rather than the then Anglo-Egyptian Sudan) and spread widely. In 1915 Niger was infected from Chad via Nigeria and in 1917 infection was again widespread in the Central African Republic and Chad having again come from 'Soudan'. By 1918 rinderpest was rampant throughout all the colonies of West Africa, causing mortality of cattle amounting to many hundreds of thousands of cattle annually and seriously reducing wild animal populations. In 1918 rinderpest spread southwards once again into what is now Zambia, causing great alarm at the prospect of re-establishing infection in South Africa. This pattern was repeated many times from then on; for example in 1939 the virus spread was halted only 60 km from the Tanganyika/Northern Rhodesia (now Tanzania/Zambia) border (Swan, 1973) and in 1951–53 there was extensive infection in southern Tanzania. Veterinary Departments in East Africa and further south repeatedly collaborated to construct immunization belts and fences to prevent a more southerly invasion (Macauley, 1973).

At the turn of the nineteenth century, Abyssinia (now Ethiopia and Eritrea) still harboured rinderpest and with the return of public security in Sudan by the British reconquest of the country and resumption of local trade across the border, rinderpest became a real threat to Sudanese livestock which had escaped infection. Trade to Egypt from Sudan, established in 1904 and reaching 37 000 cattle transported by land and sea in the year of 1918, was continually disrupted by outbreaks. Although eliminated periodically from certain areas the disease was still endemic in 1961 (Jack, 1961).

In Kenya, during the First World War, rinderpest was diagnosed in giraffes (*Giraffa camelopardalis*), African buffaloes (*Syncerus caffer*), elands (*Taurotragus oryx*), reed buck (*Redunca redunca*) and bush buck (*Tragelaphus scriptus*) at a time when the Masai herders were deliberately introducing rinderpest into their nomadic herds to immunize them; subsequently widespread outbreaks were reported in wildlife in 1934 (Macauley, 1973).

Kenya, Ethiopia, Eritrea and Sudan were clearly continuously affected, periodically and repeatedly seeding rinderpest virus infection into Uganda, Tanzania and what is now Rwanda and Burundi, with a notable epizootic occurring in 1920 and persisting in overt form until 1926 on the Kenya/Uganda border. Belgian East Africa (now Rwanda and Burundi) was affected in 1928 (Curasson, 1936). This pattern of disease occurrence continued, but by the early 1940s rinderpest rarely moved south of the Tanzanian Central Railway

Line – a line that came to assume talismanic status in the fight against rinderpest in eastern Africa. After extensive vaccination programmes, the Tanzanian veterinary authorities eventually confined rinderpest to the north of the country in a small area around Loliondo, to the north of Ngorongoro, where the last small outbreaks occurred in 1965 and 1966 (Taylor and Watson, 1967; Macadam, 1968). Thereafter Tanzania enjoyed some 14 years of freedom from the infection. Sadly this situation ended in 1982 when rinderpest was diagnosed in buffaloes in the north of the Serengeti National Park. At the time the origin of this outbreak was not satisfactorily back-traced. For a while the situation in Tanzania was extremely serious as it was found that the virus was in fact extensively distributed across the north of the country, at first in wildlife and later in cattle. After apparent rinderpest freedom of more than a decade rinderpest had re-emerged in the north-east of Uganda in 1979, rapidly spreading widely throughout the country, probably entering western Kenya in 1980 (Rossiter et al., 1983). This epizootic left in its wake a reservoir of infection, related to that in southern Sudan, which persisted in Karamoja for more than a decade until at least 1994. From there rinderpest regularly entered western Kenya (West Pokot) throughout the 1980s to the mid-1990s by trade and raiding of cattle.

Fortunately emergency vaccination campaigns undertaken in 1983 restored the Tanzanian status to one of freedom from the disease. For another 14 years this status prevailed but in 1997 northern Tanzania was again infected with rinderpest. On the latter occasion, however, it is possible to link the reappearance in Tanzania in 1997 with the reappearance in Kenya in 1994. The 1982–83 outbreak in cattle was finally halted by the application of three million doses of rinderpest vaccine in an emergency campaign facilitated by FAO. Thereafter, the EU supported nation-wide mass vaccination campaigns aimed at ensuring the eradication of the virus by the creation of a highly immune cattle population. These campaigns were undertaken in 1985, 1986 and 1987, in the course of which 23 million doses of vaccine were administered. In 1987, Tanzania became a member of the PARC project and reverted to the earlier strategy of maintaining a belt of immunized cattle in the districts along the border with Kenya. Throughout this period there were no further clinical reports of rinderpest in either domestic cattle or in ultra-susceptible wildlife species. Tanzania had apparently again become rinderpest free although this status was never subjected to the rigorous international scrutiny such a claim would nowadays require. The 1997 epizootic was again eliminated by intensive vaccination (Taylor et al., 2002b).

Somalia suffered a severe outbreak in 1928 but rinderpest was brought under a degree of control by 1930, although it was constantly re-introduced from Abyssinia (now Ethiopia) thereafter. From 1939 to 1953 there was no effective control and at that time it was considered to be widespread (Peck, 1973). The record of rinderpest in Somalia is particularly meagre but Macfarlane (1970) records that there were 25 outbreaks in Benadir region (around Mogadishu) in 1969/70. The last cases of classical rinderpest are often stated to have occurred in 1974 or 1983, when a large outbreak occurred in the south; at that time it was also detected in cattle shipped to Oman, as reported by the OIE (1983a, b). There is also clear evidence for periodic episodes of classical acute rinderpest west of the Juba River peaking in 1981, 1987, 1991–93 and 1996 (Mariner and Roeder, 2003).

## The second African panzootic

In hindsight, it is easy to see that the residual reservoirs of infection left in the Senegal River basin and in the Greater Horn of Africa would be the source of rinderpest resurgence once disease control efforts waned with the phasing-out of donor support. Serendipity dictated that this should be occurring at the same time as Nigeria's economic strength was creating a high demand for beef. Demand was met by cattle traders supplying from as far away as the Sudan and Ethiopia, and Mauritania. The inevitable re-invasion of the countries freed over the previous decades constituted the second Great African Rinderpest Panzootic of the late 1970s and early 1980s, when rinderpest from east and west converged on Nigeria. Weak disease reporting systems led to a serious under-reporting of rinderpest outbreaks and the emerging problem was not recognized until the panzootic was already well established. The livelihoods of livestock herders was devastated and, facing the loss of their herds and destitution, many Fulani herders committed suicide.

The scene had been set ten years previously in post-JP15 complacency for the convergence in the early 1980s of two rinderpest epizootics in Nigeria. One came from the west, where a retrospective study *inter alia* by Woodford (1984), together with country studies conducted in preparation for the Pan-African Rinderpest Campaign, clearly documents the covert (essentially unreported), widespread circulation of rinderpest derived from the Mauritania/Mali persisting reservoir of infection which was not eliminated until addressed by the Pan African Rinderpest Campaign in the late 1980s. Internal reports of the Malian veterinary services indicated the continuous presence of rinderpest there from 1968 to 1986. The virus responsible for this persisting reservoir and extensions from it, as typified by a virus which entered western Nigeria in 1980 (Shantikhumar and Atilola, 1990), belonged to African lineage 2.

In 1975, as JP15 phased out, and at a time that Ethiopia was generally considered to have been cleared of rinderpest, reports of giraffe (*Giraffa camelopardalis*) and lesser kudu (*Tragelaphus imberbis*) mortality in southern Ethiopia presaged the later emergence of typical rinderpest in the cattle populations of the Rift Valley and neighbouring Arssi southern highlands of Ethiopia. Initiating control of the developing epidemic was hampered for some months by misdiagnosis as 'pasteurellosis'. Subsequently, despite concerted efforts to control the disease it spread slowly but progressively northwards along the Rift Valley and around the central massif of the Ethiopian Highlands. It entered the Afar pastoralist area in 1976 and spread westwards to cross into Sudan in about 1978.

Somewhat surprisingly, characterization of rinderpest viruses obtained from eastern Ethiopia in 1994 and 1995 identified them as belonging to African lineage 1 (Dr Abraham Gopilo and Prof. Tom Barrett, personal communication) rather than African lineage 2, which might have been expected if the virus there had had its origin in the Somali pastoral ecosystem as the observations suggest. Sadly no viruses have survived from the Ethiopian outbreaks in the 1970s. However, the finding is compatible with unpublished reports of rinderpest virus from Sudan sweeping around the northern end of the highland massif to enter Afar region in the 1980s. Once in Sudan, from 1978 the virus of Ethiopian origin seems to have joined forces with a resurgence of rinderpest from the south of Sudan and it is impossible to tell whether one or other virus dominated in subsequent events. What is certain, however, is that virus from Sudan moved steadily across central Africa and on into West Africa, entering into the east of Nigeria in 1992, and it belonged to African lineage 1.

Together the epizootics originating from east and west summated to become the Second African Rinderpest Panzootic which was a cause of great concern for the international community as well as the livestock owners of affected countries. FAO provided assistance for many affected countries and worked with the Organization of African Unity and donors to organize a fresh campaign. By 1987 when PARC began operations with EU funding, rinderpest distribution had again been reduced greatly. In West Africa, rinderpest was last seen on the border between Ghana and Burkina Faso in 1988. PARC was replaced in 1999 by a third internationally coordinated programme – the PACE Programme which retained as an objective, but did not prioritize, the final eradication of rinderpest from the continent.

## The demise of African lineage 1 rinderpest virus

From the limited historical material still available it appears that African rinderpest virus lineage 1 has generally been confined to eastern Africa with a distribution stretching from Egypt through Sudan to Ethiopia, Kenya and Uganda. The only evidence of a change in this distribution occurred in the early 1980s when it crossed from Sudan to eastern Nigeria as part of the rinderpest panzootic that engulfed the whole of sub-Saharan Africa at that time. However, by 1995 African lineage 1 rinderpest virus maintenance was limited to Ethiopia and Sudan.

In Ethiopia concerted investigations from 1989 to 1992 established that reservoirs of infection were to be found in the Afar pastoral area of lowland eastern Ethiopia and in an area west of Lake Tana in western Ethiopia. The latter focus had earlier extended to the Dinder National Park in Sudan which abuts the Ethiopian border and where rinderpest was present until at least 1972 (Ali, 1974). Another focus might have persisted until as late as 1993 in the south of Ethiopia in the lowland area between the highland massif and the Somali border (Gijs van't Klooster, personal communication) and this could have been the source of the epizootic experienced from 1995. Later, it became clear that repeated outbreaks in and around the Rift Valley of Central Ethiopia and the southern highland massif arose from two sources: the first was via a linkage with the Afar reservoir whereby virus was transferred by exchange of draft oxen and heifers – characterized as African lineage 1 for viruses of 1994 and 1995. The second source for this area arose from occasional introduction from the pastoral areas of southern Sudan into trade routes moving cattle towards central Ethiopia – characterized as African lineage 1 for a 1993 virus. Rinderpest from west of Lake Tana was moved eastwards repeatedly when seasonal cattle migrations brought cattle into the contiguous western highland areas to graze on the aftermath of crop production. On the other side of Ethiopia, rinderpest regularly crossed the highland/lowland interface into the highland massif to the east as draft oxen were sold through markets to highland farmers. Not surprisingly these outbreaks tended to be initiated towards the end of the year after harvest when farmers had available cash. These rinderpest introductions into the highlands resulted in epizootics which advanced slowly spreading progressively through the highland areas, as occurred in 1992 when rinderpest spread from market to market for some months after introduction from the Afar reservoir.

Once this pattern of rinderpest enzootic persistence and extension of epizootics from the reservoirs was established this understanding could be used as a basis for developing an eradication strategy. A strong team of veterinarians working with PARC, which included, *inter alia*, Drs Gijs van't Klooster, Wondwossen Asfaw, Berhanu Admassu and Berhanu Bedane, pioneered this work. Setting aside country-wide mass vaccination as unnecessary and anyway unachievable, the new approach sought to contain rinderpest virus within the reservoirs and focus vaccination on eliminating infection from the reservoirs, establishing minimal vaccination buffer zones to protect especially vulnerable areas and strengthening surveillance and emergency preparedness in the event of infection escaping. Attempting to provide nation-wide vaccination coverage would have required the annual vaccination of some 30 million cattle. This had been attempted for many years but had never achieved more than one-third of this figure. The new strategy required vaccination of less than three million cattle per year. Key to it was the fielding of community-based animal health workers to work in insecure areas of difficult access and the use of a thermostable formulation of rinderpest vaccine to achieve high herd immunity rates (Mariner, 1996). After a major struggle for acceptance the strategy was implemented from 1993 and rapidly proved successful even if it was not without its challenges. An epizootic started by cattle from the Afar focus began in eastern Ethiopia in 1994 and provided a severe test of the strategy. Initially apparently controlled successfully by movement restriction, including market closure enforced by the army, combined with focal vaccination, the disease crossed to the western side of the highlands by illicit trade movements and even moved north to Asmara in Eritrea. In all there were some fifty outbreaks before the status quo was restored.

Resumption of mass vaccination was narrowly avoided; by the end of 1995 rinderpest had been eliminated and has not returned. The last incidents of rinderpest were reported in 1995 in Temenjayaze, Bench Zone of the Southern Nations Nationalities and Peoples Regional State in the west of Ethiopia (originating in southern Sudan) and in November 1995 in Mehoni, Southern Zone of Tigray Regional State of north-eastern Ethiopia, being the last remnant of the Afar reservoir.

The final stage in the demise of African lineage 1 rinderpest virus by elimination from its last stronghold in southern Sudan can be seen to date from 2001. For more than a decade rinderpest had essentially been contained within the extensive pastoral communities of southern Sudan. Classical severe rinderpest of African lineage 1 had last been confirmed in 1998 by the FAO World Reference Laboratory for Rinderpest[1] from samples collected in the extreme south of Sudan. These originated from an outbreak in sedentary cattle belonging to a community of agro-pastoralists living in Torit County of Eastern Equatoria Region, to where it was probably introduced with cattle traded from the neighbouring Toposa tribe. Formerly a constant and serious threat to the livelihoods of the southern Sudanese pastoralists and feared by cattle owners throughout the country to the north, rinderpest was progressively brought under control. This was achieved by an animal health programme which combined conventional veterinary services with innovative community-based approaches to animal health service delivery in remote areas marginalized from conventional services (Leyland, 1996; Mariner 1996). The coordinated approach through the United Nations Operation Lifeline Sudan (OLS) Livestock Programme with the involvement of many non-governmental organizations was so successful that progressively from the early 1990s many of the formerly severely affected pastoral communities were freed from the disease. By 2000, the government of Sudan's intensive surveillance, assisted by the OLS Livestock Programme, the African Union's Interafrican Bureau Animal Resources (AU-IBAR), through PARC and the PACE programme, and GREP, through FAO's Technical Cooperation Programme, had confirmed that suspicions of the persistence of rinderpest infection were limited to very few areas in the extreme south-east of the country.

Towards the end of 2000, persisting into 2001, reports started to be received of mortality in the cattle herded by the Murle nomadic pastoralists in the vicinity of Gumuruk in Pibor County of Jongeli State, Upper Nile Region in southern Sudan. Timely investigations were difficult to mount but despite the remoteness and insecurity of the affected area Sudanese government veterinarians supported by the FAO OLS Livestock Programme eventually reached the affected area where it was estimated that approximately 200 cattle had died. However, it was not possible to access actively infected herds and laboratory

---

[1] WRL-RP hosted by the Institute for Animal Health, Pirbright Laboratory, UK.

confirmation of rinderpest was not achieved; serological investigations were compromised by the start of emergency rinderpest vaccination. In total the Murle and closely associated Jie communities herded some 800 000 cattle with 700 000 of these belonging to the Murle. These were essentially unvaccinated populations. At that time, unlike in earlier years, there was neither evidence nor even suspicion that rinderpest was occurring in the cattle herds of any of the other major livestock-dependent ethnic groups (Dinka, Nuer, Anuak, Toposa etc.) in southern Sudan. Nor was there any real cause for suspicion elsewhere in the country further north, although it must be admitted that there were several areas in the south where the disease situation was essentially unknown because access was denied by severe civil insecurity, for example the Sobat Basin. Earlier studies in 2000 and 2001 assisted by FAO's Technical Cooperation Programme had confirmed the absence of rinderpest disease in recent years in cattle herds resident in the central sector of the country, or undertaking annual, seasonal migrations into and from the southern zone. Combined with other ongoing disease intelligence-gathering led by the NGO Vétérinaires sans Frontières (VSF) Belgium, responsible for implementing the PACE Sudan (south) project entitled '*The fight against African Lineage 1 Rinderpest*', an educated guess was that the cattle herds of the Murle and, possibly, Jie communities were the last harbouring the virus in Sudan (Figure 6.2).

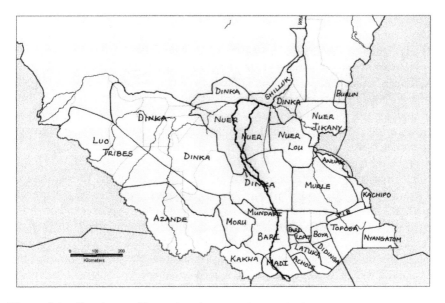

**Figure 6.2** Sketch map illustrating the approximate distribution of ethnic groups in southern Sudan used for planning at the time of the outbreak [by courtesy of Dr Bryony Jones, VSF Belgium and AU IBAR PACE].

It was considered pragmatic to act on this assumption and an intensive, focused vaccination programme was initiated by the government of Sudan under the field leadership of Dr Jacob Korok, the District Veterinary Officer, and his staff based in Pibor, who had detected the problem originally. The campaign was assisted by FAO, which had recently assumed operational responsibility for the OLS Livestock Programme, with funding from the European Commission Humanitarian Organization and the US Office for Foreign Disaster Assistance (OFDA). This was highly successful, receiving enthusiastic compliance by the livestock herders who had been seeking rinderpest vaccination. Approximately 650 000 cattle were vaccinated with quality-assured thermostable rinderpest vaccine, mainly between March and December 2001 but extending until June 2002, in the livestock populations considered to be at highest risk of rinderpest maintenance (i.e. those belonging to the Murle and Jie peoples) with another 120 000 cattle of the adjacent Toposa people being vaccinated because of their close interaction with the Jie. This was achieved by conventional and community-based animal health workers despite an ongoing civil war and the rainy season (June to October) which floods extensive areas of land annually, creating severe difficulties for access and mobility. All rinderpest vaccination had already ceased outside the extreme south-east of Sudan west of the Nile River by December 2001 and vaccination ceased everywhere in June 2002. At this time all rinderpest vaccine was withdrawn from the field and all unissued stocks were sequestered in vaccine banks in Khartoum and Lokkichoggio (in Kenya) for the northern and southern sectors respectively.

Fortunately the hypothesis that rinderpest was not present elsewhere in the ecosystem proved to be correct. Investigations in late 2001 and 2002, led by Dr Bryony Jones of PACE Sudan (south) and Dr Jeffrey Mariner for the IBAR CAPE (Community Animal Health and Participatory Epidemiology) Unit of PACE, confirmed that pastoralists in Pibor County had indeed experienced outbreaks of a cattle disease variously known as *batiboy* and *achoke*, names used for rinderpest which disease they know well. Since that time rinderpest surveillance has been strengthened considerably, using all available techniques and sometimes seizing fleeting ceasefire opportunities to access areas such as the Nuba mountains and the Sobat Basin, usually inaccessible.

The final thrust for the elimination of rinderpest from this ecosystem had taken off from a sound platform of earlier progressive rinderpest control together with demographic and disease information built up over the previous decade by NGOs working under the OLS coordination umbrella. Coordination was supported administratively and financially by UNICEF with OFDA and technically by Tufts University (Leyland, 1996). This programme had seen the geographic extent and incidence of rinderpest fall progressively to the point where a final eradication effort was feasible. Key to the latter stages of rinderpest eradication was the '*The fight against African Lineage 1 Rinderpest*' project implemented by VSF Belgium within the EU-funded PACE programme, coordinated closely with the work of FAO OLS staff in both northern and southern sectors. In addition to providing clinical services to marginalized and war-torn pastoral communities the coordinated activities maintain, *inter alia*, a disease information system capable of detecting rinderpest and reporting epidemiologically significant events requiring refutation as rinderpest suspicions. For example, in 2002, 2003 and the first five months of 2004 approximately 99, 101 and 22[2] respectively, epidemiologically significant disease events were reported of which 24, 21 and 5 respectively specifically raised a suspicion of rinderpest. Subsequently follow-up participatory disease surveillance (PDS) (Catley, 1997) by northern and southern sectors of PACE Sudan, combined with investigation of epidemiologically significant events raising suspicions of rinderpest, have uniformly failed to detect any evidence of rinderpest. In many cases outbreaks could be dismissed as not being rinderpest on clinical and epidemiological appearance, others were confirmed as being caused by a range of enzootic diseases including foot-and-mouth disease, trypanosomiasis, contagious bovine pleuropneumonia and theileriosis; in 2004 one particularly alarming report of mortality of more than 50 cattle was confirmed by the WRL-RP to be malignant catarrhal fever by PCR. None of the investigations detected rinderpest nor has there been any reason to suspect the persistence of rinderpest virus in this ecosystem which extends into the south-west lowland areas of Ethiopia, north-east Uganda and north-west Kenya. Increasingly supported by PDS programmes that record a past history of rinderpest up to 2001, but not subsequently, and complementing the disease reporting and investigation system operated by the governments of Sudan, Ethiopia, Uganda and Kenya, this progressively gives confidence that the reservoir of infection no longer exists.

## African lineage 2 rinderpest virus

The evidence suggests that African rinderpest virus lineage 2 was much more broadly distributed than lineage 1, taking in both western and eastern Africa (it was isolated in Nigeria in 1958 and in Kenya in 1962). When rinderpest re-emerged in West Africa in the early 1980s the virus that spread eastwards from Mauritania/Mali (where it had been persisting for many years) to western Nigeria belonged to African lineage 2. At that time it appeared as if West Africa was the only source of this lineage. However, we now know that in fact its distribution had not altered. All that had changed was that the virulence of the East African representative of lineage 2 had became so low as to make it clinically difficult to detect, allowing it to escape detection for more than 30 years.

A severe outbreak of rinderpest occurred in 1994 and 1995 in the kudu and buffalo populations of Tsavo National Park in southern Kenya (Barrett *et al.*, 1998;

---

[2] Reports peak during the rainy season from June onwards accounting for the low rate early in the year.

Kock *et al.*, 1999). A similar event occurred one year later in neighbouring Nairobi and Amboseli National Parks. Serological and epidemiological evidence indicates infection also in Meru National Park and in some wildlife populations outside the national parks in the east of Kenya. In the Tsavo outbreak the virus exhibited a high level of virulence in buffaloes and kudus; in the Nairobi outbreak buffaloes and eland were similarly affected with mild disease in calves. When isolates were examined by nucleotide sequencing they were shown to belong to African lineage 2, which was surprising because no representative of lineage 2 had been unearthed in eastern Africa since 1962. Furthermore, while it was now recognized that at an earlier date lineage 2 had been distributed across the continent, the last time its presence was detected was in Sokoto, Nigeria, in the early 1980s. Thus the unexpected reappearance of this lineage virus in Kenya in 1994 could not be explained in terms of spread from another well-known focus.

Although representatives of lineage 2 were isolated in central Kenya in 1958 and in northern Tanzania and north-eastern Kenya in 1962 the records of the Kenyan and Tanzanian Veterinary Services appear to show the demise of rinderpest in the Masai ecosystem of these two countries around 1966 even though rinderpest persisted further to the north (Atang and Plowright, 1969). The historical description of rinderpest in northern Tanzania is one of its shrinking distribution and fluctuating virulence and suggests that the northern Tanzanian focus from which a number of mild strains were isolated in 1962 was a relict population derived from the enzootic situation that had existed in East Africa for over 60 years. From the 1930s, outbreaks associated with a low level of field virulence were consistently observed within this enzootic area. Perhaps then, the low virulence RBT strains from Tanzanian cattle in 1962 represented viruses that had been selected for their long-term survivability under East African conditions.

In Tanzania it seems that rinderpest was capable of making a silent entry into cattle herds, apparently due to the low virulence of the infecting virus, and although this virulence gradually increased to the point of producing classic disease signs, this only occurred after the herd had been infected for 3–6 weeks. The virus was capable of transmitting to new herds in its virulent form. On at least one occasion no such increase of virulence for cattle was observed. There is also evidence that the avirulent variant was in fact virulent for game animals, which accords with the field contention that these animals were responsible for the introduction of (mild) rinderpest into uninfected herds of cattle (Robson *et al.*, 1959; Branagan and Hammond, 1965).

It has been demonstrated that the two best characterized lineage 2 viruses isolated in East Africa in 1962 have completely differing clinical effects (i.e. virulence profiles) in cattle. The Kenyan virus, RGK/1, isolated from a sick giraffe near Garissa in northern Kenya, has a high level of virulence for cattle, causing severe clinical signs and the death of 60–70% of experimental cases. It has retained this characteristic on passage in cattle and cell culture for many years. By contrast, its contemporaries from northern Tanzania and southern Kenya (of which the RBT/1 and /2 strains are the only surviving representatives) were very mild in their effects on village cattle. Under controlled laboratory conditions a number of RBT/1 infected animals failed to develop mouth lesions and could not have been clinically diagnosed as rinderpest, even by experienced observers.

When strain RBT/1 was inoculated into cattle at low dilutions the virus was virulent but when high dilutions were used it was avirulent. This has been taken to suggest the possible presence of at least two variants in the stock preparation. It was not possible to increase the virulence of another RBT/1-like virus (obtained from a sick buffalo) by back-passaging it in cattle; it remained mild in cattle.

It seems that an RBT/1-like virus could easily persist in a bovine population within a cryptic focus. Northern Tanzania supplies us evidence that such persistence did in fact happen and that an unsuspected rinderpest focus persisted in the Sonjo valley of Loliondo District, northern Tanzania from 1961 to 1965. Even after its discovery in 1965 the virus managed to remain at large until 1966. Further, evidence is recorded compatible with a residual rinderpest infection in the buffalo (1964–67) and warthog (1964–68) populations of the Serengeti National Park – this pocket of infection was not recorded clinically in cattle in the area. Disease and infection subsequently died out in the buffaloes.

After 1968 rinderpest was not recognized in East Africa until 1980 when it seems to have entered northern Tanzania from Kenya. Unfortunately the virus involved was never isolated or typed and it is not possible to draw any firm conclusions about the lineage designation. The virus appeared to possess a high level of virulence for both cattle and game animal species. It ultimately spread throughout the cattle of the Masai ecosystem of northern Tanzania and also involved the buffalo populations of Tarangire and Serengeti National Parks and the Ngorongoro Conservation Area. The outbreak lasted from 1980 to 1982; there is little evidence that the virulence of the virus changed during the course of the outbreak except that at the end, after the virus had entered the buffalo population of the Serengeti National Park, it appeared to decline in virulence and finally died out. Thereafter, there were no recorded outbreaks of rinderpest in either Kenya or Tanzania until the Tsavo outbreak of 1994. The fact that this virus belonged to lineage 2, implied persistence of a cryptic rinderpest focus over a period of nearly 30 years. The mild form of rinderpest that had persisted in Loliondo District up to 1965/66, was in fact, therefore, probably more widely dispersed than had been suspected and had persisted from that time within eastern Africa.

The bovine virulence of the re-isolated representative of lineage 2 (Nairobi Eland 1996) is not dissimilar to that of one of the RBT/1-like suite of viruses which was virulent for buffaloes but mild for cattle. This lack of cattle pathogenicity would account for the apparent ability of the virus to move between Tsavo and Nairobi National Parks, presumably by transmission among cattle, ostensibly without disclosing its presence. In experimental studies carried out by the WRL-RP, of 10 cattle experimentally infected with the Kenya/Eland/96 strain, two showed no clinical signs of disease yet seroconverted, three had pyrexia, three developed mild transient oral erosions and two died with classical acute rinderpest (Drs Euan and John Anderson, personal communication). Clinical observations during the related outbreak in the field in northern Tanzania and Kenya in early 1997 mirrored the experimental evidence. Against a background of mild to subclinical disease typical severe rinderpest was observed in a small number of herds. Similarly, clinical rinderpest was also seen in cattle in southern Kenya at the time, as it had been at the time of the outbreak in Nairobi National Park in 1996 (Rossiter, 2001). Serological evidence clearly provides evidence that infection was much more widespread than clinical disease recognizable as rinderpest, at least in northern Tanzania. Although again, unfortunately, the lineage of the infecting virus was not determined, this suggests that under an appropriate selection pressure this seemingly mild virus population could recover its lethal potential.

The detection of atypical mild rinderpest in northern Kenya in 1996, linked epidemiologically to reports of similar disease in southern Somalia, gives some clue as to the most recent location of lineage 2 virus (Mariner and Roeder, 2003). Clinical disease was seen only in calves about 4–12 months of age during a drought; even then the disease was mild and mortality was low. Somali veterinarians describe experiencing a problem for many years of 'bovine viral diarrhoea' in young cattle but their reports do not conform to the known epidemiology of that disease. This and other anecdotal reports concerning the period from the 1970s to the 1980s by expatriate veterinarians of infectious bovine rhinotracheitis and other signs suggestive of mild rinderpest in southern Somalia could well indicate the persistence of enzootic mild rinderpest.

## The enigma of mild rinderpest

When rinderpest virus of African lineage 2 was recognized as the cause of an epizootic in buffaloes in Tsavo National Park of Kenya in 1994, it was at first suspected that the source of the infection had been Sudan. This was logically correct because southern Sudan was known to constitute a reservoir of African lineage 1 rinderpest and the virus had repeatedly entered the Turkana region of Kenya from southern Sudan in the 1980s and 1990s. However, once virus characterization results were made available by the World Reference Laboratory for Rinderpest, identifying the virus as belonging to African lineage 2, it was clear that the source had to be sought elsewhere. There were many reasons to suggest that the Somali ecosystem (essentially an area west of the Juba River and spanning the Kenya/Somalia border) could at that time have constituted a reservoir of rinderpest virus infection and studies conducted in 1996 added weight to this belief (Mariner and Roeder, 2003). In this context it is of relevance to note the statement made by Plowright (1982) that 'rinderpest virus periodically invades Kenya and Uganda from the north and it is not difficult to imagine how infection could spread across the Tana and Galana Rivers down the coast and into the Tsavo, Amboseli or Kajiado Districts'; and, one could add, even further into northern Tanzania as occurred in 1980 and 1996/7. The results of extensive sero-surveillance studies conducted under the PACE Somalia programme in central and southern Somalia in 2001–03 purport to demonstrate the continuing presence of rinderpest there; unfortunately the results have not been made available for study. Working in Somalia, and especially southern Somalia, has been problematic for more than a decade. The team involved, led by Dr Stefano Tempia, also conducted surveys for clinical disease and were able to detect a syndrome compatible with mild rinderpest. Outbreaks of rinderpest in wildlife (primarily buffaloes) had been repeatedly observed in Kenya prior to and after the Tsavo epizootic and in 2003 the Kenyan epizootiologist Dr Dickens Chibeu detected foci of mild rinderpest-compatible disease outbreaks. Despite the clinical findings and to an extent suggestive serology where not compromised by ongoing sporadic vaccination, it has not proved possible to link the 'mild-rinderpest' syndrome detected in the field with rinderpest virus infection by laboratory examination. Most recently in 2004, an incident caused alarm in southern Ethiopia, reliably free from rinderpest for more than 25 years. Acting on information provided by the Kenyan Veterinary Department that a 'mild rinderpest' compatible syndrome had been detected in northern Kenya close to the junction of the borders of Kenya, Ethiopia and Somalia, the Ethiopian Veterinary Team undertook a PDS investigation in contiguous areas of Ethiopia. A similar syndrome was detected in a small area in Ethiopia. Intensive laboratory investigations for virus and antibody backed up by the World Reference Laboratory for Rinderpest provided evidence that the syndrome observed had not been caused by rinderpest. Also confounding understanding is the fact that PCR products and some tissue extracts submitted to the World Reference Laboratory for Rinderpest from the East African Regional Rinderpest Reference Laboratory at the Kenya Agricultural Research Institute (KARI) Muguga Laboratory, Kenya, contained RNA which when sequenced indicated that the virus was identical to the Kabete O vaccine/standard challenge strain. Normally one would dismiss this as evidence of laboratory contamination but for the fact that on several other occasions investigations in East Africa have given the same result – one being from clinical rinderpest in Tanzania in 1997. It is difficult to conceive how, other than by escape from laboratories or reversion to virulence of vaccine, but could rinderpest virus belonging to this ancient clade really be circulating today in Africa?

Rinderpest virus (African lineage 2) was last detected in tissues sent to the World Reference Laboratory for Rinderpest from buffaloes in Meru National Park in Kenya in 2001. All subsequent investigations of suspicious events in Kenya have not confirmed the presence of rinderpest virus. What causes the 'mild rinderpest-compatible syndrome' which has been detected repeatedly in Kenya and Somalia and recently in Ethiopia? If it is rinderpest, why do laboratory examinations which have proved so effective elsewhere fail to give the desired result? Hence the enigma against which background future events and proposed actions in eastern Africa need to be assessed. Whether or not African lineage 2 rinderpest virus is actually still extant needs to be determined urgently before implementing any more mass vaccination programmes. Could rinderpest actually have been eradicated already? One dares not believe so until proof is forthcoming and only sound and effectively executed investigations will resolve the enigma.

The determinants of the re-appearance of African lineage 2 rinderpest virus and its maintenance in East Africa have not yet been defined nor has its relationship to what is ostensibly a syndrome of mild rinderpest in cattle been established despite the excellent wildlife surveillance work conducted in eastern Africa under the auspices of PARC and PACE (see Chapter 7). Debate continues, much of it uninformed by an understanding of what has gone before. There is a strong tendency to equate mild rinderpest with African lineage 2 rinderpest, and to associate this with rinderpest maintenance in wildlife in East Africa. However, mild rinderpest has not been limited to East Africa or even to Africa; lineage 2 rinderpest virus has not been restricted to East Africa; mild rinderpest has not been restricted to East Africa; mild rinderpest does not relate only to the African lineage 2 rinderpest virus. Despite this, the assumptions are used to make pessimistic predictions about the feasibility of rinderpest eradication.

One widely held tenet of belief concerning African lineage 2 rinderpest virus in East Africa is that it is uniformly virulent for wildlife whilst being mild for cattle. However, there are numerous indications from earlier years that such viruses are not always uniformly virulent for wildlife (see for example Plowright, 1963; Branagan and Hammond, 1965) and a strain belonging to this clade but highly virulent for cattle was isolated in 1962 from a giraffe in Kenya. There is a suggestion that rinderpest in some wildlife incidents has been less than fully virulent. Robson *et al.* (1959) stated that 'the natural selection in wild game of mutants attenuated for cattle has been postulated but the hypothesis is unsupported by the presented evidence' which he discussed.

When it comes to the dilemma of rinderpest maintenance by wildlife, little progress is evident since Plowright (1963) indicated that 'the arguments crystalised into the expression of two apparently irreconcilable points of view, neither based on sound evidence, much less quantitative data'. One view, the consensus of informed veterinary opinion at the time, was that rinderpest would not be eliminated from cattle because they co-existed with large concentrations of highly susceptible wild animals whereas the other camp supported the view that if rinderpest could be eliminated from cattle it would die out completely in wildlife because it rapidly burnt itself out in the wildlife. Plowright (1963) himself was rather pessimistic at that time about the prospects of eradication. He referred to the importance of large accumulations of highly susceptible wild animal species present in parts of East Africa in which Reid (1949) described 'a reservoir of smouldering rinderpest', although at the same time the latter author indicated that the diseases died out in less dense wildlife communities in Central and Southern Tanganyika (now Tanzania) and also in large areas of Kenya and Uganda. In the current circumstances, based on studies of rinderpest epizootics in wildlife in eastern Africa in the last decade, Kock (see Chapter 7) suggests an upper limit of four years for virus circulation in wildlife, even for lesser kudus over which there is some suspicion of virus maintenance.

Rinderpest was enzootically established from at least the early 1930s in northern Tanzania and was continuously enzootic subsequently, yet immunization campaigns for rinderpest were intensified from the late 1950s onwards and seroconversion in the wild animals of the Serengeti ecosystem reduced progressively from 1959 and was not detected after 1967. This caused Plowright (1982) to conclude that 'by themselves, the large numbers of susceptible game animals in the Serengeti Region in 1962–1963 were not capable of maintaining the strains of virus current at that time'. Apart from incursions from Kenya in the early 1980s and late 1990s Tanzania has stayed free from that time.

Nowhere today are there comparable dense wildlife populations which are now reduced mainly to relict isolated populations, with the exception of the Serengeti/Mara herds which are undoubtedly free from rinderpest. Thus, the situation today has changed and the likelihood that rinderpest could 'smoulder' continuously for many years must be considered very low. However, this is not to say that rinderpest cannot 'burn' through a relatively large wildlife population for an extended period of time as it clearly did in the buffalo and eland herds of the Tsavo National Park in Kenya in 1993–95 acting as a conduit for infection between two widely separated cattle populations.

There exists an interesting similarity of historical accounts of rinderpest in Vietnam and Cambodia in the 1950s and that of rinderpest in East Africa at around the same time and now. Whilst pointing out that there was still much to learn on the subject, Hudson (1960) indicated that rinderpest in South-East Asia affected wild pigs and in diverse species of wild ruminants spread rapidly and died out spontaneously. He also pointed out varying resistance of local cattle and buffalo breeds in South-East and East Asia to rinderpest with those in Cambodia and South Vietnam being particularly resistant. Stoddard (1964) described how epizootics in cattle, buffaloes and pigs were preceded firstly by deaths in wild pigs and then in domestic swine. In some but not all areas bantengs (*Bos (Bibos) javanicus*) and gaur (*Bos (Bibos) frontalis gaurus*) experienced high mortality whereas kouprey (*Novibos sauveli*) were not affected. Stoddard (1964) observed that the virus present at that time was not causing serious damage to the domestic livestock. He did caution, however, that in his understanding the cases of atypical rinderpest in indigenous cattle were caused by a mutant of the virus which is able to transform itself rapidly into typical virulent rinderpest virus and to quickly produce typical bovine rinderpest epizootics; the virus in both forms was reported to be uniformly virulent in water buffaloes.

Of course one has to take into account genetic factors of the host in determining the outcome of virus/host interactions but mild rinderpest has been regularly encountered within and outside Africa and with all three lineages of rinderpest virus. For African lineage 2 the evidence is briefly described above and for African lineage 1 this has been recorded, in Kenya in the mid-1980s (Wamwayi *et al.*, 1992) and in Egypt (*vide infra*). In Egypt mild rinderpest was recognized in the 1980s (*vide infra*), but dated back to the early years of the twentieth century related to cattle from Iraq (notorious as 'Baghdadlis') (Littlewood, 1905). As mentioned elsewhere, incidents of mild rinderpest were a feature of rinderpest in the then 'Indo-China' (now referred to generally as South-East Asia) in the 1950s.

So what can one conclude? As it is unlikely that the East African virus will die out spontaneously in cattle, its hidden presence poses a grave risk for the rest of the continent and eventually the world. Low virulence seems not to be a fixed characteristic and reversion to full virulence is to be expected should movement into suitable susceptible populations occur. Given that its distribution seems not definable on the basis of clinical reporting, planning and implementing the use of vaccination and zoo-sanitary procedures to remove rinderpest from the Somali pastoralist's herds poses a major problem. The issue is one of finding both the will and the means to define its geographic distribution and undertake the concerted action necessary.

Is mildness the result of a chance mutation of a rinderpest virus or is it possible that mildness is an attribute of certain viruses which is induced by selecting strains for dominance from within a quasi-species swarm (Smith *et al.*, 1997) of rinderpest virus within animals in an outbreak situation. The latter would tend to be compatible with field observations that virulence is not a fixed attribute of rinderpest viruses and can evolve in either direction. Pragmatically, the latter assumption has been adopted by GREP. Fortunately, the history of East Africa and South-East Asia in the 1950s and 1960s suggests that the circulation of rinderpest between domesticated livestock and a susceptible wildlife population does not preclude area-wide elimination of the virus.

# Concluding remarks: global eradication by 2010 – a dream or reality?

The first years of the twenty-first century are in sharp contrast with any period during the previous decade or even millennia. Remarkably there has been no re-emergence of rinderpest in any of the countries/regions cleared of rinderpest in the past ten years, indeed all accruing evidence tends to confirm the understanding that both the Asian and African 1 lineages of rinderpest virus have been extinct since 2001. Rinderpest has not been detected in Asia (neither disease nor serological evidence of infection) since cases were found in the year 2000 in the Indus River buffalo tract of Sindh province in Pakistan. Although there is suspicion from participatory epidemiological studies that the last cases might actually have occurred in early 2001 this is really of little significance since subsequent intensive investigations in Pakistan serve only to continue to confirm the absence of infection, not just disease (Martinez *et al.*, 2003). Evidence from Afghanistan confirms that that country has remained free since the 1995 incursion was eradicated in 1997. India continues to confirm that it eliminated rinderpest by eliminating the reservoir of infection in Tamil Nadu, Kerala and Karnataka in the southern peninsula in 1995. South-East Asia and the archipelagic area of East Asia has undoubtedly been free from rinderpest since the late 1950s except for an area of Vietnam where the virus might have persisted until as late as 1977. Elsewhere in Asia, surveillance exercises summate to construct an understanding that the other reservoirs of infection had also been resolved at about that time. There can be little doubt that China, Mongolia and Russia have been free from 'wild' infection for many decades. Enigmatic rinderpest outbreaks in Georgia (1989), Russia/Mongolia (1991) and Amur region of Russia (1998) can almost certainly be ascribed to reversion to virulence of the vaccine used in an attempt to create an immunized buffer zone on the borders of the USSR and later the Russian Federation with neighbouring countries and therefore do not indicate areas of persisting endemicity. The Kurdish triangle (Turkey, Iran and Iraq) experienced its last infection in 1996 and Yemen last detected infection in 1997. Again formal surveillance data tend to confirm rinderpest absence. Accreditation of rinderpest freedom is progressing reasonably well and is gaining pace.

In Africa there is growing confidence that the West and Central African countries have been free from rinderpest since the last cases occurred on the Burkina Faso/Ghana border in 1988. The OIE accreditation process is providing confidence in the fact that West and Central African countries have been free from rinderpest since then. Rinderpest virus of African lineage 1 persisted in Ethiopia until 1995 and in Sudan until 2001. In both countries there is convincing evidence for the absence of virus circulation since then. These were the last strongholds of African lineage 1 rinderpest virus, which has almost certainly joined the Asian lineage in being consigned to history in the wild.

It is only the possible persistence of a supposedly mild form of rinderpest in the Somali pastoral ecosystem of Kenya, Somalia and Ethiopia that prevents one from suspecting that rinderpest has been eradicated from Africa, and the world. There is, however, no cause for complacency for there exists a significant body of experience recording the recent presence in Kenya and Somalia of a disease syndrome in cattle compatible with the concept of 'mild rinderpest' close to the area in which 'mild' rinderpest virus strains were described in the 1950s and 1960s with rediscovery in the 1990s. The last definitive detection of rinderpest virus was in African buffalos (*Syncerus caffer*) adjacent to the Somali pastoral ecosystem in eastern Kenya in 2001. This was unequivocally identified as virus of African lineage 2 by the World Reference Laboratory for Rinderpest. Yet, all subsequent investigations of what could be a mild form of rinderpest in cattle in Kenya and Somalia (and most recently in a contiguous area of southern Ethiopia in 2004) have failed to provide clear evidence of rinderpest virus presence whether by virus detection or serology. Even wildlife serosurveillance, a valuable indicator of rinderpest virus circulation, has suggested that seroconversion of wildlife sentinels is no longer occurring in the high risk area of eastern Kenya (see Chapter 7). The current situation is an enigma and failure to resolve it threatens to compromise the ultimate success of GREP.

Due attention must be given to the involvement of wildlife in virus maintenance highlighting the need for wildlife surveillance to continue at an appropriate level. If indeed rinderpest is still present, as one must assume until proven otherwise, it seems to be able to infect cattle without provoking the clinical syndrome typical of classical rinderpest; it might not be readily detectable clinically. Nothing in the account presented here suggests that the 'wildlife/mild rinderpest' phenomenon encountered in the eastern Africa scenario, if indeed that is what it is, should necessarily compromise eradication provided that due account is taken of previous experience and sound principles of investigation and control are applied.

Encouraging progress in accreditation of rinderpest freedom across most of the territories in which rinderpest used to damage the livelihoods of livestock farmers suggests that finalizing this process will not be a major constraint for GREP once all foci of infection have been eliminated. The major challenge remains timely resolution of the Somali ecosystem enigma and elimination of this last reservoir of infection if it is present. A successful and timely outcome to GREP will not be assured unless all the countries, agencies, organizations and other stakeholders involved re-dedicate themselves to eradicating rinderpest and to a coordinated, transboundary strategy which seeks to resolve the suspicions about rinderpest presence before re-instituting vaccination. Unless a strong and sound coordinating focus is established for eastern Africa a successful outcome will remain in jeopardy.

# References

Ali, B.E.H. (1974) The isolation of rinderpest virus from an oribi and reedbuck in an outbreak involving wild animals. *Sudan J. Vet. Sci. Anim. Husband.* **15**, 1–10.

Anon (1971) Report of Activities of the Government Veterinary Services. *Refuah Veterin.* **28**, 121–7.

Atang, P. and Plowright, W. (1969) Extension of the JP-15 rinderpest control campaign to Eastern Africa: the epizootiological background. *Bull. Epizoot. Dis. Afr.* **17**, 161–70.

Barrett, T., Amarel-Doel, C., Kitching, R.P. and Gusev, A. (1993) Use of the polymerase chain reaction in differentiating rinderpest field virus and vaccine virus in the same animals. *Rev. Sci. Techn. Office Int. Epizooties*, **12**, 865–72.

Barrett, T., Forsyth, M., Inui, K., Wamwayi, H.M., Kock, R., Wambua, J., Mwanzia, J. and Rossiter, P.B (1998) Rediscovery of the second African lineage of rinderpest virus: its epidemiological significance. *Vet. Rec.* **142**, 669–71.

Boldrini, G. (1954) Un episodio di pesta bovina su una nave del 'Lloyd Triestino'. *Veterin. Ital.* **5**, 1182–3.

Branagan, D. and Hammond, J.A. (1965) Rinderpest in Tanzania: a review. *Bull. Epizoot. Dis. Afr.* **13**, 225–46.

Brüning, A., Bellamy, K., Talbot, D. and Anderson, J. (1999) A rapid chromatographic strip test for the pen-side diagnosis of rinderpest virus. *J. Virol. Methods* **81**, 143–54.

Catley, A. (1997) Adapting participatory appraisal (PA) for the veterinary epidemiologist: PA tools for use in livestock disease data collection. Proceedings of the Society for Veterinary Epidemiology and Preventive Medicine, Chester, UK, pp. 246–57.

Curasson, G. (1936) La peste bovine. In: *Traité de pathologie exotique vétérinaire et comparé*, Volume 1. Paris: Vigot Frères, ch. 3.

Edwards, J.T. (1949) The uses and limitations of the caprinised virus in the control of rinderpest (cattle plague) among British and Near-Eastern cattle. *Br. Vet. J.* **105**, 209–53.

FAO (1984) *Rinderpest Eradication in South Asia – Requirements and Action Plans.* FAO/APHCA Publication 3, Expert Consultation on Requirements for the South Asian Rinderpest Eradication Campaign, Izatnagar, India, December 1983. FAO Regional Office for Asia and the Pacific.

FAO (1993) *The Success of Operation Rinderpest by the West Asia Rinderpest Eradication Campaign Coordination.* Rome: FAO.

FAO (1996) *The World Without Rinderpest.* Animal Production and Health Paper 129. Proceedings of the FAO Technical Consultation on the Global Rinderpest Eradication Programme, Rome, Italy, 22–24 July.

FAO (1998) *Rinderpest: The Challenge Ahead.* Report of the FAO Technical Consultation on the Global Rinderpest Eradication Programme, Rome, 28–30 September.

FAO (1999) Emergency Prevention System for Transboundary Animal and Plant Pests and Diseases (EMPRES) – Livestock Programme Fourth Expert Consultation: Early Warning Systems for Transboundary Animal Diseases and Review of the Global Rinderpest Eradication Programme, Rome, 24–26 May.

Hafez, S.M., Abou-Zeid, A.A., Osman, F.S., Fadle, N.E. and Abdul-Rahim, S.A. (1985) Factors contributing to the occurrence of rinderpest in Saudi dairy farms. *Proc. Saudi Biol. Soc.* **8**, 309–22.

Hambridge, G. (1955) *The Story of FAO.* New York: Van Nostrand, pp. 149–51.

Hudson, D.R. (1960) Lutte contre les maladies animales. Rapport aux gouvernements de la Birmanie, du Cambodge, du Laos, de la Thailande et du Viet-nam. FAO Programme Elargi d'Assistance Technique, Rapport no. 1202, Rome.

Hussain, M., Iqbal, M., Taylor, W.P., and Roeder, P.L. (2001). Pen-side test for the diagnosis of rinderpest in Pakistan. *Vet. Rec.* **149**, 300–2.

Jack, J.D.M. (1961) Part V: The Sudan. In: G.P. West (ed.), *A History of the Overseas Veterinary Services*, Part 1. London: British Veterinary Association, pp. 123–43.

Kakizaki, C. (1918) Study on the glycerinated rinderpest vaccine. *Kitasato Arch. Exp. Med.* **2**, 59–66.

Kock, R.A., Wambua, J.M., Mwanzia, J., Wamwayi, H., Ndungu, E.K., Barrett, T., Kock, N.D. and Rossiter, P.B. (1999) Rinderpest epidemic in wild ruminants in Kenya 1993–97. *Vet. Rec.* **145**, 275–83.

Kurchenko, F.P. (1995) Prophylaxis and actions to eliminate rinderpest. *Veterinariya-Moskva*, No. 8, 27–31.

Kurchenko, F.P., Nikishin, I.V., Karpov, G.M., Vishnyakov, I.F., Bakulov, I.A., Buzun, A.I., Balabanov, V.A., Mitin, N.I., Arkhipov, N.I., Malakhova, M.S. and Kopteva, A.A. (1993) Isolation and identification of rinderpest virus in Georgia. *Veterinariya-Moskva* No. 3, 19–22.

Laktionov, A.M. (1967) The Prevention of Rinderpest. *Trudy Vsesoyuznogo Instituta Eksperimental 'noi Veterinarii*, **34**, 302–11.

Lepissier, H.E. (1971) General Technical Report on OAU/STRC Joint Campaign against Rinderpest in Central and West Africa, pp. 1–203.

Leyland, T. (1996) The world without rinderpest: outreach to the inaccessible areas. The case for a community-based approach with reference to Southern Sudan. Proceedings of the FAO Technical Consultation on the Global Rinderpest Eradication Programme, FAO Animal Production and Health Paper 129, 109–122. Rome: FAO.

Littlewood, W. (1905) Cattle plague in Egypt in 1903–04–05. *J. Comp. Pathol.* **18**, 312–21.

Macadam, I. (1968) Transmission of rinderpest from goats to cattle in Tanzania. *Bull. Epizoot. Dis. Afr.* **16**, 53–60.

Macauley, J.W. (1973) Kenya. In: *A History of the Overseas Veterinary Services*, Part 2. London: British Veterinary Association, pp. 139–61.

Macfarlane, I.M. (1970) Proceedings of the Second Technical Review Meeting of the Joint Campaign against Rinderpest Phase IV. Kampala, Uganda, 1–2 December 1970, p. 102.

Majok, A.A., Roeder, P.L., Ward, D.E., Barker, T.J., Osmani, A., Mohammed, D., Salemi, M.A. and Sayedi, N. (2000) Could war-torn Afghanistan be a sanctuary for rinderpest virus? In: Proceedings of an International Symposium on Veterinary Epidemiology and Economics (ISVEE), Breckridge, Colorado, pp. 844–46.

Mariner, J.C. (1996) The world without rinderpest: outreach to marginalized communities. Proceedings of the FAO Technical Consultation on the Global Rinderpest Eradication Programme, FAO Animal Production and Health Paper 129. Rome: FAO, pp. 97–107.

Mariner, J.C. and Roeder, P.L. (2003) The use of participatory epidemiology in studies of the persistence of rinderpest in East Africa. *Vet. Rec.* **152** (21), 641–7.

Mariner, J.C., Hussain, M., Roeder, P.L. and Catley, A. (2003). The use of participatory disease searching as a form of active surveillance in Pakistan for rinderpest and more. In: Proceedings of the 10th International Symposium on Veterinary Epidemiology and Economics, Viña del Mar, Chile, 17–21 November.

Nawathe, D.R. and Lamorde, A.G. (1982) Recurrence of rinderpest in Nigeria. *Vet. Rec.* **111**, 203.

Nawathe, D.R. and Lamorde, A.G. (1985) Rinderpest in Nigeria: the unfinished story. *Vet. Rec.* **117**, 669.

Nawathe, D.R., Lamorde, A.G. and Kumar, S. (1983) Recrudescence of rinderpest in Nigeria. *Vet. Rec.* **113**, 156–7.

OIE (1983a) Confirmed outbreak rinderpest on dhow 'Yaqoobi' ex Somalia. Epizootiological information Number OM 83/2/88. Paris: Office International des Epizooties.

OIE (1983b) Rinderpest outbreaks reported at Sumail. Epizootiological information Number OM 83/3/113. Paris, Office International des Epizooties.

OIE (2004) Terrestrial Animal Health Code Appendix 3.8.2: Surveillance Systems for Rinderpest. Paris: OIE [http://www.oie.int/eng/normes/mcode/en_chapitre_3.8.2.htm].

Peck, E.F. (1973) Somaliland Protectorate. In: *A History of the Overseas Veterinary Services*, Part 2. London: British Veterinary Association, pp. 255–65.

Plowright, W. (1963) The role of game animals in the epizootiology of rinderpest and malignant catarrhal fever in East Africa. *Bull. Epizoot. Dis. Afr.* **11**, 149–62.

Plowright, W. (1982) The effects of rinderpest and rinderpest control on wildlife in Africa. *Symposium of the Zoological Society of London*, No. 50, 1–28.

Reid, N.R. (1949) In: *Report of the Department of Veterinary Science and Animal Husbandry*, Tanganyika 1948. Cited by Plowright (1963).

Robson, J., Arnold, R.M., Plowright, W. and Scott, G.R. (1959) The isolation from an eland of a strain of rinderpest virus attenuated for cattle. *Bull. Epizoot. Dis. Afr.* **7**, 97–102.

Roeder, P.L. and Reichard, R. (1999) Report to the OIE of a Mission to the Russian Federation Concerning the Outbreak of Rinderpest in Amur Region in 1999. Paris: OIE.

Rossiter, P.B. (2001) Morbilliviral diseases: Rinderpest. In: E.S. Williams and I.K. Barker (eds), *Infectious Diseases of Wild Mammals*. Ames, IO: Iowa State University Press, pp. 37–45.

Rossiter, P.B., Hussain, M., Raja, R.H., Moghul, W., Khan, Z. and Broadbent, D.W. (1998) Cattle plague in Shangri-La: observations on a severe outbreak of rinderpest in northern Pakistan 1994-1995. *Vet. Rec.* **143**, 39–42.

Rossiter, P.B., Jessett, D.M., Wafula, J.S., Karstad, L., Chema, S., Taylor, W.P., Rowe, L. Nyange, J.C., Otaru, M., Mumbala, M. and Scott, G.R. (1983) Re-emergence of rinderpest as a threat in East Africa since 1979. *Vet. Rec.* **113**, 459–61.

Scott, G.R. (2000) The murrain now known as rinderpest. *Newsletter of the Tropical Agriculture Association, UK* **20**, 14–16.

Semenikhin, A., Vishnyakov, I., Avilov, V., Kolomitsev, A. and Mickolaichuk, S. (1995) Rinderpest Epizootic in Tuva. In: M. Schwyzer, M. Ackermann, G. Bertoni, R. Kocherhans, K. McCullough, M. Engels, R. Wittek and R. Zanoni (eds), *Immunobiology of Viral Infections*. Proceedings of the Third Congress of the European Society of Veterinary Virology, pp. 451–4.

Shaila, M.S., Purushothaman, V., Bhavasar, D., Venugopal, K. and Venkatesan, R.A. (1987) Peste des petits ruminants in India. *Vet. Rec.* **125**, 602.

Shantikhumar, S.R. and Atilola, M.A. (1990) Outbreaks of rinderpest in wild and domestic animals in Nigeria. *Vet. Rec.* **126**, 306–7.

Singh, K.V. and Ata, F. (1967) Experimental rinderpest in camels – a preliminary report. *Bull. Epizoot. Dis. Afr.* **15**, 19–23.

Smith, D.B., McAllister, J., Casino, C. and Simmonds, P. (1997) Virus 'quasispecies': making a mountain out of a molehill? *J. Gen. Virol.* **78**, 1511–19.

Stoddard, H.L. (1964) La campagne de lutte contre la peste bovine. Rapport au gouvernement du Cambodge. FAO Programme Elargi d'Assistance Technique, Report no. 1749, Rome.

Swan, J.F.C. (1973) Northern Rhodesia (Zambia) 1932–1943. In *A History of the Overseas Veterinary Services*, Part 2. London: British Veterinary Association, pp. 228–9.

Taylor, W.P. (1990) Achievements, difficulties and future prospects for the control of rinderpest in Africa. In: Kuil, Paling and Huhn (eds), *Livestock Production and Diseases in the Tropics* (Proc. 6th. Int. Conf. Inst. Trop. Vet. Med.). Wageningen, 28 Aug–1 Sept, 1989, pp. 84–90.

Taylor, W.P., Diallo, A., Gopalakrishna, S., Sreeramalu, P., Wilsmore, A.J., Nanda, Y.P., Libeau, G., Rajasekhar, M. and Mukhopadhyay, A.K. (2002a) Peste des petits ruminants has been widely present in southern India since, if not before, the late 1980s. *Prev. Vet. Med.* **52**, 305–12.

Taylor, W.P., Roeder, P.L., Rweyemamu, M.M., Melewas, J.N., Majuva, P., Kimaro, R.T., Mollel, J.N., .Mtei, B.J., Wambura, P., Anderson, J., Rossiter, P.B., Kock, R., Melengeya, T. and Van den Ende, R. (2002b) The control of rinderpest in Tanzania between 1997 and 1998. *Trop. Anim. Hlth Prod.* **34**, 471–87.

Taylor, W.P. and Watson, R.M. (1967) Studies on the epizootiology of rinderpest in blue wildebeest and other game species of Northern Tanzania and Southern Kenya, 1965–7. *J. Hyg. (Cambr.)* **65**, 537–45.

Throssel, G.L. (1980) The rinderpest outbreak in Western Australia in 1923: Australia's debt to farrier sergeant W.E.F. Burton, licensed veterinarian. *Aust. Vet. J.* **56**, 200–1.

Wamwayi, H.M., Fleming, M. and Barrett, T. (1995) Characterisation of African isolates of rinderpest virus. *Vet. Microbiol.* **44**, 151–63.

Wamwayi, H.M., Kariuki, D.P., Wafula, J.S., Rossiter, P.B., Mbuthia, P.G. and Macharia, S.R. (1992) Observations on rinderpest in Kenya, 1986–1989. *Rev. Sci. Off. Int. Epizoot.* **11**, 769–84.

Woodford, M.H. (1984) Rinderpest in wildlife in Sub-Sahelian Africa. Consultant Report (TCP/RAF/2323) for OAU-IBAR. Rome: FAO.

# Rinderpest and wildlife

# 7

## RICHARD A. KOCK

African Union, Interafrican Bureau for Animal Resources, Pan African Programme for the Control of Epizootics (AU–IBAR PACE), Nairobi, Kenya

## Introduction

As indicated in previous chapters, rinderpest is a serious disease of cattle and other large ruminants. It can also affect many wildlife species with devastating effects and these have become crucial in monitoring the disease in the region of Africa where it is thought to still exist, namely in the Kenya/Somalia ecosystem (Roeder and Taylor, 2002). Rinderpest has not been seen in the field for several years. The last laboratory confirmed case occurred in buffalo in Meru National Park in Kenya in 2001. As the story of rinderpest draws to a conclusion, the result of over a century of effort by veterinarians and others, we should not be too quick to congratulate ourselves but remain cautious for some considerable time. Near elimination in Africa was reached before following the JP15 campaign but unfortunately the programme no more than reduced the disease to a few residual foci from which, a decade later, the virus re-emerged with calamitous results (see Chapter 6).

Authorities believed that this resurgence was merely evidence of an incomplete vaccination campaign in cattle, a result of the inability to access many remote pastoral herds harbouring the virus in West, Central and East Africa and that the scientific basis for eradication was still sound (Provost, 1982). In response, the international community redoubled its efforts in the late 1980s and 1990s through the Pan African Rinderpest Campaign (PARC), to be managed by the Interafrican Bureau for Animal Resources (IBAR) as part of the Organization of African Unity (OAU). The experts believed that the new strategy with focused coverage of infected populations, an improved capacity for the delivery of vaccines, better vaccine preparation and stability (less reliant

ISBN-13: 978-0-12-88385-1
ISBN-10: 0-12-88385-6

on the cold chain), and sensitive seromonitoring tools would succeed in eradicating the virus. In addition a process of verification was put in place by the
Office International des Epizooties (OIE) for countries to follow – the OIE
Pathway. It was designed to ensure the absence of viral persistence through
active clinical and serological surveillance of cattle. Later wildlife was
included in the process as it became more evident how important a sentinel
they provided for rinderpest virus during this process.

# Rinderpest in African wildlife, 1994–2004

The above strategy has proven to be effective in most regions of Africa (and
Asia) (see Chapter 6), but PARC epidemiologists were surprised by a major
epidemic in the Tsavo National Park (Tsavo) Kenya in the mid-1990s, not in
cattle but in wildlife (Barrett et al., 1998; Kock et al., 1999a). The origin of the
virus was unclear as no cattle disease was reported at the time and no transboundary disease epizootics were evident. The fact that the outbreak came to
light through routine disease investigation undertaken by the Kenya Wildlife
Services and not through the surveillance system of the Kenyan Veterinary
Department was also noted. As a result it was decided to increase the coordination and integration of disease investigation in susceptible wild animals
under PARC. In 1998 a project was developed to improve liaison between
wildlife and livestock authorities and to undertake wildlife serosurveillance in
nine priority countries, where the virus was known to persist based on recent
history of livestock or wildlife disease or where these were considered at risk
due to their proximity to recent infections. The methodology included disease
investigation, and retrospective and purposive serosurveillance using approved
serological tests for rinderpest and peste des petits ruminants virus (PPRV)
antibody detection in livestock (OIE, 2001, 2003) as well as partially validated
tests for screening and research purposes (Libeau et al., 1992, 1995).
Interpretation of results for rinderpest antibody were based strictly on the use
of both the anti-RPV H C-ELISA (BDSL Kit) and the virus neutralization test
(VNT – performed in an FAO reference laboratory for any given sera). The
project, which concluded surveillance in June 2000, produced data on the
activity of the virus (CIRAD, 2001), including evidence for the historic infection of wildlife in West and Central Africa and, as recently as 1999, the infection of buffaloes Syncerus caffer in Eastern Africa. It also demonstrated the
absence of rinderpest antibodies from the largest African wildlife concentration
in the Greater Serengeti ecosystem in all animals born since approximately
1985. Additionally, antibodies to PPR infection were unequivocally identified
in wildlife sera from all sampled countries in West and Central Africa and in
Ethiopia in eastern Africa. The data also supported the hypothesis that there
was rapid extinction of the virus after an epidemic from buffalo and other
species (the data showed a high rate of transmission at the herd (Ro ~ 10) and

population levels), i.e. that wildlife were not acting as a reservoir. Comparison of the observed and serological data showed that the standard OIE tests appeared to be valid at least for buffalo but the work raised some questions about their relative sensitivity, specificity and applicability (when used alone) for detecting rinderpest virus-induced antibody amongst susceptible wildlife species. There was also the complication of apparent cross-reaction with the serological tests between PPR and rinderpest antibody with sera from areas where both diseases were or had recently been present. There were also concerns about the role of some species in the epidemiology of the disease amongst wildlife.

Wildlife surveillance continued after PARC under the Pan African Programme for the Control of Epizootic disease (PACE), with improved methodologies (e.g. serial testing of all wildlife sera with both RPV anti-H cELISA and VNT and N C-ELISA for PPR with cross-neutralization if sera were positive to ensure differentiation between the antibodies) and with a focus on buffalo populations. This programme was developed with European Union (EU) funding to improve networks for epizootic disease surveillance and is discussed in Chapter 6. Results from the wildlife surveillance (Kock *et al.*, 2005) provided much-needed clarification of the likely rinderpest virus circulation at a time when vaccination was ceasing in many countries but when it was also difficult to monitor the status of the virus in the concerned cattle populations – the problem being that recently vaccinated cattle cannot be serologically surveyed for natural virus infection, as the virus and vaccine antibody in serum are indistinguishable with the available tests. Monitoring for episodes of cattle disease in countries still practising vaccination was dependent on passive or active clinical surveillance. With mild expression of disease in cattle this was a major constraint to monitoring virus activity, especially in eastern Africa. Fortunately through spatial and temporal analysis of the wildlife data, it was possible to unequivocally show the time and distribution of past and recent epidemics in a number of countries in the region and this result is illustrated by the data from eastern Africa (Figure 7.1). This shows the spatial distribution and locations where positive antibodies were identified from wildlife species over a ten-year period. Analysis of this data (Kock *et al.*, 2005) showed historical infection in many East and Central African countries as well as areas where the virus was persistent with recent infection, within or adjacent to the so-called Somali ecosystem. Infection was confirmed (virus isolation or PCR) in buffalo, eland and kudu in the Tsavo and Nairobi National Parks during the epidemic reported in the 1990s (Kock *et al.*, 1999a), with evidence of a recurrence of infection in a sector of the Tsavo East National Park in 1998–99 (based on serology) and an isolated outbreak confirmed (PCR and serology) in Meru National Park in 2001, the latter despite two emergency blanket cattle vaccination campaigns in Kenya (1997–1999) after the Tsavo epidemic. Other ecosystems across East, West and Central Africa were either free of disease or antibody in wildlife whilst younger cohorts of the population were negative.

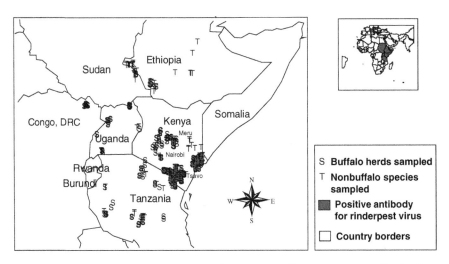

**Figure 7.1** Spatial distribution of positive and negative rinderpest antibody from buffalo and other wildlife in eastern Africa 1994–2004.

These results were also consistent with known historical livestock epidemics but there were some confusing data from certain locations (Chad, Central African Republic, Ethiopia, Tanzania and Mauritania), which proved to be either a result of cross-reaction in the tests for rinderpest with PPR antibody or false-positive test results in individual sera. False results were interpreted when a single test was positive without the support of another OIE approved test and/or not consistent with the expected sero-epidemiological picture at the herd level. In all cases either cross-neutralization tests were performed to differentiate between PPR and rinderpest antibody or repeat sampling and serial testing (anti-H C-ELISA and VNT) were undertaken and in all cases the situation was clarified. No other foci of virus or recently acquired antibody in sera were detected in the zones surveyed other than in the Somali ecosystem.

The results of studies on the virus isolated during the wildlife epidemic in Kenya (Barrett *et al.*, 1998) showed it belonged to African lineage 2 and that records of lineage 2 virus activity in Eastern Africa were last published in the 1960s (Plowright, 1963). The virus from the cattle and wildlife outbreak that occurred in Tanzania in the early 1980s (Nyange *et al.*, 1985) was not isolated or characterized, so its relationship with the RBT/1, RBT/2 & RGK/1 viruses from the 1960s and the Tsavo and Meru outbreaks of 1995 and 2001 remains uncertain.

The so-called Tsavo outbreak in 1994–97 (Kock *et al.*, 1999a) is central to understanding the recent patterns of viral circulation in the East African region and some background is useful. The impact of PARC in Kenya by 1993 was evident with an apparent reduction in reports of rinderpest in livestock (Wamwayi *et al.*, 1992). Levels of immunity in the cattle population in Kenya were relatively high as a result of annual vaccination but the wildlife population was, as shown by some studies, increasingly susceptible (Rossiter *et al.*, 2005). The source of the Tsavo epidemic is not known but anecdotal information suggests Orma cattle during the drought in 1993 made incursions along the Tiva River in Northern Tsavo East National Park and introduced the virus. Many buffalo died but this was initially put down to drought until lesser kudu started dying some months later and results of investigation suggested rinderpest as a cause. The disease spread through the Tsavo Park westwards in slow (1994) and fast phases (1995), involving many species with high mortality, especially in buffalo and kudu. The virus was finally isolated in 1995. The disease continued to spread and reached buffalo in Amboseli National Park in 1995, wildlife in Nairobi in 1996 and cattle in northern Tanzania in 1997 (Taylor *et al.*, 2002). Nairobi receives livestock from all regions of the country, so an epidemic spread to this location cannot be certain but as there are contiguous wildlife populations between Amboseli and Nairobi, this scenario was possible. In a separate part of the country in Meru National Park, wildlife were also affected during 1995 but again the source of virus is unknown, but without contiguous wildlife between Tsavo and Meru, again cattle was most likely. From observation, the epidemic was over by 1997 in all areas.

At the time of the Tsavo epidemic is was assumed that any likely incursion of virus would be from Sudan but the observations suggested virus came from North Eastern Kenya and most probably from Somali and/or Orma cattle, which occupy this region. After this epidemic there was extensive vaccination of cattle and levels of immunity in all host species were likely relatively high. There were no reports of disease for a few years. The evidence for viral circulation in Kenya subsequently is described in more detail below but the most important question is whether these later reports relate to the tail of the Tsavo epidemic or fresh incursions of virus to wildlife populations from the as yet unconfirmed reservoir in cattle of the Somali ecosystem.

# The role of wildlife in the maintenance of rinderpest virus in East Africa

The role of wildlife in the persistence of rinderpest virus has been reviewed over the years (Plowright, 1982; Woodford, 1984; Anderson, 1995). Debate as to their importance continues simply because the disease continues to emerge in wildlife populations and the detailed virology and epidemiology of rinderpest in most non-domestic species is largely unknown. While this might be considered a constraint in the development of a strategy for rinderpest eradication, and given the impossibility of experimentally establishing all the facts for all animal species, common sense, available data and field observations continue to be the basis for assessing the risks of persistence due to wildlife. Laboratory studies remain few, the most recent being transmission experiments between cattle and buffalo using an isolate of virus obtained from kudu in Tsavo (Wamwayi, 2003). The results confirmed that this strain of virus can transmit readily between buffalo and cattle kept in adjacent pens (aerosol transmission), with buffalo showing severe disease symptoms and cattle only a mild syndrome, subclinical in many cases without apparently seroconversion in all contacts.

Assuming that rinderpest virus is being maintained amongst the mosaic of wildlife and livestock in the Somali ecosystem, the question is how? This chapter examines the evidence.

# Rinderpest disease in wildlife under epidemic conditions

Wildlife epidemics associated with rinderpest in cattle have been reported since the disease was first seen in Africa in the nineteenth century. Significantly there are a number of reports of the disease associated with a mild syndrome in cattle (Robson et al., 1959; Branagan and Hammond, 1965). In wildlife, species susceptibilities were more or less consistent, with buffalo, the tragelaphine (bovine) antelopes (eland *Taurotragus oryx*, bushbuck *Tragelaphus scriptus*, and lesser kudu *Tragelaphus imberbis* spp.), giraffe (*Giraffa camelopardalis*) and warthog (*Phaecocherus* spp.) most severely affected but other species were involved, significantly the migrating wildebeest in the vast Serengeti–Mara plains in Tanzania and Kenya. Prior to the successful use of the vaccines developed at the Muguga laboratory in the 1950s and 1960s, scientists believed that the virus was indeed maintained in large wildlife populations and that this would prevent eradication of the virus in the future (Plowright, 1987). This fear proved false, at least within the cattle of the Masai steppe, as the disease was successfully eradicated here by the end of the 1960s by the vaccination of cattle (Plowright and McCulloch, 1967; Taylor and Watson, 1967), with a cattle-associated recurrence on only one occasion in the 1980s (Rossiter et al., 1983a; Anderson et al., 1990), and this was despite the lack of control measures against wildlife disease. The current population of wildebeest (*Connochaetus taurinus*) has grown to over 1.25 million animals as a result of the eradication of rinderpest (East, 1998) and there has been no recurrence. This provided the main argument for ignoring wildlife in the vaccination strategy. However, in order to understand the epidemiology of rinderpest in wildlife we need to examine all the available data and look at the role that buffalo and other species might play.

The most consistently and visibly affected species is buffalo. Reported data show that rinderpest is a highly infectious disease in this species, with clinical signs not dissimilar to those seen classically in cattle, as it affects all in-contact individuals within a short period of time. It is probable that, prior to vaccination, the maintenance of the virus in many regions was dependent on cattle and to a lesser extent buffalo populations (Plowright, 1968a; Rossiter, 2001; Kock *et al.*, 2005). In the case of buffalo with an average herd size of between 200 and 300 individuals, the disease can be present in a single herd for about three months irrespective of the prior immune status of the herd (Kock *et al.*, 2005). The buffalo either die or recover with a serum antibody produced, which is potentially detectable for life. To survive in nature the virus depends on a continuous supply of new susceptible animals there being no re-infection and no carrier state (Plowright, 1968a). The recently reported data (Kock *et al.*, 2005) support this, providing evidence for the disappearance of the virus after epidemics in buffalo. These results are from retrospective serology repeated in known infected herds and populations, showing absence of antibody in animals born after epidemics. Illustrations of data that support this argument are reproduced in Figures 7.2 and 7.3 from buffalo in the Tsavo ecosystem. The sera (53) collected in Tsavo towards the end of the epidemic in 1994–95 (Figure 7.2) show all age groups to have antibody to rinderpest virus, confirming the high rate of transmission within and between buffalo herds. Negatives included two buffalo sampled from a herd in the Chuyulu hills, located near the head of the epidemic, and this herd was healthy. The other two negative cases were lone bull buffalo. Excluding these four sera, the prevalence was 100% in this sample. Figure 7.3 shows data collected in 1999–2000 from a number of discrete herds (9) in the north and west region of the Tsavo ecosystem. These samples were from a proportion of the same herds sampled in 1994–95 and by extrapolating from the age of the animals, the data show a point in time after which herds were apparently no longer exposed to the virus. In the chart, the animals aged less than 4 years were all seronegative and all animals older than 8 years were seropositive. Calculation from this result suggests that from 1993 to 1996 the virus was dying out and no

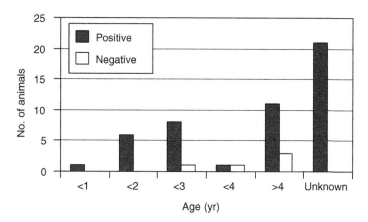

**Figure 7.2**  Tsavo: rinderpest antibody status of buffalo, 1994–1995.

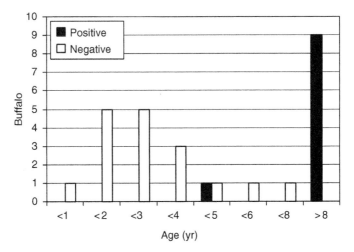

**Figure 7.3** Tsavo: rinderpest antibody status of buffalo in the north and west sectors, August 1999 – December 2000.

further circulation took place after 1996 in these herds. This is consistent with the observations and reports of clinical disease at the time. It is further supported by a sample (5) in 1997 from one herd in Kamboyo, Tsavo West known to have been infected in 1994, including buffalo aged 2 years or less, of which all sera were negative. With a high rate of transmission within and between herds this is the expected epidemiological result. The virus burnt out. It is nevertheless remarkable how from 1994 to 1997 rinderpest virus spread over an area of 60 000 square miles affecting all the buffalo herds within the ecosystem (>10 000 individuals) despite relatively low densities of wildlife in between discrete buffalo herds. In Tsavo alone the buffalo mortality was conservatively estimated at 60% (Kock *et al.*, 1999a) based on total counts undertaken in 1994 (Douglas-Hamilton *et al.*, 1994) and 1996. Survey data of Tsavo based on a sample count were also consistent with this finding (Census, 1994, 1997) with an estimated decrease of 65% over the period of the epidemic. From the data the overall period the virus persisted in the Tsavo ecosystem was approximately three years and this is consistent with other reports of historical outbreaks in the Serengeti reported by Rossiter *et al.* (1983a, 1983b, 2005), but the period for which populations of other species might be infected is unknown, although in Tsavo the last animal observed with rinderpest was a lesser kudu.

In the Tsavo (naive) epidemic many species and the whole population of buffalo was involved but this is not always the case. For example in the Meru National Park outbreak, reported in 2001 (OIE, 2001; Kock *et al.*, 2005), where the eligible proportion of buffalo in each herd was estimated at 40% (i.e. the young born to surviving buffalo after the last known infection in 1995), only a

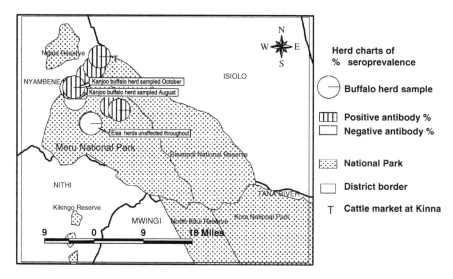

**Figure 7.4**    Rinderpest serology of buffalo herds, Meru National Park, 2001.

part of the whole population in Meru (~60%) was affected (Figure 7.4), while the disease was also cryptic and only detected by routine serosurveillance. The herds in the north of Meru were affected and the disease spread from east to west. The epidemic was confined to the National Park within the protected area system of 1000 sq miles affecting an estimated 1000 animals out of a population of approximately 1500. The origin of the virus was unknown but many cattle were present in the park during a drought in 2000–2001 and the first buffalo herds to seroconvert were closest to the areas of incursion of these cattle into Meru Park from the Kinna and Korbessa locations to the east.

The samples taken in 2002–2004, after the epidemic (Figure 7.5) were from eland, waterbuck, hartebeest and buffalo, including those in the adjacent Bisinadi reserve. These sera from eligible animals were all negative, showing that the virus had burnt itself out in buffalo while other species had been unaffected since the 1995 epidemic.

Another set of data, which supports the hypothesis that in partially immune populations an epidemic can be limited in its extent, was obtained in Tsavo, where there was an apparent recurrence of infection in 1998 in buffalo. This hypothesis was based on results from routine serosurveillance in 1999 to February 2000 (Figure 7.6), which showed positive antibody in all sera (except from an aged lone bull) but only from the south-eastern sector of Tsavo, and the majority of these sera were from animals born since the end of the outbreak in 1994–95. This is in contrast to the findings in Figure 7.3. These herds sampled from the south-east had had no history of disease since 1994. These infections

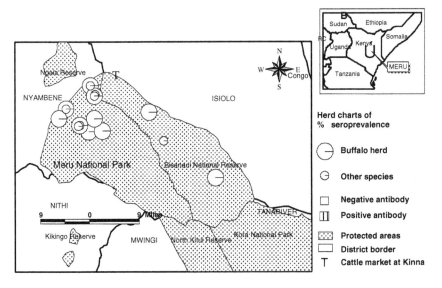

**Figure 7.5**   Rinderpest serology of wildlife, Greater Meru ecosystem, 2002–2004.

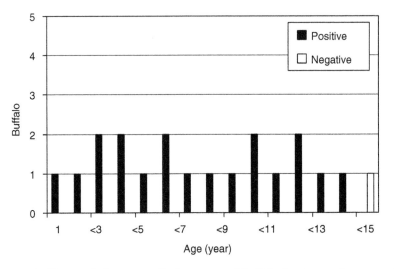

**Figure 7.6**   Tsavo: rinderpest antibody status of buffalo in the south-east sector, February 2000.

were most likely a result of a single introduction of virus from in-contact cattle migrating from the Somali ecosystem, to ranches adjacent to the National Park. Species other than buffalo remained unaffected, which is consistent with the findings from Meru in 2001.

It is well known that all cloven-hoofed mammals are susceptible to rinderpest virus infection but, as noted above, in observed outbreaks not all species appear to have been clinically affected or affected at the same time. From the above examples and from earlier reports (Carmichael, 1938; Branagan and Hammond, 1965; Kock *et al.*, 1999a, 2005) it appears that the proportion of the population that are diseased or seroconvert, even in a naive outbreak, is less in species other than buffalo. The reason for this is perhaps a lower rate of transmission amongst and between these species as a result of lower contact rates or perhaps some resistance to infection inherent in some species to the strain of virus. This is illustrated from data (Figure 7.7) taken from sampling in 1999 in Tsavo, which shows the seroprevalence at 22% overall. Seropositive results were obtained in eland (1/2), impala (1/8), lesser kudu (0/5), warthog (0/6) and giraffe (5/10), and 78% of these animals were alive at the time of the epidemic. These data also show that the virus did not persist and reinfect animals beyond 1995 with all (22% of the sample) animals born since the epidemic remaining seronegative.

These data are intuitively correct for rinderpest virus based on the conventional understanding of the epidemiology of the virus. These species are at lower herd and population densities than buffalo. This pattern, however, was not always in evidence. For example, wildebeest in the Nairobi National Park outbreak in 1996 (Kock *et al.*, 1999a) did not show a high rate of infection or seroconversion. This was despite the fact that wildebeest population densities were relatively high and animals were seen in close contact with infected buffalo and eland during the height of the Nairobi epidemic. This is in contrast to reports from the Serengeti in the 1960s (Taylor and Watson, 1967) and 1980s (Rossiter *et al.*, 2005), where high seroprevalence was recorded, although in

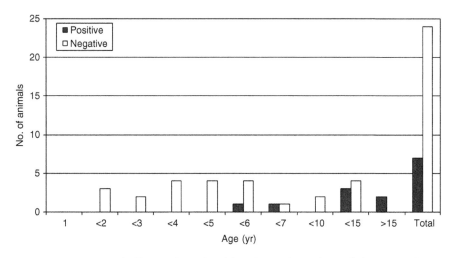

**Figure 7.7**    Tsavo: giraffe, warthog, eland, impala and lesser kudu rinderpest antibody status, 1999.

Loliondo, an area where a persisting focus of rinderpest virus in cattle was confirmed in 1965, no evidence for transmission of virus to wildebeest was found.
Another example of apparent resistance to infection occurred with Grant's
gazelle (*Gazella granti*), seen in contact with infected buffalo herds in Tsavo
East National Park in 1994, and these animals did not seroconvert (Kock *et al.*,
1999a).

Two other species worth mentioning are the warthog and the lesser kudu. A
number of the common warthog (*P. africanus*), which were sampled in Tsavo
and Nairobi National Parks, close to areas where infected buffalo were resident, did not seroconvert yet this species is reported to be highly susceptible
(Plowright, 1968b, 1987). Population survey data from Tsavo (Census, 1994,
1997) showed a 55% decline over this period, so perhaps it was affected with
few survivors, although disease was never reported. Lesser kudu appeared to
be affected during the Tsavo epidemic but over a different time period to buffalo (i.e. in any given location kudu were observed sick some months after buffalo were affected), which is evidence that in this species there was an
independent epidemic. Kudu were severely affected with obvious clinical disease (blindness) and high overt mortality based on field observations (Kock *et
al.*, 1999a), supported by a reported 42% decrease in population for the ecosystem from aerial survey results over the period of the epidemic. Yet this species
lives at low densities (home range of 60–500 ha in females and 650 ha in
males), in small female groups (comprising around three long-term associates),
which are loosely aggregated sometimes in larger groupings of up to 24 individuals. Males are more independent and avoid each other wandering in search
of oestrus females (Kingdon, 2003). Being highly secretive, they do not often
come into contact with other groups or species. It is therefore surprising that
the virus spreads at all in this species and yet it appears to readily do so from
the observations in Tsavo. Male behaviour might in part provide the explanation but it would appear that even given this behavioural character, persistence
of virus in individual kudu would theoretically need to be much longer than for
cattle or buffalo to ensure sufficient probability of transmission across a population in an area of several thousands of square kilometres. The other interesting observation is that antibodies were only detected from samples taken from
dying animals. No retrospective samples from surviving kudu in the population
have yet proven to be positive but the dataset for kudu is too small to make any
firm conclusions. It is also worth noting that in this species, and to a degree in
others (buffalo, giraffe and bushbuck), the pathology appears to differ from that
seen in cattle (Kock *et al.*, 1999b; Rossiter, 2001), the main lesions occurring
in the eye while buffalo frequently also showed extensive dermatoses in addition to diarrhoea.

If buffalo populations alone cannot maintain the virus and other species (in
general) are even less affected, this supports the hypothesis that new wildlife
epidemics require incursion of virus from another source, presumably cattle.
The only possible anomaly in this regard is the kudu where the virus was

observed to persist longer in the population than expected from what is known of the epidemiology of rinderpest, but it would appear that under epidemic conditions the virus also burns out in this species through high mortality.

Given these findings, the role of cattle in these reported wildlife epidemics is of considerable importance as they are believed to have been the source of the virus in every event. However, during the Tsavo episode there was no unequivocal diagnosis of rinderpest in cattle although there was supportive data from a mild disease syndrome detected around Nairobi and in the Kajiado and Mandera districts of Kenya where rinderpest antigen was detected by the agar gel immunodiffusion test (Rossiter, 2001) and a rinderpest-like disease in cattle in northern Tanzania was detected based on positive results using a pen-side test (Taylor *et al.*, 2002). Unfortunately, as no genomic material was isolated and sequenced, rinderpest in cattle was never officially reported to OIE. The proposed link in Tsavo and more generally with wildlife over this period therefore remains unsubstantiated.

## Rinderpest in wildlife under endemic conditions

The other scenario that needs discussion is endemic maintenance, where virus is continuously cycling through a single or multiple host population. Currently, it is proposed that this is the situation in the Somali ecosystem and that cattle are the principal hosts (Mariner and Roeder, 2003; Kock *et al.*, 2005). For this system the questions that need to be asked are: what is the evidence for persisting infection, and what is the role of wildlife in the epidemiology and maintenance of the virus? To attempt to answer these we need to identify the population and the potential host species for the virus in the ecosystem and re-visit available data.

The Somali ecosystem is generally now defined as an area spanning north-eastern Kenya, southern Somalia and south-eastern Ethiopia within which the Somali pastoral community and their livestock range. It is a vast area covering some 200 000 square kilometres and on the periphery includes the second largest wildlife protected area systems in Kenya – the Greater Meru Conservation Area (GMCA), encompassing Meru and Kora National Parks and the game reserves on their periphery. In recent years the system might also be considered to have extended into the Tsavo ecosystem, as Somali livestock are increasingly being moved into ranches on the edge of the national park for fattening prior to sale. The region is lowland (<4000 feet) with a variety of vegetation zones (tropical and sub-tropical broad-leafed forests, grasslands and shrub lands). Except for the coastal belt in the south, the area is arid or semi-arid with few rivers. There is little agriculture and the various habitats are more or less intact with wildlife present throughout the zone. There are some endemic susceptible wildlife species in the ecosystem including hirola antelope (*Beatragus hunteri*), dibitag (*Ammodorcas clarkei*) and desert warthog

(*Phaecocherus aethiopicus*), while the area contains the largest population and distribution of the lesser kudu in Africa. There are also large numbers of resident buffalo and migrating coastal topi (*Damaliscus lunatus topi*), and oribi (*Ourebia ourebia haggardi*) in the southern range; giraffe (*Giraffa camelopardalis reticulata*), Grant's gazelles, bushbuck, eland, duiker (*Cephalophus* spp.), waterbuck (*Kobus ellipsyprimnus*), gerenuk (*Litocranius walleri*), dikdik (*Madoqua* spp.) and oryx (*Oryx gazella beisa*) are widespread. It is a pastoral livestock system with nomadism and seasonal migration. The wildlife and livestock freely mix on pasture and at watering points. There has been little settlement or development, although during the past 20–30 years there has been a rapid decline in wildlife numbers, especially within Somalia, associated with the proliferation of automatic weapons. Except for warthogs, wildlife densities are low when compared to the Kenyan Masai lands. Desert warthog are of particular interest as they are a species endemic to the Somali ecosystem, present in good numbers, locally resident, widely distributed and in close daily contact with livestock. Rinderpest antibody-positive samples were detected in samples collected during 2000 but only in 15% of the warthogs examined (Kock *et al.*, 2005), the positive animals being clustered around the highest livestock density in the area. It was also observed from the cluster that the virus was not affecting all warthogs sampled in that sub-population or even amongst all family members. This might suggest that in each case direct transmission had occurred either from another wildlife species or from cattle, without subsequent intra-specific transmission. The dataset is small and there is also the question of sensitivity and specificity of the tests used in warthog so conclusions are difficult to make. However, if the latter hypothesis were true this would make warthog a useful sentinel for the presence of the virus in cattle, the presumed main host for rinderpest virus in this ecosystem.

Wildlife serosurveillance data over the past decade are only available from Kenya as Somalia has been in the midst of a civil war while sampling has not been possible in the south-eastern sector of Ethiopia. In Kenya then, individual herds of a range of species within the Somali ecosystem were sampled under the recent PARC and PACE programmes between 1995 and 2004, with some known resident buffalo populations sampled repeatedly to provide longitudinal data.

Buffalo serological data from a sample taken in 1999–2000 outside of GMCA (Figure 7.8) show 50% of the population with antibody with only the 3–4-year-old age group unaffected. This finding might be due to the mixing of infected and uninfected herds or to two periods of virus activity in the population, the first before 1994 and the second but perhaps less extensive episode, in 1997–98. These would pre-date the two epidemic periods recorded in Tsavo (1993–96, ~1998) and Meru (1995, 2001). In addition, giraffe, eland, bushbuck, hirola, topi and warthog in the Somali ecosystem (outside the GMCA) were shown by retrospective sero-surveillance to have antibodies to rinderpest (Figure 7.9). The distribution of antibody in this wildlife again excludes the 3–4-year age cohort (5–6 and 7–8), but on average there is a lower seroprevalence than in buffaloes across all age groups.

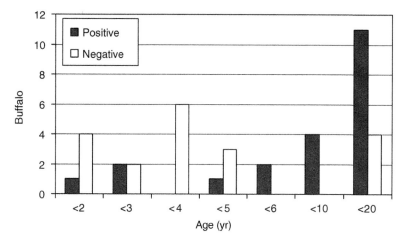

**Figure 7.8** Somali ecosystem excluding Meru: rinderpest antibody status of buffalo, 1999–2000.

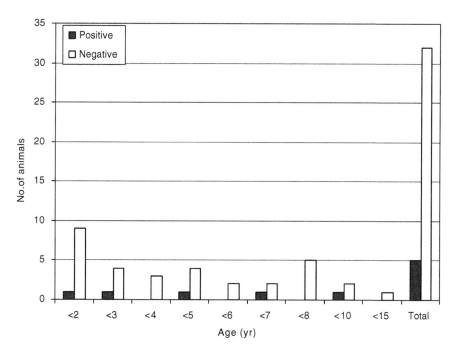

**Figure 7.9** Somali ecosystem excluding Meru: giraffe, warthog, eland, topi and lesser kudu rinderpest antibody status, sampled 1999.

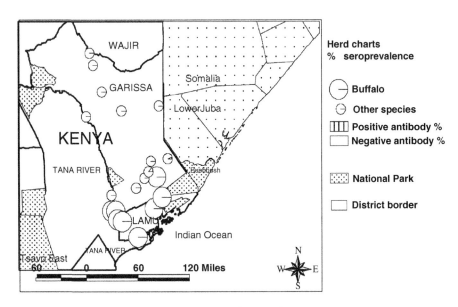

**Figure 7.10** Rinderpest serology of wildlife, Somali ecosystem, 2002–2004.

This could be interpreted as for buffalo but perhaps suggests sporadic but regular exposure of individuals to the virus up to 1998, i.e. there is no temporal pattern, which might be associated with a defined epidemic.

More recent data (2002–2004) (Figure 7.10) show that the eligible population of buffalo, giraffe and warthog in the ecosystem (i.e. mainly those born since 1998) has not continued to seroconvert, which suggests that the wildlife are no longer being exposed as regularly as before. Even if this apparent absence of virus in wildlife since 1998 proves to be correct there needs to be some epidemiological explanation for the difference in seroprevalence patterns between Tsavo, Meru and the rest of the Somali ecosystem over the period 1993–99. Perhaps it is a sampling anomaly, e.g. in terms of timing of surveys in relation to the circulation of virus, but the suggestion presented here is that these data reflect the difference between a zone of endemic maintenance and an epidemic zone.

For this probable zone of endemic maintenance there are still important questions to be answered. Where was the virus being maintained over the 30 years after the last phylogenetically related virus (RGK/1) was isolated? Over this period there was no official report of rinderpest-like disease or epidemics in this ecosystem although there is evidence that the virus was active in the intervening period based on virus isolation from a sick eland in the Isiolo region in the 1970s (Rossiter *et al.*, 1987), and from wardens' reports indicating possible infection of wildlife in the 1970s–80s in at least the Meru region. Could this virus have been present in the cattle population but cryptic or so mild as to be undetected by the government veterinarians in the field and the pastoralists themselves?

The role of livestock remains to be clearly demonstrated for the proposed area of endemic maintenance, as indeed it does for the historical epidemics mentioned above. Data on this aspect are limited but do suggest that cattle could be the reservoir for the virus. These include participatory disease surveillance data (Mariner and Roeder, 2003) and data from cattle surveys in 2003 in which an outbreak was reported (OIE, 2003) but never confirmed. The presence of rinderpest antibody averaging 17% of the cattle in southern Somalia (district prevalence varying from 0 to 26.5%) and a similar percentage in cattle from across the border in Kenya, are all supportive data. However, regarding serology it must be remembered that in both these areas vaccination, albeit at a relatively low rate, was practised up to 2003.

It is suggested in this paper that the area of endemic maintenance depends on the integrated system described above, which increases the overall host population size (multi-host system) and creates a unique environment (different to that found elsewhere in Africa) conducive to virus persistence. These conditions might have created circumstances where only a few wildlife and cattle herds are infected at any one time, allowing susceptible animals to build in other herds before they in turn contribute to the movement of virus around the ecosystem. This multi-host system might also explain the mild nature of the disease in cattle. Under these conditions blanket vaccination of cattle once or even twice may be insufficient to eliminate the virus as some infected herds may not be reached, allowing continued transmission to other eligible cattle and wildlife to continue. It might take a much more targeted vaccination strategy than used hitherto with intensive and continuous surveillance in all species to achieve the goal of eliminating the virus.

## Conclusions

Despite the considerable progress made under the PARC and PACE programmes, the rinderpest virus only persists in Africa, and probably within the Somali ecosystem. Here, since the last outbreak in Meru, no control action, i.e. vaccination, of any significance took place, so it must be assumed until proven otherwise that the virus is still present. The question still remains as to exactly where (or what) this area of endemic maintenance is. A general zone has been identified and reported as infected to the OIE by Kenya but as the origin of the last confirmed virus (Meru) was probably trade cattle, which could have come from almost anywhere within the ecosystem, it is still an enigma. Significantly, data to the end of 2004 show an absence of virus circulation amongst wildlife in the southern part of the (Kenya) Somali ecosystem, most probably since 1998, and on the periphery (Meru and Tsavo), since the last reported or suspected epidemics. This zone has the highest numbers of cattle and livestock in the Somali ecosystem, so logically is the likely area of maintenance. Can we assume therefore that the virus either has become very limited in distribution or eliminated or somehow latent and is not being transmitted to wildlife? The reported (but unconfirmed) outbreak in cattle in Garissa, Kenya in 2003 (OIE, 2003) offered a glimmer of hope of coming to grips with the so-called mild rinderpest of cattle but the failure to provide a clear laboratory diagnosis adds to the confusion as does the absence of antibody in this district in wildlife in 2004. So the area of endemic maintenance remains ill-defined and we may simply be currently observing an inter-epidemic period in the ecosystem. These possible cyclical epidemic periods in the region have also been suggested by other authors (Mariner and Roeder, 2005).

The virus or viral RNA isolated from the last two confirmed epidemics in wildlife in eastern Africa are of one strain of African lineage 2 and the transmission between buffalo and cattle has been proven experimentally, if not in the field. Mild rinderpest-like disease has been identified in cattle within the ecosystem and the possibility of rinderpest virus circulating is accepted even without the necessary field confirmation of virus and all countries involved are increasing efforts to confirm the presence or absence of the virus.

Irrespective of the circumstantial evidence of cattle as the reservoir of virus, concerns about the role of wildlife need to be addressed. Buffalo in the Somali ecosystem can be considered to be part of the maintenance host population but as they are restricted to the southern portion in the coastal zone, their overall impact is probably limited and there is no evidence that the species is maintaining the virus, in the absence of cattle or another source of infection. They remain, however, the main sentinel for disease within and on the periphery of the ecosystem. The role of other species appears to be as dead-end hosts but that of lesser kudu and warthog is still unclear. A multi-host epidemiological mechanism for persistence may exist, and this virus may well prove to have adapted to the unique conditions of the Somali ecosystem remaining cryptic, and only causing a mild subclinical syndrome in cattle. If this is the truth, a new case definition for a novel rinderpest-like disease may be required.

The fact that virus disappeared in the Kenyan and Tanzanian Masai lands and more recently in the Sudan grasslands and in all other African regions without recourse to control of the disease in wildlife is a strong argument for the current policy (delineating the area of endemic maintenance, followed by vaccination of cattle within this zone), but should not be a reason for complacency. The Masai lands differ from the Somali ecosystem in that wildlife and livestock are less integrated (with the majority of wildlife within the Greater Serengeti protected areas), with mainly seasonal contact. In Sudan, where the virus is apparently now eradicated, it is worth noting that the massive wildlife populations of eastern Equatoria (more abundant historically even than the Greater Serengeti, with some 2 million migrating white-eared kob in the 1980s), have all but disappeared. Was it vaccination (which never reached the theoretical levels necessary for eradication across the whole population of cattle), or was it wildlife destruction that was the driving force in eradication of rinderpest from the Sudan?

With our current knowledge, there are more questions than answers and the rinderpest story may be set to continue for some years to come.

## Acknowledgements

The author would like to thank the many colleagues who have contributed to the information presented in this paper and specifically the Director of the African Union – Interafrican Bureau for Animal Resources for permission to publish this chapter.

## References

Anderson, E.C. (1995) Morbillivirus infections in wildlife (in relation to their population biology and disease control in domestic animals). *Vet. Microbiol.* **44** (2–4), 319–32.

Anderson, E.C., Jago, M. *et al.* (1990) A serological survey of rinderpest antibody in wildlife and sheep and goats in northern Tanzania. *Epidemiol. Infect.* **105** (1), 203–14.

Barrett, T., Forsyth, M.A. *et al.* (1998) Rediscovery of the second African lineage of rinderpest virus: its epidemiolgical significance. *Vet. Rec.* **142**, 669–71.

Branagan, D. and Hammond, J.A. (1965) Rinderpest in Tanzania: a review. *Bull. Epizoot. Dis. Afr.* **13**, 225–46.

Carmichael, J. (1938) Rinderpest in African game. *J. Comp. Pathol.* **51**, 24–8.

Census (1994) Census 9702. Ministry of Planning and National Development, Department of Resource Surveys and Remote Sensing, Summary of Aerial Survey(s): For Tsavo Ecosystem. Nairobi, Kenya, DRSRS.

Census (1997) Census 9403. Ministry of Planning and National Development, Department of Resource Surveys and Remote Sensing, Summary of Aerial Survey(s): For Tsavo Ecosystem, Nairobi, Kenya, DRSRS.

CIRAD (2001) Final report of the African Wildlife Veterinary Project. Montpellier, France, CIRAD EMVT.

Douglas-Hamilton, I., Cachago, S., Litoroh, M. and Mirangi, J. (1994) *Tsavo Elephant Count.* London: E. Consultants.

East, R.E. (1998) African Antelope Database IUCN/SSC Antelope specialist group. *Occ. paper of the IUCN Species Survival Commission.* IUCN, Switzerland, pp. 209–14.

Kingdon, J. (2003) *The Kingdon Field Guide to African Mammals.* London: A&C Publishers, pp. 357–8.

Kock, N.D., Kock, R.A. *et al.* (1999a) Pathological changes in free-ranging African ungulates during a rinderpest epizootic in Kenya, 1993 to 1997. *Vet. Rec.* **145** (18), 527–8.

Kock, R.A., Wambua, J.M. *et al.* (1999b) Rinderpest epidemic in wild ruminants in Kenya 1993–97. *Vet. Rec.* **145** (10), 275–83.

Kock, R.A., Wamwayi, H.M., Rossiter, P.B., Libeau, G., Wambwa, E., Okori, J., Shiferaw, F. S., Mlengeya, T.D. (2005) Rinderpest in East Africa: continuing re-infection of wildlife populations on the periphery of the Somali ecosystem. *Prev. Vet. Med.* (in press).

Libeau, G., Diallo, A. *et al.* (1992) A competitive ELISA using anti-N monoclonal antibodies for specific detection of rinderpest antibodies in cattle and small ruminants. *Vet. Microbiol.* **31**, 147–60.

Libeau, G., Prehaud, C. *et al.* (1995) Development of a competitive ELISA for detecting antibodies to the peste des petits ruminants virus using a recombinant nucleoprotein. *Res. Vet. Sci.* **58** (1), 50–5.

Mariner, J.C. and Roeder, P.L. (2003) Use of participatory epidemiology in studies of the persistence of lineage 2 rinderpest virus in East Africa. *Vet. Rec.* **152** (21), 641–7.

Mariner, J.C., McDermott, J. *et al.* (2005) A model of lineage-1 and lineage-2 rinderpest virus transmission in pastoral areas of East Africa. *Prev. Vet. Med.* **69**, 245–63.

Nyange, J.F.C., Otaru, M.M.M. and Mbise A.N. (1985) Incidences of abnormal wild animal mortality in northern Tanzania 1979–82. *Bull. Anim. Hlth. Prod. Afr.* **33**, 55–7.

OIE (2001) World Animal Health in 2001. Paris: Office International des Epizooties.

OIE (2003) World Animal Health in 2003. Paris: Office International des Epizooties.

Plowright, W. (1963) Some properties of strains of rinderpest virus recently isolated in E. Africa. *Res. Vet. Sci.* **4**, 96–108.

Plowright, W. (1968a) Rinderpest virus. *Monogr. Virol.* **3**, 25–110.

Plowright, W. (1968b) Inter-relationships between virus infections of game and domestic animals. *E. Afr. Agr. Forestry J.* Special issue, pp. 260–3.

Plowright, W. (1982) The effects of rinderpest and rinderpest control on wildlife in Africa. *Symp. Zool. Soc. Lond.* **50**, 1–28.

Plowright, W. (1987) Investigations of rinderpest antibody in East African wildlife 1967–1971. *Rev. Sci. Tech. Off. Int. Epiz.* **6** (2), 497–513.

Plowright, W. and McCulloch, B. (1967) Investigations on the incidence of rinderpest virus infection in game animals of N. Tanganyika & S. Kenya 1960–3. *J. Hyg.* **65** (3), 343–58.

Provost, A. (1982) Scientific and technical bases for the eradication of rinderpest in intertropical Africa. *Rev. Sci. Tech. Off. Int. Epiz.* **1** (3), 619–41.

Robson, J., Arnold, R.M., Plowright, W. and Scott, G.R. (1959) The isolation from an eland of a strain of rinderpest virus attenuated for cattle. *Bull. Epizoot. Dis. Afr.* **7**, 97–102.

Roeder, P.L. and Taylor, W.P. (2002) Rinderpest. *Vet. Clin. North Am. Food Anim. Pract.* **18** (3), 515–47, ix.

Rossiter, P.B. (2001) Morbilliviral diseases: rinderpest. In: E. Williams and I.K. Barker (eds), *Infectious Diseases of Wild Mammals*. Iowa State University Press, pp. 37–45.

Rossiter, P.B., Jessett, D.M. *et al.* (1983a) Re-emergence of rinderpest as a threat in East Africa since 1979. *Vet. Rec.* **113** (20), 459–61.

Rossiter, P.B., Karstad, L., Jessett, D.M., Yamamoto, T., Dardiri, A.H. and Mushi, E.Z. (1983b) Neutralising antibodies to rinderpest virus in wild animal sera collected in Kenya between 1970 and 1981. *Prev. Vet. Med.* **1**, 257–64.

Rossiter, P.B., Taylor, W.P. *et al.* (1987) Continuing presence of rinderpest virus as a threat in East Africa, 1983–1985. *Vet. Rec.* **120** (3), 59–62.

Rossiter, P.B., Wamwayi, H.W. and Ndungu, E. (2005) Rinderpest surveillance in East African wildlife 1982–1993: transient infection of the Serengeti–Mara ecosystem. *Prev. Vet. Med.* (in press).

Taylor, W.P., Roeder, P.L. *et al.* (2002) The control of rinderpest in Tanzania between 1997 and 1998. *Trop. Anim. Hlth. Prod.* **34** (6), 471–87.

Taylor, W.P. and Watson, R.M. (1967) Studies on the epizootiology of rinderpest in blue wildebeest and other game species of northern Tanzania and southern Kenya, 1965–7. *J. Hyg. (Lond.)* **65** (4), 537–45.

Wamwayi, H.M. (2003) Chapter 6.2, East African Workshop on Mild Rinderpest. Nairobi, Kenya, Maendeleo House Nairobi, Kenya.

Wamwayi, H.M., Kariuki, D.P. *et al.* (1992) Observations on rinderpest in Kenya, 1986–1989. *Rev. Sci. Tech.* **11** (3), 769–84.

Woodford, M.H. (1984) Rinderpest in wildlife in Sub-Sahelian Africa. Consultant Report (TCP/RAF/2323) for OAU-IBAR. Rome: FAO.

# Diagnosis of rinderpest virus and peste des petits ruminants virus

**8**

## JOHN ANDERSON,* MANDY CORTEYN* AND GENEVIEVE LIBEAU†

*World Reference Laboratory, Institute for Animal Health, Pirbright Laboratory, Surrey, UK
†CIRAD–EMVT, Montpellier, France

## Introduction

For generations rinderpest was diagnosed purely by observation of clinical signs. During this period rinderpest regularly caused continent-wide epidemics in Europe, Asia and Africa which devastated the livestock population and led to the establishment of the first Veterinary Faculty in an attempt to overcome the problem. As technology evolved over the years, techniques were developed to assist in the diagnosis, control and eradication of the disease. This chapter gives an overview of the current diagnostic methods used to detect and differentiate rinderpest and PPR infections in ruminant species. Both antibody and antigen detection methods are described, the former used extensively for evaluating the success of vaccination campaigns and serosurveillance and the latter for the detection of virus in clinical samples.

## Sample collection

A rapid response to reports of suspect rinderpest/PPR is essential if good diagnostic samples are to be obtained. The selection of sample donors is also critical as samples from recovered animals rarely, if ever, give positive results for

ISBN-13: 978-0-12-88385-1
ISBN-10: 0-12-88385-6

virus isolation or genome detection. Excellent protocols for sample collection are given in the FAO Manual on the Diagnosis of Rinderpest (Anderson *et al.*, 1996) and in the FAO/PACE guidelines for confirming suspect outbreaks of rinderpest by Roeder and van't Klooster (2004). The main points are summarized below.

Ideally, samples should be collected for:

- Virus isolation
- Detection and characterization of viral RNA by reverse transcription–polymerase chain reaction (RT–PCR)
- Detection of viral antigen by immunocapture ELISA
- Detection of viral antigen in fixed tissue by immunohistochemisty.

At least five animals from each affected herd should be sampled and as much material as possible collected. Samples should be collected as follows.

*Post-mortem* samples taken from freshly slaughtered animals or overnight deaths:

- Mesenteric lymph nodes: collect aseptically, fill one universal container (collect further lymph node material for RT–PCR in Trizol/RNA later)
- Spleen: collect aseptically, fill one universal container
- Eye swabs: collect three from each eye, moisten each with two to three drops of sterile saline and place in universal container (collect further eye swabs for RT–PCR in Trizol/RNA later)
- Uncoagulated blood in EDTA: fill one 5 ml vacutainer tube
- Further eye swabs, nasal swabs, swabs of necrotic debris from the buccal mucosa and lymph node may be collected for immunocapture testing
- Small pieces of each tissue sampled should be preserved in 10% formaldehyde for immunohistochemistry.

Store samples in a cool box with cold packs (not required for formaldehyde preserved tissues) and transport to the laboratory as quickly as possible. Samples should be stored at 4–8 °C during transit using ice or cool packs. Screw-cap drinking water bottles make effective cool packs when filled with water and frozen and are less prone to leakage than ice-filled plastic bags.

*Samples from live animals* should be taken from animals with a high fever (more than 40 °C, preferably 41 °C), watery eye discharge, erosive mouth lesions and without diarrhoea. Samples from animals with severe diarrhoea are unlikely to give positive results as they are normally in a late stage of infection when the virus is being cleared. Eye swabs, nasal swabs, swabs of necrotic debris and uncoagulated blood in EDTA (as described above) and prescapular lymph node biopsies may also be collected. A 10 ml blood sample should provide sufficient serum for c-ELISA or virus neutralization test (VNT) testing. Clot retraction should start after about 2 hours at ambient temperatures, when the samples can be stored vertically in a refrigerator or cool box until the next day and serum should be removed by pipetting or centrifugation the following day to avoid haemolysis of the red cells affecting the sera.

It is vital that each animal sampled is given a unique identifier, e.g. date/sequential number for that day/place/age/sex. The location of the sampling area should also be recorded (ideally the latitude and longitude obtained using GPS). A full set of information should be sent to the laboratory to assist in their interpretation of the results. All labelling should be indelible and avoid markers which can be rubbed off in transit, particularly when wet. Indelibility is often accomplished using adhesive surgical tape and a permanent marker pen or biro.

The Institute for Animal Health, Pirbright was designated the FAO World Reference Laboratory for Rinderpest in 1994. Since then it has provided a free diagnostic service world-wide. In 2003 it was re-designated the FAO World Reference Laboratory for Morbilliviruses. Samples submitted by air must be packed in accordance with IATA regulations in a double-layered, leak-proof container with either dry ice or freezer packs. Wet ice must not be used since any leakage will be treated as a suspect infected material and may be destroyed by the airport authorities.

# Virus isolation and identification

Until recently, rinderpest virus isolation and identification were considered an imperative to diagnosis but newer molecular techniques, especially the polymerase chain reaction (PCR) and nucleotide sequencing, not only allow a more rapid diagnostic result but they also can identify the lineage of the virus concerned and give a clear picture of the epidemiological situation. Virus isolation is still important, however, and should be attempted whenever possible, but with the increase in the prevalence of extremely mild strains of rinderpest, the clinical signs may be very slight (if any), and the diagnostic window very small. Unlike the situation in the past when dealing with 'cattle plague' where clinical signs were severe and tissues from infected animals easy to collect, the chance of isolating virus from samples collected from animals infected with mild strains is much lower.

Primary and secondary cell cultures of calf kidney have been used for virus isolation for many years. Cell lines such as Vero and Madin Darby bovine kidney (MDBK) cells have also proved suitable. In many cases two to three blind passages may be needed to adapt the virus to a particular cell culture. Cytopathic effect may take 7–10 days to develop and media must be replaced regularly every 2 days.

Subsequently bovine T lymphoblast cells transformed with the protozoa *Theileria parva* were used for rinderpest virus isolation. They were shown to be more sensitive and recover a wider range of rinderpest virus strains than either calf kidney, or Vero cells (Rossiter *et al.*, 1992). Cytopathic effect (CPE) develops within 24 hours, considerably faster than the 7–10 days' culture required when using calf kidney, Vero or MDBK cells. These cells may be obtained from the International Livestock Research Institute (ILRI), Nairobi, Kenya. The use of these lymphoblastoid cell lines for rinderpest diagnosis, although promising, has not been widely adopted, possibly because of the presence of the parasite.

More recently, Kobune *et al.* (1991) showed that the Nakamura strain of lapinized rinderpest virus, which previously had been difficult to grow in cell cultures, would grow in a tamarind lymphoblastoid cell line, B95a. Typical CPE begins at 24 hours and consists of syncytia and ballooning cells. Mild strains of rinderpest virus, such as those currently circulating in part of eastern Africa, also grow well in B95a cells. For virus isolation, peripheral blood mononuclear cells (PBMC) from a suspect infected animal are mixed with lymphoblastoid cells at a ratio of 1:5 ($10^6$: $5.0 \times 10^6$) in a $25\,cm^2$ flask. Extracts of tissues made in PBS (10% w/v) can also be added to cell cultures. In this case, the extracts should be added for a period of 1–2 hours only before they are removed and fresh culture medium added as the tissues can contain toxic substances.

For PPR virus isolation, Vero cells continue to be used as the virus does not grow readily in B95a cells. Several blind passages are usually required before virus-specific CPE is observed. Primary lamb kidney cells and goat and sheep skin cells can also be used to isolate the virus.

However, it should be noted that virus isolation can only be attempted in well-equipped laboratories and on freshly collected specimens and the main drawbacks of the technique are:

- It is time-consuming, requiring 2 weeks or more if blind passage is needed.
- It requires tissue culture and sterile test samples, which are not always possible to find in field situations in developing countries.
- It is labour-intensive in that it requires a laboratory skilled in supporting tissue culture techniques.

Once virus-induced CPE is observed, the cells can be frozen at –80°C to preserve the virus stock. It can then be amplified and identified using the tests described below but these techniques can also be used to detect virus antigen directly from infected secretions or tissue homogenates.

# Antigen detection

## Agar gel immunodiffusion (AGID)

One of the earliest diagnostic techniques for the detection of rinderpest virus antigens was the agar gel immunodiffusion test (White, 1958). Reaction wells in the shape of a rosette are cut into agar gel-coated Petri dishes or slides and suspect antigen homogenates and anti-rinderpest antisera added to adjacent wells.

The antigen and antibody diffuses through the gel and forms a precipitin band where they meet. The technique was greatly improved when high titre hyperimmune rabbit serum was introduced. This was produced using a protocol which did not induce antibodies to cellular proteins thus reducing non-specific reactions. The AGID technique was widely used for many years in endemic regions and is still used in many developing countries where facilities do not exist for undertaking more complex tests. The sensitivity and speed of this assay were later modified by the incorporation of an electrophoretic step (Rossiter and Mushi, 1980). When an electric current is applied across the gel, the antigen migrates towards the anode and the antibody towards the cathode and speeds up the reaction. This was termed counter-immunoelectrophoresis (CIEOP). Although more sensitive, this was never widely adopted due to the cumbersome nature of the equipment.

Both of the above tests detect RPV and PPRV antigens in animal secretions (Wafula et al., 1986) but the identification of the virus relied on the isolation of the infectious agent in tissue culture and its further characterization by animal inoculation since PPRV, unlike RPV, is non-pathogenic for cattle (Zwart and Macadam, 1967a, b; Macadam, 1968; Gibbs et al., 1979), or virus by neutralization using virus-specific sera (Taylor, 1979; Rossiter et al., 1988).

## Immunocapture ELISA

The advent of monoclonal antibodies (mAbs) made possible accurate differential diagnosis of many virus diseases. Monoclonal antibody profiling can be used to differentiate between RPV and PPRV (McCullough et al., 1986; Libeau et al., 1997), however, enzyme-linked immunosorbent assay (ELISA) technology offered the opportunity to develop simple, rapid and highly specific diagnostic assays to identify RPV and PPRV. These tests are carried out in 96-well plates and are suitable for large-scale sample analyses.

In the immunocapture ELISA the sample to be analysed is allowed to react with the detection antibody and a second antibody (capture antibody), previously absorbed onto the ELISA plate surface, captures the immunocomplex formed. One of the antibodies can be a polyclonal (capture antibody) and the other a mAb (reaction antibody). Saliki (1993) adopted this approach to identify PPRV in tissues and secretions. The use of a polyclonal capture antibody increases the sensitivity of the assay because of its high avidity for the antigen but the use of mAbs for both capture and detection, as developed by Libeau et al. (1994), increases the specificity of the assay.

The principle of the mAb-based immunocapture test is illustrated in Figure 8.1. Monoclonal antibodies were essential for the development of this assay since they react with a single defined epitope or antigenic determinant. The test utilizes a combination of RPV-specific, PPRV-specific and RPV and PPRV cross-reactive mAbs. The RPV-specific and PPRV-specific mAbs used were directed against the nucleoprotein (N) of the viruses and differentiated

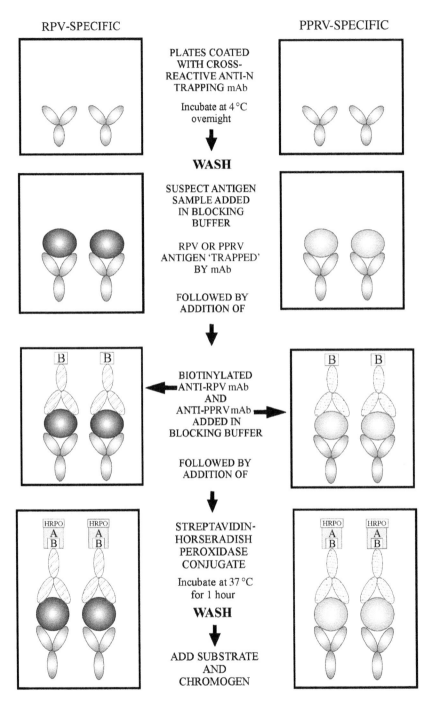

**Figure 8.1** Principle of immunocapture ELISA.

unambiguously RPV from PPRV (Libeau and Lefèvre, 1990). The capture mAb, which is also directed against the N protein, is broadly cross-reactive and recognizes the N protein of all viruses in the *Morbillivirus* genus. The detector mAbs specific for each virus are biotinylated with biotin-XX-ester to allow a coloured reaction with a peroxidase-streptavidin conjugate. All three mAbs are directed against non-overlapping antigenic domains on the N protein of RPV and PPRV, as demonstrated by competitive binding assay (Libeau *et al.*, 1997).

Absence of reciprocal competition between these mAbs allows a single step incubation reaction and illustrates that accuracy and specificity can be maintained in rapid diagnostic tests based on such pairs of mAbs (Ehrlich and Moyle, 1986; Nikkari *et al.*, 1989). Indeed, if this were not the case, the accessibility of the site recognized by one antibody would be a function of the incubation time of the second, and also of the affinity of each of them that forms the complex. In addition, when captured, the nucleoprotein is orientated in such a way that the epitopes for the detector antibodies are accessible. The mAb-based immunocapture ELISA is now accepted by OIE as an alternative to virus isolation for the diagnosis of RPV and PPRV.

## Sensitivity and specificity

The specificity of the immunocapture was first established on the supernatants from infected cell cultures by comparing the results obtained from 31 viral strains representative of the variability of the morbillivirus group. Supernatants from three viruses that mimic the clinical signs of rinderpest, namely infectious bovine rhinotracheitis, bovine viral diarrhoea virus and bovine papular stomatitis virus, were also tested. The specificity of the test is complete *vis-à-vis* RPV and PPRV and distinguishes them from the other ruminant viruses giving rise to similar clinical manifestations as indicated above. On the other hand, the test does not allow a distinction between PPRV and some laboratory viral strains of measles and canine distemper. The host specificity of these viruses is such that it has no consequence for the test applied to ruminants. All the RPV strains were found positive in the test with optical density values ranging from 0.2 to 2.8 when N protein was detected by the RPV-specific mAb, whereas values less than 0.013 were obtained with the PPRV-specific mAb. PPRV gave opposite values when tested with the same mAbs.

The sensitivity of the assay for both RPV and PPRV was determined by using virus preparations with known titres of infectious particles and known amounts of protein using the recombinant N protein of PPRV expressed in a baculovirus system. The limit of RPV detection is $10^{2.2}$ $TCID_{50}$/well while the PPRV assay detects as little as $10^{0.6}$ $TCID_{50}$/well. The discrepancy in the sensitivity for the two viruses may be due to a disparity in the affinity of the detecting antibody towards N-RPV and N-PPRV. In addition to a high sensitivity, the test was shown to work on samples maintained at room temperature over a period of one week. Although it is known that the N protein is particularly sensitive to degradation by cellular proteases, this demonstrated that the diagnostic test, based on the use of mAbs to the N protein, was valid even if not carried out immediately after sampling. One can assume therefore that, while the N protein is present in huge quantity in the tissues or secretions, the epitopes recognized by the mAbs have a relatively high stability. This has a very important epidemiological significance, knowing the difficulty of obtaining fresh samples from outbreaks in developing countries. It also alleviates the difficulty of isolating the viruses, particularly PPRV for which several blind passages are often required (Saliki, 1993). To ensure maximal isolation efficiency, the samples must be collected during the onset of pyrexia (Bourdin and Doutre, 1976; Lefèvre, 1987).

## Field validation

The introduction of the immunocapture technique as a diagnostic procedure to regions where both RPV and PPRV are endemic strengthened the diagnostic and surveillance capabilities of the veterinary teams and assisted them in the disease control programmes. Abraham and Berhan (2001) compared the performance on field samples of the AGID test that was routinely used in their laboratory with the immunocapture ELISA. The ELISA detected RPV antigen in 64% of the samples compared to 32% with AGID. The study also showed that the type of specimen was an important factor in the ability to detect positive reactors: the ELISA detected antigen in 100% of the gum scraping, in 73% of the eye swabs and in 43% of the lymph nodes while the AGID test was positive on the same specimens in only 33%, 46% and 0% respectively. The ELISA detected PPRV in 70% of the nasal swabs and 50% of the lung samples, but none in lymph nodes or spleen. The study demonstrated, as also shown by Wafula *et al.*, (1986) using the AGID test, that gum scraping and ocular swabs from infected animals are the most suitable samples for this test as large quantities of virus antigen are present. Furthermore, the stability of the antigen in clinical samples was monitored for 4 days and the RPV and PPRV antigen was still detected in specimens left at 4 °C or at room temperature.

## Impact

The immunocapture ELISA is simple, rapid and highly specific and has been adopted as a routine technique in many laboratories involved in the Global Rinderpest Eradication Programme (GREP). The fact that the test reagents are very stable and can be delivered freeze-dried has facilitated the development of a kit and its introduction in developing countries. Epidemiosurveillance, with the aim of detecting rinderpest at or below 1% prevalence in the national herd, is one of the main activities of the Pan African Control of Epizootics (PACE) programme along with the ability also to detect PPRV and contagious bovine pleuropneumonia (CBPP) antigen to help in their control. The immunocapture ELISA is a prescribed OIE test and is an essential tool to GREP. The rationale for RPV/PPRV surveillance is to enable the detection of new outbreaks as rapidly as possible allowing a quick response and subsequent reduction in stock losses.

# Pen-side test for rinderpest

Although in the past the AGID kit has been used as a field test, it does not have the required sensitivity, specificity and rapidity to give a fast accurate diagnosis in the presence of the suspected infected animal (at pen-side). As indicated above, at the current stage of the GREP a rapid response to any emerging outbreak is essential to prevent further spread of disease. This is particularly pertinent in the areas where the remaining foci of endemic rinderpest persist, areas of social unrest and insecurity, such as the Somalia ecosystem.

Chromatographic strip-test technology (Clearview™) has existed for many years and is most widely used in human pregnancy testing. Until recently, it had rarely been applied to veterinary diagnostics, the first example being the use of a pen-side test developed for the detection of *Chlamydia* antigens in humans, which was shown to be suitable for use with sheep (Wilsmore and Davidson, 1991).

## Principle of the test

The principle of the chromatographic strip test is shown in Figure 8.2. The test device consists of a plastic case, approximately the size of a microscope slide, which encases a nitrocellulose membrane and has three 'windows' cut into the top surface: a 'sample' window, 'test' window and 'control' window (Plate 7). Virus-specific monoclonal antibodies are bound to blue latex particles and applied to an absorbent pad (situated under the sample window) in direct contact with a nitrocellulose membrane. The nitrocellulose membrane has an immobilized band of specific monoclonal antibody (situated under the test window) and a further band of immobilized anti-mouse antibody (situated under the control window). Addition of the sample to the sample window hydrates the latex particles and if antigen is present, the mAb on the particles 'captures' the antigen. The particles, complexed with antigen, move along the nitrocellulose membrane by a wick effect until they reach the band of specific mAb. The immobilized mAb 'captures' the antigen already bound to the particle, in a similar manner to an immunocapture ELISA, and there is an accumulation of blue particles which can be seen by the naked eye. Excess mAb-labelled particles migrate further along the nitrocellulose until they reach the immobilized anti-mouse antibody where

1. Dry strip

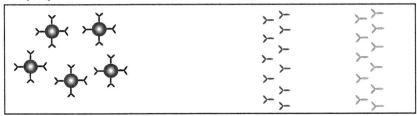

2. Add sample (containing antigen) in sample buffer

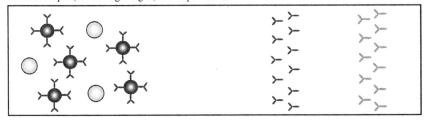

3. Antigen-antibody-particle complex moves due to wick effect

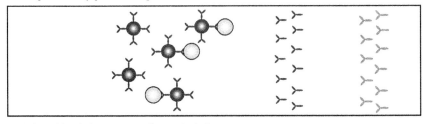

4. Coloured bands form at test and control windows

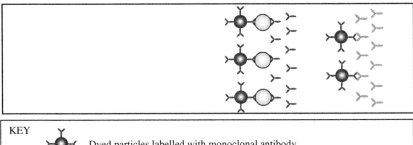

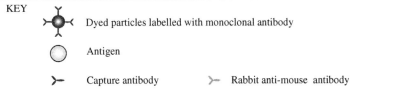

**Figure 8.2** Chromatographic strip test (Clearview) technology for pen-side diagnosis of rinderpest.

the mAb bound to the particle is captured by the anti-mouse antibody. This again leads to a build-up of blue particles visible to the naked eye. The whole process takes approximately 5–10 minutes. In negative samples a blue line is seen only at this position and its appearance indicates that the test is complete.

## Development

A panel of 100 rinderpest-specific mAbs were screened for their reactivity with a panel of rinderpest virus antigens. An mAb was selected based on its range of reactivity with the different RPV strains and the lack of cross-reactions with PPRV antigens. Optimal binding of the mAbs to the particles and nitro-cellulose is dependent on pH, molarity, type of buffer and antibody concentration. Binding conditions were optimized using pH and molarity gradients with different buffers and at different antibody concentrations. Once binding conditions were optimized, prototype devices were constructed to select the optimal sample buffer and evaluate their performance against a range of RPV infected tissue culture supernatants. Again this involved pH and molarity gradients of a range of buffers.

## Validation

The specificity and detection range of the prototype devices were tested against representatives of all three RPV lineages and also against PPRV strains (Bruning *et al.*, 1999). They were also tested against antigen preparations of bluetongue (BT), bovine virus diarrhoea (BVDV), canine distemper (CDV), epizootic haemorrhagic disease (EHDV) and foot-and-mouth disease (FMDV) viruses, all of which may be confused with rinderpest on clinical signs. The devices were capable of detecting all three lineages of rinderpest virus and showed no cross-reactions or non-specific results with antigens to PPRV, BTV, BVDV, CDV, EHDV or FMDV. Test sensitivity was evaluated by testing a dilution range of rinderpest viruses which had been pre-titrated in tissue culture. The minimum detection level for the strip-test using the attenuated variant of Kabete O was found to be $10^{2.5}$ $TCID_{50}$ while for all other RPV isolates the level of detection ranged from $10^{2.1}$ to $10^{4.3}$ $TCID_{50}$.

Test sensitivity and specificity were further examined using eye swabs collected daily from cattle either infected with virulent RPV or vaccinated with the attenuated RBOK vaccine strain. Positive strip-test results were found from 4–5 days post infection and continued until 9 days post infection, when the animals were killed. Similar results were obtained with immunocapture ELISA and confirmed by RT/PCR (see below). As expected, animals vaccinated with the attenuated RBOK vaccine had no detectable RPV antigen in the eye swabs since the vaccine virus is not transmissible. The test was also shown to be suitable for testing homogenates of a wide range of tissues from the lymphatic, respiratory and digestive system including tongue, gums, abomasum, ileum, liver and spleen tissues collected *post mortem*. Field samples submitted to the FAO World Reference Laboratory for Rinderpest and subsequently stored at $-70°C$ were also examined where the strip-test proved to be slightly more sensitive than the immunocapture ELISA.

## Field validation

Field trials of the prototype devices were carried out in Pakistan. The Pakistani veterinary officers and technicians found the test easy to use in the field and results overall indicated that the strip-test was more sensitive than the immunocapture ELISA but less sensitive than the PCR. Although the strip-test missed some individual PCR-positive samples, on a herd basis, the strip-test identified all the individual infected premises. Devices left behind after the field trial were subsequently used to detect some remaining foci of infection and assisted greatly in the RPV eradication campaign in Pakistan (Hussain *et al.*, 2001). Prototype devices were also used in Tanzania to confirm the presence of a mild strain of rinderpest (Wambura *et al.*, 2000).

Although the prototype was successful, it was felt that the intensity of the result band could be increased. Concerns regarding the test sensitivity to detect lineage 2 rinderpest virus also needed addressing. As a result an alternative mAb was adopted, which gave a wider range of detection, particularly of lineage 2 viruses. After further validation this has now been adopted in the final product (Svanova, Sweden) and these Mark II devices have been used successfully in Pakistan and are currently being used in the Somali ecosystem.

## Impact

The main impact has been to give local animal health officers and community-based animal health workers the ability to diagnose RPV at pen-side, without the delays incurred in sending samples back to national or international laboratories. They also have irrefutable evidence, in the form of the positive device, to attach to their reports.. An unexpected benefit is the ability to extract the RNA from the test device and sequence the PCR product, thus allowing the virus genotype to be determined if no other samples are available. The Mark II device has a greater range of detection and consequently shows a lower specificity resulting in cross-reactions with PPRV antigens. This should not pose a problem since PPRV is subclinical in cattle and complementary devices have been developed which are capable of specifically detecting PPRV antigen.

The ability of PPRV (but not RP) to haemagglutinate has led to the development of a haemagglutination test to detect PPRV antigen (Ezeibe *et al.*, 2004). This simple, specific, inexpensive diagnostic test is currently being evaluated in Nigeria, India and Pakistan.

# Genome detection for RPV and PPRV

The advent of the polymerase chain reaction (PCR) offered the possibility of extreme sensitivity and the ability to adjust test specificity. Initially, a broadly reactive test was required which was capable of detecting all strains of RPV and PPRV followed by highly specific assays to allow a differential diagnosis. Since these viruses have RNA genomes they must first be copied into DNA using an enzyme known as reverse transcriptase (RT), the RT step. The copy DNA (cDNA) is then amplified by PCR, the whole process being commonly known as RT–PCR (Forsyth and Barrett, 1995). Unfortunately, the high sequence variability found in RNA viruses makes it difficult to design a unique set of primers for RT-PCR amplification that are guaranteed capable of detecting all new field isolates. To overcome this problem and to allow differential diagnosis of RPV and PPRV several sets of primers were designed, based on well-conserved sequences in the N, P and F genes. The 'universal primers' for all morbilliviruses were derived from the N and P genes while RPV- and PPRV-specific primers were designed using F gene sequence data. Control primers to check the RNA quality were based on the highly conserved $\beta$-actin gene which is abundantly expressed in all cells and will be present even in negative samples (Forsyth and Barrett *et al.*, 1995). This strategy allowed the detection of field isolates from every region in the world where RPV and PPRV are known to exist. To facilitate the multiple PCR analyses, the RT step is performed using random hexanucleotide primers and aliquots of cDNA are then amplified using a panel of primer sets to identify and differentiate between the virus nucleic acids in the samples.

Initially, the test was optimized and validated using known positive RNA samples. A positive control must be included in every test as a qualitative measure of the RT and PCR amplification steps. Human measles virus RNA is used as the positive control to reduce any risk of cross-contamination and a resulting false-positive result. A negative control must also be performed to detect any possible contamination of reagents. A positive test produces DNA fragments of the expected size and their authenticity is confirmed either by direct sequence analysis of the DNA fragments or by a so-called nested PCR. In this a sample of the putative positive DNA is re-amplified using a primer set which is internal to the original set. This primer set will not be capable of amplifying any false-positive DNA fragments which may be produced in some cases and be close to the size expected for the positive sample.

RT–PCR was further validated using samples collected from experimentally infected animals. There was a difference between the results obtained from animals infected with two different strains of RPV. Viral RNA was detected as early as 2 days post infection in cattle infected with the virulent Kabete 'O' strain of virus compared to 4–6 days post infection in animals infected with the Saudi 1/81 strain. Similar strain variations were noted in PPRV infected goats.

Further test validation was carried out using field samples submitted to the WRLR from the Indian sub-continent, the Middle East and Africa. These represented 15 sets of diagnostic samples from nine countries totalling 68 individual samples. Of these, seven sets (23 samples) were examined by RT–PCR, virus isolation and AGID. Five sets of these (12 samples) were RT–PCR positive and none were positive for virus isolation or AGID. The need for employing multiple primer sets was highlighted in examining samples from an outbreak of PPRV in Pakistan where the field strain did not amplify with the 'universal' P gene primer set but did amplify with the F gene PPRV-specific primer set and the nested primers.

A major advantage of RT–PCR is the ability to sequence the PCR products and gain invaluable insight into the relationships between various isolates which can give some indication of the possible geographic origin of the virus. Over the years this has been built up into a database of sequences which show that there have been three distinct lineages of rinderpest, excluding the vaccine which forms a separate lineage, circulating in the world in the last 30 or so years. Similar sequence analyses have allowed the grouping of many PPRV field isolates into four distinct lineages based on F gene sequence data (Figure 8.3). The usefulness of this technology first proved itself in 1993 when an unusual outbreak of RPV occurred on the Russian–Mongolian border and the lineage was identified as being of Asian origin (Barrett *et al.*, 1993). Similarly in 1994, when an unexpected outbreak of RPV was diagnosed in wildlife, mainly buffalo (*Syncerus caffer*) and lesser kudu (*Tragelaphus imberbis*) in the Tsavo National Parks in the south of Kenya, away from the usual route of infection from Sudan in the north-west of the country, sequence analysis showed that it was from a second lineage of the virus which had previously been identified 30 years previously in the same region of Kenya and which was thought to have become extinct. This important finding indicated the presence of another, previously hidden, endemic focus in the region (Barrett *et al,* 1998; see also Chapter 7).

# Rinderpest antibody detection

## Virus neutralization test

The VNT for the detection of antibodies to rinderpest virus was developed by Plowright and Ferris (1961) using bovine kidney cell cultures as the indicator system and a constant virus dose/variable serum dilution technique. Originally performed in test tubes, this was later converted to a 96-well micro-plate assay using Vero or MDBK cells. Although used for many years to monitor the humoral antibody response to rinderpest vaccination, the VNT has now been replaced in most laboratories by the ELISA. This is due to the need for maintaining tissue culture and the requirement for sterile serum samples, both of which are extremely difficult in many developing countries.

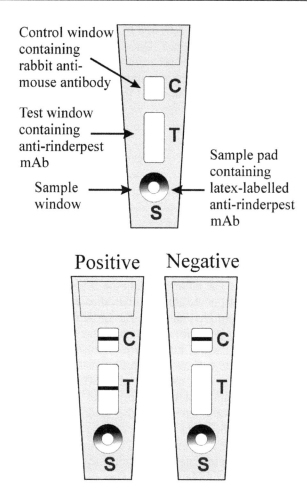

**Figure 8.3**  Pen-side test device.

The VNT still has a role in the examination of sera from game animals. Insufficient rinderpest-positive sera from the various game animal species have been tested by ELISA to ensure accurate determination of negative/positive cut-off points and background non-specific values; therefore it is recommended that game sera should be examined or at least confirmed by the VNT.

## Indirect ELISA

Due to the resurgence of rinderpest in Africa in the 1980s a massive rinderpest vaccination campaign was planned as a major part of the Pan African Rinderpest Campaign. The aim was to eradicate rinderpest from Africa using blanket vaccination to attain levels of sterilizing immunity (believed to be between 70–85% herd immunity) followed by cessation of vaccination, active disease search and serum surveillance. Due to the thermolabile nature of the live attenuated RBOK vaccine after reconstitution it was essential to carry out seromonitoring to evaluate the herd immunity and, indirectly, to monitor the performance of the vaccination teams and the cold chain (essential to maintaining the integrity of the attenuated vaccine). Most of the laboratories involved in the PARC had no tissue culture facilities; therefore an indirect ELISA was developed (Anderson *et al.*, 1982). This was field-trialled in Tanzania as part of their pre-PARC emergency programme by testing 20 000 sera each year. Results were initially compared with VNT results and the test was found to have a diagnostic sensitivity of 97% and diagnostic specificity of 97% (Anderson *et al.*, 1991a).

The assay was produced jointly as a kit by the Institute for Animal Health (IAH) and the Joint FAO/IAEA Animal Health Section in Vienna, Austria, being introduced to all countries involved in the PARC by a series of multinational training courses followed up with individual country visits and troubleshooting where necessary. The laboratories in the 'IAEA Rinderpest Network' were supplied with quality controlled, standardized kits and regular training and updates from staff from IAH and CIRAD–EMVT. The test was used successfully from 1986 to 1990 for seromonitoring throughout the PARC. However, the indirect ELISA was not rinderpest-specific and gave cross-reactions with antibodies to PPRV. This caused problems in PPRV endemic regions when examining sheep sera and also with cattle which had been exposed to PPRV and developed a humoral antibody response. The test was also significantly affected by poor water quality in the laboratories which sometimes required the use of bottled drinking water for the preparation of blocking buffer until the distillation plant or de-ionizer could be replaced. Sera which had been frozen and thawed many times (due to electricity cuts at local laboratories) also gave some problems. These problems resulted in a reduced differential between positive and negative samples that was overcome through the development of a monoclonal antibody-based competitive ELISA that allowed testing of all animal species with a single conjugate.

## Competitive ELISA

A competitive ELISA (c-ELISA) (Figure 8.5) for the detection of antibodies to RPV was developed in 1994 (Anderson *et al.*, 1991b) and was adopted for use throughout the PARC in 1995. The principle of the test (see Figure 8.4) was the interruption of the reaction between RPV antigen and mAb against RPV by the addition of test serum samples. The presence of antibodies to RPV in the test serum sample blocked the reactivity of the mAb resulting in a reduction of the expected colour, following the addition of enzyme-labelled anti-mouse antibody and substrate/chromogen. The mAb used in the test was RPV-specific, directed against the viral haemagglutinin (H), and gave no cross-reactions with

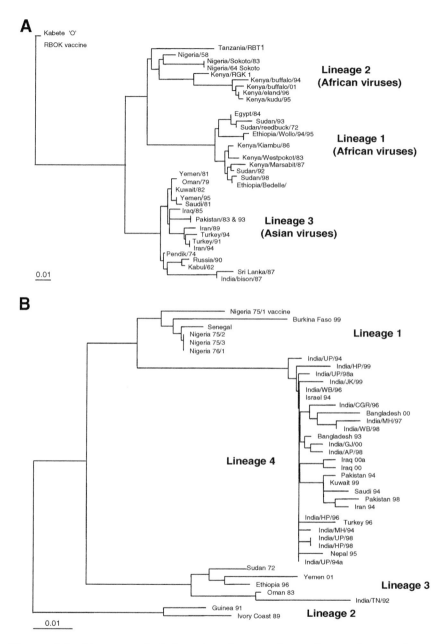

**Figure 8.4** Lineages of rinderpest and peste des petits ruminants viruses. Phylogenetic trees for rinderpest viruses (A) and peste des petits ruminants viruses (B). The trees were derived using the PHYLIP DNADIST and FITCH programmes (Felsenstein, 1997). The branch lengths are proportional to the genetic distances between the viruses and the hypothetical common ancestor that existed at the nodes in the tree. The bar represents nucleotide changes per position.

antibodies to the closely related PPRV. Other workers (Libeau *et al.*, 1991) developed competitive assays based on mAbs directed against the N protein of RPV, but these showed cross-reactivity with PPRV antibodies which precluded their use for seromonitoring, particularly in areas with endemic PPRV.

The anti-H c-ELISA was validated by comparison with the indirect ELISA and the VNT. Overall there was a 98% agreement between the anti-H c-ELISA and the VNT but the most significant improvement was in comparison with the indirect ELISA. Serum samples which had been frozen and thawed many times and gave poor results by indirect ELISA still showed clear negative and positive populations when the anti-H c-ELISA results were subject to frequency distribution analysis. Another major advantage was the ability to test sera from any animal species without the need for species-specific conjugates. A complementary assay was also developed for the detection of antibodies to PPRV (Anderson *et al.*, 1991a).

The assay is still used throughout Africa, Asia and the Middle East and has proved to be extremely reliable and robust. The test was less affected by poor water quality and the use of an mAb-based assay allowed a very high level of standardisation. Regular external quality assurance testing for the c-ELISA, organized by the Joint Division FAO/IAEA, showed a 99% agreement between all laboratories in the Rinderpest Network.

As the Global Rinderpest Eradication Programme started to take effect, more countries ceased vaccination as they moved through the OIE Pathway for rinderpest eradication. This meant a transition from rinderpest seromonitoring (the detection of antibody response following rinderpest vaccination) to serum surveillance (the detection of antibodies following infection). The c-ELISA had originally been developed for the detection of antibodies to the rinderpest vaccine strain and doubts were expressed as to the sensitivity of the assay to detect antibodies to other field strains of virus. Sera collected from experimentally infected animals showed that although the assay had a lower sensitivity for detecting antibodies to other lineages of rinderpest virus the assay was still capable of detecting them, albeit at a later stage post infection. Some suggested that the c-ELISA based on the rinderpest N protein would offer greater sensitivity and another alternative was the baculovirus expressed N protein indirect ELISA (Yilma *et al.*, 2003). However, at a GREP Technical Consultation, the consensus was that test sensitivity is not the most important factor for serum surveillance. Test specificity is the most important, since false-positive results will stimulate too many suspect rinderpest investigations for which the countries involved lack the resources or manpower to carry out. The anti-H c-ELISA was shown to have the highest specificity. Over a number of years, following cessation of vaccination in Ethiopia, the number of 'false-positive' results was calculated. Initially, the numbers were slightly higher, due to inaccuracies in ageing animals based on dentition, but after 3–4 years the numbers found were approximately 0.5%. This gives the anti-H c-ELISA a specificity of 99.5% under field conditions (personal communication, Van't Klooster).

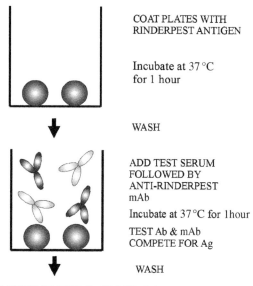

COAT PLATES WITH
RINDERPEST ANTIGEN

Incubate at 37 °C
for 1 hour

WASH

ADD TEST SERUM
FOLLOWED BY
ANTI-RINDERPEST
mAb

Incubate at 37 °C for 1 hour

TEST Ab & mAb
COMPETE FOR Ag

WASH

**ADD ANTI-MOUSE HRPO CONJUGATE**

Incubate at 37°C for 1 hour, wash, add substrate/chromogen

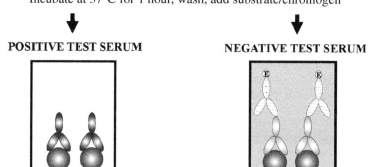

**POSITIVE TEST SERUM**

**NEGATIVE TEST SERUM**

TEST ANTIBODY BINDS TO ANTIGEN

DETECTING Ab (mAb)
CANNOT BIND

CONJUGATE (ANTI-MOUSE)
CANNOT BIND

NO ENZYME PRESENT

**NO COLOUR**

TEST ANTIBODY DOES NOT BIND

DETECTING Ab (mAb)
BINDS TO ANTIGEN

CONJUGATE (ANTI-MOUSE)
BINDS

ENZYME PRESENT

**COLOUR**

**Figure 8.5**   Principle of competitive ELISA.

A figure of 100% specificity was quoted by Geiger, Wamwai and Ndungu in an independent evaluation reported at the FAO-EMPRES Technical Consultation on GREP 2002 and a similar figure was derived from testing 11 982 serum samples from cattle and buffalo in Thailand, all of which were found to be negative. An excellent summary of all available data on anti-H c-ELISA specificity and sensitivity is included in a document prepared by Roland Geiger (2004) for the Animal Production and Health Section of the Joint Division FAO/IAEA. He states that at a cut-off of 50% test sensitivity may range from 60 to 70% in some groups of animals infected with lineage 2 RPV to close to 100% in animals vaccinated with the RBOK vaccine. The specificity of the test being close to 100%, it is expected that not more than five samples will give false-positive results if sera from 1000 genuinely negative animals are tested. This drastically reduces the number of follow-up investigations needed compared to other assays of lower specificity.

The aim of GREP is to declare the world free of rinderpest by 2010. Before this declaration can be made, a global serological survey will have to take place to demonstrate the lack of any circulating rinderpest virus. The use of the anti-H c-ELISA will allow standardization and comparability between all the testing laboratories, a situation which is the envy of many medical health programmes.

# References

Abraham, G. and Berhan, A. (2001) The use of antigen-capture enzyme-linked immunosorbent assay (ELISA) for the diagnosis of rinderpest and peste des petits ruminants in Ethiopia. *Trop. Anim. Hlth Prod.* **33** (5), 423–30.

Anderson, J., Anderson, E.C., Chiduo, F., Joshua, G.E., Loretu, K., Mpelumbe, I.E. and Kavishe, T.E. (1991a) Field evaluation of the indirect ELISA for sero-monitoring during the rinderpest eradication campaign in Tanzania. In: *Seromonitoring of Rinderpest throughout Africa: Phase One.* Proceedings of a meeting held in Bingerville, Cote d'Ivoire 19–23 November 1990. IAEA-TECDOC-623. Vienna: International Atomic Energy Agency, pp. 87–101.

Anderson, J., Barrett, T. and Scott, G. R. (1996) *Manual on the Diagnosis of Rinderpest*, 2nd edn. Rome: FAO Animal Health Manual 1.

Anderson, J., McKay, J.A. and Butcher, R.N. (1991b) The use of monoclonal antibodies in competitive ELISA for the detection of antibodies to rinderpest and peste des petits ruminants viruses. In: *Seromonitoring of Rinderpest throughout Africa: Phase One.* Proceedings of the Final Research Coordination Meeting of the IAEA Rinderpest Control Projects, Cote d'Ivoire, 19–23 November 1990. IAEA-TECDOC-623. Vienna: International Atomic Energy Agency.

Anderson, J., Rowe, L.W., Taylor, W.P. and Crowther, J.R. (1982) An enzyme-linked immunosorbent assay for the detection of IgG, IgA and IgM antibodies to rinderpest virus in experimentally infected cattle. *Res. Vet. Sci.* **32**, 242–7.

Barrett, T., Amarel-Doel, C., Kitching, R.P. and Gusev, A. (1993) Use of the polymerase chain reaction in differentiating rinderpest field virus and vaccine virus in the same animals. *Rev. Sci. Tech.* **12**, 865–72.

Barrett, T., Forsyth, M.A., Inui, K., Wamwayi, H.M., Kock, R., Wambua, J., Mwanzia, J., Rossiter, P.B. (1998) Rediscovery of the second African lineage of rinderpest virus: its epidemiological significance. *Vet. Rec.* **142** (24), 669–71.

Bourdin, P. and Doutre, M.P (1976) Rinderpest in small ruminants in Senegal. Current data. *Rev. Elev. Med. Vét. Pays Trop.* **29**, 199–204.

Bruning, A., Bellamy, K., Talbot, D. and Anderson, J. (1999) A rapid chromatographic strip test for the pen-side diagnosis of rinderpest virus. *J. Virol. Methods* **81**, 143–54.

Ehrlich, P.J. and Moyle, R.W. (1986) Ultrasensitive cooperative immunoassays with mixed monoclonal antibodies. *Methods Enzymol.* **121**, 695–702.

Ezeibe, M.C.O., Wosu, L.O. and Erumaka, I.G. (2004) Standardisation of the haemagglutination test for peste des petits ruminants (PPR). *Small Ruminant Res.* **51** (3), 269–72.

Felsenstein, J. (1997) An alternative least squares approach to inferring phylogenies from pairwise distances. *Syst. Biol.* **46**, 101–11.

Forsyth, M.A. and Barrett, T. (1995) Evaluation of polymerase chain reaction for the detection and characterisation of rinderpest and peste des petits ruminants viruses for epidemiological studies. *Virus Res.* **39** (2–3), 151–63.

Geiger, R. (2004) Towards the OIE recognition of freedom of infection from rinderpest. Guidelines for serological surveillance and the laboratory testing of rinderpest; results of an FAO/IAEA consultants Meeting. IAEA-TECDOC (in press).

Gibbs, L.P.J., Taylor, W.P., Lawman, M.J.P. and Bryant, J. (1979) Classification of the peste des petits ruminants virus as the fourth member of the genus Morbillivirus. *Int. Virol.* **11**, 268–74

Hussain, M., Iqbal, M., Taylor, W.P. and Roeder, P.L. (2001) Pen-side test for the diagnosis of rinderpest in Pakistan. *Vet. Rec.* **149** (10), 300–2.

Kobune, K., Sakata, H., Sugiyama, M. and Sugiura, A. (1991) B95a, a marmoset lymphoblastoid cell line, as a sensitive host for rinderpest virus. *J. Gen. Virol.* **72**, 687–92.

Lefèvre, P.C. (1987) Peste des petits ruminants et infection bovipestique des ovins et des caprins. *Études et synthèses de l'Institut d'Elevage et de Médecine Vétérinaire des Pays Tropicaux*, 2nd edn.

Libeau, G. and Lefèvre, P.C. (1990) Comparison of rinderpest and peste des petits ruminants viruses using anti-nucleoprotein monoclonal antibodies. *Vet. Microbiol.* **25**, 1–16.

Libeau, G., Diallo, A., Calvez, D. and Lefevre, P.C. (1991) A competitive ELISA using anti-N monoclonal antibodies for specific detection of rinderpest antibodies in cattle and small ruminants. In: *Seromonitoring of Rinderpest throughout Africa: Phase One.* Proceedings of a meeting held in Bingerville Cote d'Ivoire, 19–23 November 1990. IAEA-TECDOC-623. Vienna: International Atomic Energy Agency, pp. 55–66.

Libeau, G., Diallo, A., Colas, F. and Guerre, L. (1994) Rapid differential diagnosis of rinderpest and peste des petits ruminants using an immunocapture ELISA. *Vet. Rec.* **134**, 300–4.

Libeau, G., Saliki, J.T. and Diallo, A. (1997) Caractérisation d'anticorps monoclonaux dirigés contre le virus de la peste bovine et de la peste des petits ruminants: identification d'épitopes conservés ou de spécificité stricte sur la nucléoprotéine. *Rev. Elev. Méd. Vét. Pays Trop.* **51**, 181–90.

Macadam, I. (1968) Transmission of rinderpest from goats to cattle in Tanzania. *Bull. Epizoot. Dis. Afr.* **16**, 53–60.

McCullough, K.C., Sheshberadaran, H., Norrby, E., Obi, T.U. and Crowther, J.R. (1986) Monoclonal antibodies against morbilliviruses. *Rev. Sci. Tech. Off. Int. Epizoot.* **5**, 411–27.

Nikkari, S., Halonen, P., Kharitonenkov, I., Kivivirta, M., Khristova, M., Waris, M. and Kendal, A. (1989) One-incubation time-resolved fluoroimmunoassay based on monoclonal antibodies in detection of influenza A and B viruses directly in clinical specimen. *J. Virol. Methods* **23**, 29–40.

Plowright, W. and Ferris, R.D. (1961) Studies with rinderpest virus in tissue culture. III. The stability of cultured virus and its use in virus neutralisation tests. *Arch. Virol.* **11**, 516–33.

Roeder, P. and van't Klooster, G. (2004) Guidelines for confirming suspected outbreaks of rinderpest by laboratory examination. In: PACE Common Services Technical and Workshop Reports, 9th Advisory Committee Meeting of the PACE Programme, 5–7 April 2004, Nairobi, Kenya.

Rossiter, P.B., Herniman, A.J. and Wamwai, H.M. (1992) Improved isolation of rinderpest virus in transformed bovine T lymphoblast cell lines. *Res. Vet. Sci.* **53**, 11–18.

Rossiter, P.B. and Mushi, E.Z. (1980) Rapid detection of rinderpest virus antigen by counter-immuno-electrophoresis. *Trop. Anim. Hlth Prod.* **12**, 209–16.

Rossiter, P.B., Taylor, W.P. and Crowther, J.R. (1988) Antigenic variation between three strains of rinderpest virus detected by kinetic neutralisation and competition ELISA using early rabbit antisera. *Vet. Microbiol.* **16**, 195.

Saliki, J.T. (1993) Structure and functional characterization of various isolates of peste des petits ruminants virus using monoclonal antibodies. PhD, Cornell University.

Taylor, W.P. (1979) Serological studies with the virus of peste des petits ruminants in Nigeria. *Res. Vet. Sci.* **26**, 236–42.

Wafula, J.S., Mirangi, P.K., Ireri, R.G. and Mbugua, N. (1986) Development and stability of rinderpest virus antigens in cattle tears and lymph nodes. *Trop. Anim. Hlth Prod.* **18**, 26–30.

Wambura, P.N., Moshy, D.W., Mbise, A.N., Mollel, G.O., Taylor, W.P., Anderson, J. and Bruning, A. (2000) Diagnosis of rinderpest in Tanzania by a rapid chromatographic strip-test. *Trop. Anim. Hlth Prod.* **32**, 141–5.

White, G. (1958) A specific diffusible antigen of rinderpest virus demonstrated by the agar double-immunodiffusion precipitation reaction. *Nature (Lond.)* **181**, 1409.

Wilsmore, A.J. and Davidson, I. (1991) Clearview rapid test compared with other methods to diagnose chlamydial infection. *Vet. Rec.* **128**, 503–4.

Yilma, T., Aziz, F., Ahmad, S., Jones, L., Ngotho, R., Wamwai, H., Beyene, B., Yesus, M., Egziabher, B., Diop, M., Sarr, J. and Verardi, P. (2003) Inexpensive vaccines and rapid diagnostic kits tailor-made for the global eradication of rinderpest, and technology transfer to Africa and Asia. *Dev. Biol. (Basel)*, **114**, 99–111.

Zwart, D. and Macadam, I. (1967a) Transmission of rinderpest by contact from cattle to sheep and goats. *Res. Vet. Sci.* **8**, 37–47.

Zwart, D. and Macadam, I. (1967b) Observation of rinderpest in sheep and goats and transmission to cattle. *Res. Vet. Sci.* **8**, 53–57.

# Old prophylactic methods

# 9

## JEAN BLANCOU
*Paris, France*

## Introduction

According to the *Dictionary of Veterinary Epidemiology*, prophylaxis is a set of measures employed to prevent the occurrence of a disease. It can be applied at the level of the individual or population and involve medical (e.g. biological or pharmaceutical) or sanitary (e.g. isolation or disinfection) measures. When the objective of treatment is to reduce pathogen excretion and consequently reduce the risk of exposing naive animals to infection, treatment of the infected individuals constitutes a prophylactic measure for the population (Toma, 1999).

In very early times, prophylactic measures were targeted to individuals rather than populations, the successful *treatment* of a single animal benefiting the rest of the herd and contributing to control the spread of the epizootic. Later *sanitary* and *medical measures* were applied at the herd level and, where necessary, at the regional level. These two approaches were used either to compete with or complement each other, depending on the situation. As far as rinderpest is concerned, many of the measures described above have been recommended or used since ancient times, when this disease was widespread in many regions of the world.

This chapter will deal with these prophylactic methods as applied to rinderpest infections, focusing on those used up until the beginning of the twentieth century, before the discovery of modern prophylactic tools. These new methods are described at length in other chapters of this monograph (see Chapters 8 and 11).

## Individual animal treatment

The *Veterinary Papyrus of Kahun (El-Lahun)*, written between 2130 and 1930 BC, contains descriptions of diseased bulls suffering from enteritis, suppurating eyes and abdominal pain. An in-depth analysis of these descriptions by Walker convinced the author that the cause of such disease was likely to be rinderpest (Walker, 1964). The treatment recommended was generally aimed at lowering the body temperature by pouring cold water on the sick animal. Such therapy was of course unlikely to cure the disease and was unable to prevent its spreading in the herd, but it at least shows that the Egyptians did not want to let sick animals just die, or possibly contaminate each other.

In the Graeco-Roman period, more attention was paid to the diseases of sheep or horses rather than those of cattle. The different disease conditions seen in these species were not clearly distinguished, the same treatments being applied to all species. This probably led to mis-diagnosis of the many different diseases of bovids, for example rinderpest and contagious bovine pleuropneumonia.

Cato the Elder (234–149 BC) recommended that, in the case of any disease of cattle (*bos*), the sick animal should be made to swallow a raw egg, followed the next day by wine poured from a wooden bowl in a which an onion had been rubbed, both the patient and the attendant being in a state of fasting and 'standing above the ground'. Most of these recommendations are tainted with magic: the wood, as well as standing above the ground (i.e. standing on a board, as represented in some Roman *bas-reliefs)*, was thought to help avoid the bad influence of the earth, the source of disease. The same recommendations were repeated 200 years later by Columella, who suggested pouring the wine directly into the nostrils of the sick animal (*'in naribus infundas'*), which is potentially very dangerous to the animal being treated (Columella, translated 1954).

The isolation of animals, before or after treatment, was also recommended by Columella and this quarantine of sick animals was much more effective in controlling the epizootics. Unfortunately, from the Middle Ages to the eighteenth century, the wise statement of Columella was forgotten. This period was the golden age of curative procedures based on magic, superstition or religious practices, which for centuries were the only means available to treat human or animal diseases. Around the year AD 1000, the Anglo-Saxon Leech Books recommended that 'if cattle were dying' a concoction made from groundsel, springwort, cockspur grass and cleavers should be poured into the mouth of the sick animal, making five crosses of hassuck grass (set on four sides of the cattle), and singing the *Benedicam* etc. around the cattle (Spinage, 2003). The resort to prayers tended rather to encourage contagion, by calling meetings in front of the church and bringing large numbers of animals together to be blessed. In Belgium such gatherings were officially prohibited in 1745 on pain of excommunication (Société des Médecins de Genève 1745; Curasson, 1942; Mammerickx, 1994).

When rinderpest was again introduced into Europe from eastern countries in 1711, new attempts were made to treat disease using animal, vegetable or mineral polypharmacy. 'Theriaca', a potion containing the flesh of a viper, in favour since Nero's time, mercury, salt, and wine or a more unusual medication containing urine and pigeon droppings were said to be 'effective on one animal in two' and came into fashion again around this time (Paulet, 1775). Of course bleeding, purgatives, enemas and setons were also recommended 'to reduce the raging action of the venom' (Theves, 1994). These treatments are described at length in some historical reviews (Mammerickx, 1994; Blancou, 2003; Spinage 2003).

It is sufficient to say that none of them was effective, and Lancisi, as early as 1715, was one of the first to protest against them stating that 'it was better to kill all sick and suspect animals, instead of allowing the disease to spread in order to have enough time and the honour to discover a specific treatment that is often searched for without any success' (Leclainche, 1955; Mantovani and Zanetti, 1993). This statement was repeated for centuries: in 1746 the English King's Privy Council stated again that 'all the methods of cure which have been put in practice, both at home and abroad, have proved so unsuccessful, that they have rather contributed to propagate than stop the infection'. This statement is still valid today, as nobody in almost 300 years has succeeded in curing the cattle plague.

# Sanitary measures

## Isolation

Columella was the first Roman author to recommend that, if the plague falls upon a herd, the cattle must be divided up, into a number of groups, and sent to distant places with infected animals being segregated from the healthy (*segregandi a sanis morbidi*) so that no infected animal may come into contact with the rest and destroy them with contagion (Columella, translated 1997). During the Byzantine period, Vegetius in his *Mulomedicina* (written at the end of the fourth century) made exactly the same recommendation, but did not agree with the previous Roman authors who imputed the contagion to 'divine displeasure'. Contrary to what is stated erroneously by most of the veterinary historians, Vegetius criticized these practices and stated that this divine origin was invoked 'only by fools, as is often the case' (*a sultis, ut solet*) (Blancou, 2003).

Undoubtedly, the most comprehensive descriptions of effective prophylactic measures taken against rinderpest were provided by Giovani Maria Lancisi (1654–1720). He is considered as the 'co-inventor', along with Thomas Bates, of the process of sanitary prophylaxis for this disease (Bates, 1718). Although Lancisi is the one who paved the way for the eradication of cattle plague in Europe (Wilkinson, 1992; Mantovani and Zanetti, 1993), perhaps being afraid to appear too modern, he refers to Virgil and Columella's recommendations to control contagious diseases in sheep.

When rinderpest was first introduced to Padua in 1711, Lancisi, as an archiater, was charged with coordination of the control of rinderpest in the Papal States. In his famous book *De Bovilla Peste* (published in 1715) he made 11 precise recommendations to eliminate the disease. These included the confinement of: infected bovines (recommendation no. 2), dairy cows (recommendation no. 9), recovered animals (recommendation no. 10) and farmers and dogs from the affected premises (recommendation no. 11) (Lancisi, 1715) (Figure 9.1).

# JO: MARIÆ LANCISII

A' Secretiori Cubiculo , & Archiatri Pontificii

## DISSERTATIO HISTORICA

### D E

# BOVILLA PESTE,

Ex Campaniæ finibus anno MDCCXIII
Latio importata:

## D E Q U E   P R Æ S I D I I S

PER SANCTISSIMUM PATREM

# CLEMENTEM XI.

## PONTIFICEM MAXIMUM

Ad avertendam aëris labem , & Annonæ caritatem
opportunè adhibitis .

Cui accedit Confilium de Equorum Epidemia , quæ Romæ
graffata eft Anno M D C C X I I.

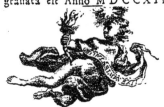

ROMÆ   MDCCXV.

Ex Typographia Joannis Mariæ Salvioni
In Archigymnafio S Apientiæ.

SVPERIORVM PERMISSV.

Melchior · Magius · S. Domus · et · Ciuit: Lauretanæ.
· ∽ · Gubernator · 1715 · ∽ ·
· ∽ · ∽ ·

**Figure 9.1**   Facsimile of the original *Dissertatio* of Giovani Maria Lancisi.

In July 1714 Bates was nominated by the Lords Justices to investigate the first outbreak of rinderpest in England. In his initial report to the King, he started by recommending the separation of animals when any sickness was detected (Spinage, 2003). Subsequently, all the official measures for isolation taken in Europe were directly inspired by the original advice of Bates and Lancisi, for example in Germany (1714), France (1745), Luxembourg (1769). Additional measures were also taken to ensure the proper enforcement of these regulations. These included branding the horns of suspect cattle (the first attempt to ensure the traceability of live animals), establishing sanitary cordons around the infected farms, and controlling these cordons with the help of the army. In the case of severe episodes of the disease (e.g. in 1745 in the county of Oldenburg, Germany) even pigs, sheep and geese were to be confined (Greve, 1927).

## Import restrictions and quarantine measures

The importation of cattle from an infected country was prohibited for the first time in 1599 by the cities of Venice and Padua. At that time rinderpest was raging in Hungary and Dalmatia, putting Western Europe at risk. Leclainche commented that this decision marked the birth of veterinary sanitary policing (Leclainche, 1955).

A decree of 20 October 1716 promulgated by Friedrich Wilhelm I of Prussia stipulated quarantine measures for animals imported from foreign countries. These measures were later adopted by most of the other European countries. In 1714 the Governor of the Austrian Low Countries stipulated that a health certificate be required for imported cattle as well as for meat and fresh or salted hides. On 6 January 1739, an Order of the King of France banned the importation of foreign cattle without such a certificate and a health certificate was also required for persons accompanying the animals.

An order of the French Royal Council made on 31 January 1771, which regulated trade in animals in the event of an epizootic, was rigorously applied during a rinderpest episode in the south of France in 1774: even the export of pigs and sheep to foreign countries was banned, no doubt to avoid people or material becoming contaminated and bringing the pathogen back on their return. (Caput, 1966). During the nineteenth century, a quarantine period of 20 days was required for the 'Steppe cattle' imported into Western Europe from Eastern Europe (Scott, 1996).

## Slaughter and compensation

Lancisi and Bates simultaneously were the first to recommend stamping-out as the most effective measure available to combat the cattle plague. Lancisi recommended sacrificing cattle that were definitely contaminated by 'hitting them with a lead ball so as to not spill a single drop of infected blood'. The original text, in low Latin, unfortunately does not clearly state how to kill the animal, since the Latin word *glandis* refers to a lead ball used in a catapult (Lancisi, 1715) Bates recommended that the owners of sick cows should bring them to be slaughtered at the first signs of the disease (quoted in Spinage, 2003).

According to Leclainche, the first example of direct compensatory measures for livestock owners in the event of slaughter of their diseased animals was during the epizootic of rinderpest which killed more than 5000 head of cattle between July and December 1714 in England. At that time, Bates recommended the killing and destruction of sick cattle, and a reward of 5–40 shillings, depending on the age of the animal, was allocated from the Civil List of King George I. As can always happen, this kind of reward had unwanted effects and fraudsters were denounced in a satirical poem of John Morphew in 1717: 'some cunning huxters, who had cows old, dry and lean ... knock'd 'em on the head ... and claimed the sum of forty shillings'! (Fleming, 1871). In 1716, Friedrich Wilhelm I also made the sacrifice of sick animals compulsory. They were to be separated immediately from the healthy cattle and branded on the horn. Those who disobeyed were to be flogged and hanged (Torner, 1927). In 1745, in the German county of Oldenburg, dogs and cats were also ordered to be killed by being shot or beaten to death (Greve, 1927).

## Destruction of carcasses

The earliest recommendations to destroy the carcasses of cattle that had died from contagious disease are to be found again in the writings of Vegetius: he advised the farmers to bury these cadavers deeply, and far from their house, to avoid contagion by their viscera (*'usque eo etiam mortua cadavera ultra fines villae projicienda sunt, et altisimae obruenda sunt sub terris'*) (cited by Layard, 1757; Simonds and Brown, 1868). The same recommendation was repeated 1000 years later by health officers in Lyons (France), when farmers were obliged to bury their dead animals at a depth of 6 feet, in quicklime, during an epizootic in 1604 (Hours, 1957).

During the first outbreak of rinderpest in England in 1714, Bates recommended that all cattle from affected herds should be destroyed and burnt. Later, because too many cattle were required to be burnt, he changed his mind and recommended burial in a hole 4½–6 feet deep and covered in quicklime (Spinage, 2003).

Interestingly, the same story was repeated in Great Britain some three centuries later, during the epizootic of foot-and-mouth in 2001: the cost of the first huge and polluting blazes convinced the government to change to using mass burial sites for the carcasses. Lancisi, in 1715, recommended burying the cadavers deeply, without removing so much as a hair, and at the same time burying all their excreta and 'any drop of virulent material' (Lancisi, 1715; Mantovani and Zanetti, 1993).

## Destruction or decontamination of other virulent material

Carcasses were not the only source of contagion that was targeted during the fight against rinderpest in the past. In 1559, rinderpest in cattle and dysentery in humans were raging at the same time in the States of Venice. The sale or distribution of meat, butter or cheese obtained from cows affected by rinderpest was therefore prohibited, and these had to be destroyed, under pain of death (Leclainche, 1955).

Again, the 11 recommendations of Lancisi in 1715 were the most appropriate and pragmatic regarding the decontamination of infected material. After the sacrifice of the affected animals, he tried to eliminate every remaining source of virulence. This started with the walls and the floor of the cowshed and the mangers being scraped and cleaned of all dirt and litter which were then to be burnt: Lancisi referred specifically to the laws of Moses, applied in case of human leprosy, as a precedent.. Decontamination measures were also applied to containers and drinking troughs, which were to be washed with strong lye obtained with quicklime, as well as to the clothing of the farmers, which were to be disinfected by fumigation with sulphur and aromatic chemicals (Lancisi, 1715). This advice was later followed by other authorities, for example in France where walls and floor of infected cowsheds were to be washed with lime water or vinegar, stables fumigated with juniper, sulphur etc., or in Germany where contaminated objects were disinfected by fumigation with sulphur or with caustic soda, and live pigs, sheep and geese were washed with vinegar (Greve, 1927).

It was not until 1775 that scientific trials were carried out to check the actual resistance of the contagious agent to such treatments. Vicq d'Azyr, a French physician, demonstrated that the fresh hides of bovines that had died from rinderpest were unable to transmit the disease to naive animals if treated with lime for six days, or even less. Twenty years later, Abilgaard in Denmark showed that the contagion in infected material could be destroyed when exposed to a temperature of at least 150 °C (Curasson, 1942).

# Medical measures

## Religion, magic and drugs

When many centuries ago rinderpest was widespread in Eurasia, farmers as well as human and animal healers were powerless to prevent it and, as in the case of many other diseases, the religious authorities implored the heavens. In the year 376, Cardinal Baronius said that no animal was safe unless it was branded on the forehead with a red-hot iron in the form of a cross (Fleming, 1871). In the thirteenth century, the Arabs (Asthahoursis) favoured magic, and hung elephant or camel teeth around the necks of their cattle to prevent the cattle plague (Moulé, 1896).

During the Middle Ages drugs that were considered to be efficacious were used to prevent the disease. Even as late as 1648, Gervase Markham described 'a medicine which never failed to preserve as many (cattle) as have taken it: take of old urine a quart, and mix it with a handfull of Hens dung dissolved therein, and leat your beast drink it' (Swabe, 1997). In 1759, Danish farmers attempted (without great success) to preserve their cattle from the infection by the fumes of tobacco, which they continually smoked in the cowsheds, even sitting up the whole night in turns in the midst of the herd for that purpose (Fleming, 1871).

## Inoculation

The idea that rinderpest in animals was a similar disease to smallpox in humans led to the idea that it could be controlled by 'variolation' (or 'variolization'). Recommendation of this treatment was published for the first time in 1711 in Geneva in *Dissertatio*: *De contagiosa epidemia, quae in Patavino Agro, & tota ferè veneta dicione in Boves irrepsit* by Bernardino Ramazzini. According to Karasszon and Scott, Ramazzini tried to protect healthy cattle by threading through their dewlap setons soaked in morbid effluents of sick animals (Karasszon, 1988; Scott, 1996), but no mention of this trial can be found in his original *Dissertatio* (Mantovani and Zanetti, 1993). In any case, the idea of inoculation was not really new to Europe, where many attempts had already been made to protect ovines and caprines against sheep pox by inoculating them with infectious material (Hurtrel d'Arboval, 1839). In the case of rinderpest, the idea came from the observation that, although more than 75% of animals died from the disease when naturally contaminated, the mortality rate was only 25% when they were experimentally inoculated with infectious material (Theves, 1994).

Little is known about the results of Ramazzini's first trials and if they really achieved their objective. He died soon afterwards and Spinage raises doubts about their reality (Spinage, 2003). Nevertheless, such trials were later undertaken by others in an attempt to avoid sacrificing the animals. Attempts were made in Brunswick (Germany) in 1746, then in England by Sir William St Quintin (1754) and Layard (1757), in France by Vicq d'Azyr (1774), in Germany again by Bulow, in Switzerland by Berg, in the Netherlands by Nozeman, Kool, Swencke, Tak and later by Sandiford, van Doeveren and Camper (1755–69) (see also Chapter 5). Most of these research workers recognized that preventive inoculation could be dangerous under certain circumstances, and should not be practised in disease-free herds. Layard, in particular, stated that 'no one will think of bringing the infection into any place free from it ... but, if the contagious distemper be in the neighbourhood of a herd ..., by inoculating his cattle ... the grazier or farmer may secure his flock' (Layard, 1757). Vicq d'Azyr, after unsuccessful trials in France, also concluded that inoculation was undesirable since all farm animals died of it (Cavrot, 1999; Vallat, 2001). Fleming, in 1871, stated that: 'many able men have asserted that to the adoption of this remedy [the inoculation] Holland was longer in getting rid of the plague than any other country'.

The interest shown throughout Europe in this technique had nevertheless convinced the Russian authorities to verify its validity. Trials were organized in seven experimental stations, using several hundred cattle of different breeds and ages. The results of these trials were analysed by a Commission which concluded, in January 1863, 'that their [negative] observations obtained with the most meticulous care and with exact controls were more convincing than a thousand experiments performed without any critical assessment and without any appreciation of accidental circumstances'. The experimental stations were, therefore, shut down in Russia and inoculations were abandoned in that country as well as in most of the other European countries.

## Serum and vaccines

Other approaches were taken to protect cattle from rinderpest; for example at the end of the eighteenth century Petrus Camper tried inoculations with lung fragments containing small worms, which he found in dead animals and believed to be the causal agents of the disease (Leclainche, 1955). Trials were continued in the nineteenth century when experts in the disease realized that the stamping-out method was not applicable in the free-ranging herds of Eastern Europe, Asia or Africa. Therefore, in 1896 Koch was invited to South Africa to study the problem of rinderpest and there he carried out a series of experiments in an attempt to protect the cattle by subcutaneous injection of 5–10 ml of bile from infected animals. A few years later, Kolle and Turner replaced this method, which probably spread more disease than it prevented, by inoculating serum obtained from recovered individuals, which had been shown by Semmer, in 1893, to prevent rinderpest, along with blood obtained from sick animals (Spinage, 2003; see also Chapter 11).

The first true vaccines were obtained by serial passages *in vivo* of the bovine virus through other animal species, first in goats by Edwards in 1927 and then in rabbits by Nakamura in 1942, which was followed by serial passages *in ovo*. The currently used vaccine was developed by serial passage of the virus *in vitro* in bovine kidney cell cultures by Plowright in the 1950s. By these means the virus thus lost its virulence for cattle but retained its immunogenicity (see Chapters 11 and 12 for a more extensive description of vaccine development).

# Conclusions

This short overview of the history of attempts to control rinderpest shows that, even if detailed research on the aetiology of animal diseases could not begin before the advent of microbiology, whatever the period, effective sanitary prophylaxis could be applied. However, almost a century and half were lost in disputes about whether or not to use 'variolation' to combat the cattle plague. In the end a 'stamping-out' policy proved to be the most effective measure in Western Europe. As soon as safe and efficient vaccines were available it was possible to prevent disease in free-ranging herds in Asia and Africa and this approach has been highly successful in reducing the incidence of rinderpest to almost negligible levels.

With modern diagnostic tools and vaccines new strategies can be developed to combat diseases such as rinderpest. However, should an outbreak of rinderpest occur again somewhere in the world, most veterinary services could still follow the principles set forth by Lancisi some 300 years ago to eliminate it. Indeed, there is still no specific treatment for rinderpest, and vaccination is not compatible with free international trade of animals and animal products in the twenty-first century.

# References

Bates, T. (1718) A brief account of the contagious disease which raged among the milch cowes near London, in the year 1714; and the methods that were taken for suppressing it. *Phil. Trans. R. Soc.* **30**, 872–85.

Blancou, J. (2003) *History of the surveillance and control of transmissible animal diseases.* Paris: Office International des Épizooties.

Caput, J. (1966) La grande épizootie de 1774–1775 en Béarn. *Bull. Soc. Sci. Lett. Arts Pau* **5**, 75–98.

Cato (1975) *De agricultura* (trans. with commentary by Raoul Goujard). Paris: Les Belles Lettres.

Cavrot, C. (1999) La participation d'un académicien, F. Vicq d'Azyr, à la résolution de l'épizootie de 1774. Thesis doctorat vétérinaire, University of Nantes.

Columella, L.J.M. (1954) *De re rustica*, Books V–IX (trans. E.S. Forster and E.H. Heffner). Cambridge, MA: Harvard University Press.

Columella, L.J.M. (translated 1997) *De re rustica*, books V-IX. Edited and translated by E.S. Forster and E.H. Heffner. Harvard University Press.

Curasson, G. (1942) *Traité de pathologie exotique vétérinaire et comparée. Tome I: Maladies à ultra-virus*, 2nd edn. Paris: Vigot Frères.

Fleming, G. (1871) *Animal Plagues: Their History, Nature and Prevention.* London: Chapman & Hall.

Greve, O. (1927) Oldenburger Verordnung bei der Rinderpest. Anno 1745. *Vet.-hist. Mitt.* **7**, 25–7.

Hours, H. (1957) *La Lutte contre les épizooties et l'Ecole vétérinaire de Lyon au XVIII siècle.* Paris: Presses universitaires de France.

Hurtrel d'Arboval, L.H.J. (1839) Dictionnaire de médecine, de chirurgie et d'hygiène vétérinaires, 2nd edn, Tome VI. Paris: Baillire.

Karasszon, D. (1988) *A Concise History of Veterinary Medicine.* Budapest: Akademiai Kiado.

Lancisi, G.M. (1715) *Dissertatio historica de bovilla peste, ex campaniae finibus anno MDCCXIII Latio importata.* Rome: Ex Typographia Joannis Mariae Salvioni.

Layard, D.P. (1757) An essay on the nature, causes and cure of the contagious distemper among the horned cattle in these Kingdoms. London: J. Rivington, Ch. Bathurst & T. Payne.

Leclainche, E. (1955) Histoire illustré de la médecine vétérinaire. Tome II. Paris: Editions Albin Michel.

Mammerickx, M. (1994) Les anciennes méthodes de prophylaxie des maladies animales en Belgique. *Rev. Sci. Tech. Off. Int. Epiz.* **13** (2), 487–98.

Mantovani, A. and Zanetti, R. (1993) Giovani Maria Lancisi – De Bovilla Peste and stamping out. *Hist. Med. Vet.* **18**, 97–110.

Moulé, L. (1896) *Histoire de la médecine vétérinaire. Deuxième période. Histoire de la médecine vétérinaire au moyen âge (476–1500). Première partie: la médecine vétérinaire arabe.* Paris: Imprimerie Maulde, Doumenc et Cie.

Paulet, J.-J. (1775) *Recherches historiques et physiques sur les maladies épizootiques avec les moyens d'y remédier dans tous les cas.* Part 2. Paris: Ruault Éd.

Scott, G.R. (1996) The history of rinderpest in Britain. Part 1: 809–1799. *State Vet. J.* **6**, 8–10.

Simonds, J.B. and Brown, G.T. (1868) History of the early outbreaks of malignant disease of cattle, including the progress of the cattle plague in the continent to the end of 1867. In: *Report on the cattle plague in Great Britain during the years 1865, 1866 and 1867.* London: HMSO, pp. 237–68.

Société des Médecins de Genève (1745) *Réflexions sur la maladie qui a commencé depuis quelques annés à attaquer le gros bétail en divers endroits de l'Europe.* Paris: Piget Imprimeur.

Spinage, C.A. (2003) *Cattle Plague: A History.* New York: Kluwer Academic/Plenum Publishers.

Swabe, J. (1997) *The Burden of Beasts: A Historical Sociological Study of Changing Human–Animal Relations and the Rise of the Veterinary Regime.* Academisch Proefschrift. Universiteit van Amsterdam.

Theves, G. (1994) De 'la maladie des bêtes à cornes' au Duché de Luxembourg pendant le XVIII^eme siècle. Traitement et prophylaxie. *Ann. Méd. Vét.* **138**, 81–8.

Toma, B. *et al.* (1999) *Dictionary of Veterinary Epidemiology.* Ames, IO: Iowa State University Press.

Torner, W. (1927) Eine veterinärpolizeiliche Verordnung, Friedrich Wilhelm I von Preussen aus dem Jahre 1716 zur Bekämpfung des Sterbens unter dem Horn-Viehe. *Tierärztl. Rdsch.* **33**, 345–6.

Vallat, F. (2001) Les épizooties en France de 1700 à 1850, inventaire clinique chez les bovins et les ovins. *Histoires et Sociétés Rurales* **15**, 67–104.

Walker, R.E. (1964) The Veterinary Papyrus of Kahun: a revised translation and interpretation of the ancient Egyptian treatise known as the Veterinary Papyrus of Kahun. *Vet. Rec.* **76** (7), 198–200.

Wilkinson, L. (1992) *Animals and Disease: An Introduction to the History of Comparative Medicine.* Cambridge: Cambridge University Press.

# Immunology of rinderpest – an immunosuppression but a lifelong vaccine protection

# 10

## S. LOUISE COSBY,* CHIEKO KAI† AND KAZUYA YAMANOUCHI‡

*Microbiology, School of Medicine, Queen's University Belfast, UK
†Laboratory Animal Research Center, Institute of Medical Science, University of Tokyo, Japan
‡Nippon Institute for Biological Sciences, Tokyo, Japan

## Introduction

Individuals who recover from morbillivirus infections including rinderpest develop lifelong immunity to reinfection despite the ability of these viruses to cause severe immunosuppression. Understanding the mechanisms which morbilliviruses use to induce a protective immune response on one hand and inhibition of immune function on the other is therefore of considerable interest. While mechanisms of immune suppression have been examined in cattle, information is lacking with regard to the immune response necessary for recovery from natural or experimental wild-type virus infection with rinderpest virus (RPV), as a comparison of the immune response in cattle that recover with those that succumb due to wild-type infection has not been directly examined. Particular RPV proteins involved in immune protection and immunosuppression are indicated based on comparison with other natural morbillivirus host systems as well as RPV small animal models and *in vitro* systems. In addition valuable information has been obtained from the study of vaccination with both attenuated and non-replicating vaccines.

ISBN-13: 978-0-12-88385-1
ISBN-10: 0-12-88385-6

# Recovery from rinderpest infection

## Humoral immunity

Although the humoral immune response in recovery has not been directly examined for RPV, Lund *et al.*, (2000) showed that animals infected with the virulent Saudi 1/81 strain of RPV failed to develop an antibody response, suggesting that this may contribute to the severity of disease. The humoral immune response has been shown to be important for infection outcome with other morbilliviruses. A correlation has been shown between the serum antibody titre and recovery from canine distemper infection of the CNS in both hamsters and dogs as well as phocine distemper infection of seals (Cosby *et al.*, 1983; Rima *et al.*, 1990; Rima *et al.*, 1991). Cosby *et al.* (1983) also reported that acute encephalitis caused by large plaque CDV infection in hamsters can be reduced in the presence of maternal antibody while Schlereth *et al.* (2003) has shown that after passive antibody transfer to cotton rats, MV vaccine-induced immunity and protection from later challenge is inhibited. Maternal antibodies may also have a protective effect for RPV. Low levels of maternal antibody have been detected in the sera of cattle, sheep and goats born to RPV- and PPRV-infected mothers (Ata *et al.*, 1989; Libeau *et al.*, 1992), although the protective effects of this maternally derived antibody were described by Geert Reynders (see Chapters 1 and 5); and an early report also describes the protection against RPV of calves born to mothers vaccinated with an MV vaccine (Provost *et al.*, 1968) (see also Chapter 1). Measles vaccine is not effective in the first 9 months to a year because of the presence of maternal antibodies and is also probably important in the context of RPV vaccination.

## Cell-mediated immunity

There is no direct evidence for the role of cell-mediated immunity in recovery from wild-type RPV infection in cattle. However, as discussed in the following section this arm of the immune response is clearly of major importance for protection by vaccination against challenge. The only study to directly examine recovery without prior vaccination was carried out by Yamanouchi *et al.*, (1974b) in rabbits infected with the lapinized strain of RPV and using an experimental immunosuppressive approach. Treatment of rabbits with anti-thymocyte serum (ATS) or combined treatment with adult thymectomy and ATS, both of which were confirmed to significantly suppress cell-mediated immunity, failed to alter the recovery process, in terms of clinical signs, of virus clearance from the blood and lymphoid tissues, and of repair of the lymphoid lesions (Kobune *et al.*, 1976). On the other hand, whole body irradiation with 800 R of r-ray aggravated the clinical course of RPV infection in rabbits, resulting in an increased fatality rate. Histological examinations revealed marked necrosis and haemorrhages in the lymphoid tissues, haemorrhages and ulcers in the gastrointestinal tract, and decrease of haematopoietic cells and haemorrhages in the bone marrow. In contrast, rabbits whose femur was shielded with a thick lead plate during r-ray irradiation recovered from RPV infection. Histological changes in these irradiated animals under shielding were also similar to those in untreated rabbits except for slight atrophy of the thymus in the former.

These results suggest an important role of the radiosensitive bone marrow cells in recovery from RPV infection (Yamanouchi, 1980). The relative role of neutrophils and macrophages as bone marrow-derived cells was investigated in selective suppression experiments. Suppression of neutrophils by the intravenous administration of nitrogen mustard failed to modify the clinical course of RPV infection. In contrast, suppression of macrophages by the intravenous administration of carageenan or silica resulted in fatal infection with histological lesions essentially similar to those observed in the r-ray experiment. Delayed treatment with carageenan later than 4 days post inoculation, however, was ineffective in aggravation of the clinical course and all animals survived. These results indicate the essential role of macrophages probably as an early defence mechanism.

The findings in the rabbit RPV model appear to conflict with studies in CDV and MV, which suggest a major role for the cytotoxic T lymphocyte (CTL) response in recovery from infection. It has been demonstrated in dogs infected with a wild-type strain of CDV that the extent and duration of the CTL response was crucial in determining the outcome of infection. Also a delayed CTL response correlated with persistent infection of the CNS (Appel *et al.*, 1982). However, in studies with RPV in cattle and CDV in dogs it is not possible to distinguish the relative importance of cell-mediated and humoral immunity as suppression of both appear to correlate with severity of disease. The contribution of each has been examined more specifically in animal models with MV. Niewiesk *et al.* (1993) showed that the susceptibility of mice to develop measles encephalitis is related to the ability of particular mouse strains to mount an efficient CTL response. The relative importance of the CTL response for protection against measles infection has also been demonstrated more recently in rhesus monkeys where treatment with monoclonal antibodies against both B cells and CD8+ lymphocytes resulted in prolonged duration of viraemia and development of a desquamating skin rash, whereas B cell depletion alone had no effect (Permar *et al.*, 2004). Further experiments in both cattle and rabbits are necessary to determine which aspects of the immune response are associated with recovery.

# Vaccination

## Attenuated vaccines

Knowledge of the immune response and protection against RPV infection is primarily from vaccine studies. Plowright (1984) examined the duration of immunity in cattle vaccinated with the RBOK strain and kept for 6–11 years in rinderpest-free environments and then challenged with wild-type virus by parenteral or intranasal inoculation or by contact exposure to cattle with clinical signs. Nasal excretions were examined for virus and blood for viraemia over 10–14 days following challenge. The neutralizing antibody was followed for 6-month periods over the whole vaccination period and daily up to 3 weeks after challenge and then at longer intervals. All 33 animals which were exposed to wild-type virus failed to react clinically, a rinderpest viraemia was not detected and no transmission of virus from the challenged vaccines to susceptible controls occurred. Clear-cut serological responses to challenge were seen in six cattle challenged after 7 years or more, although the reactions were delayed to 9–10 days, which is not typically anamnestic.

An early report describes protection of cattle against rinderpest challenge following vaccination with the MB113 strain of measles virus, supporting the view that morbilliviruses are immunologically cross-protective and that this is related to the similarity between individual proteins (Provost *et al.*, 1968). The major MV proteins which induce a humoral response are the nucleocapsid (N), fusion (F) and haemagglutinin (H) proteins (Niewiesk *et al.*, 1993). Rinderpest infection is much more readily amenable than MV for studying the immunity to individual morbillivirus antigens in the natural host. Lund *et al.* (2000) examined the CD4+ T cell response in cattle, inoculated with either RBOK or KS-1 capripox control vaccine and challenged with the virulent Saudi 1/81 strain of RPV. The proliferative response to whole RPV or individual structural proteins expressed using recombinant adenoviruses was determined. Infection with the vaccine strain was found to induce a strong CD4+ response to all proteins tested, namely the H, F, N and matrix (M) proteins in animals inoculated with the attenuated strain (Figure 10.1). No protein was found to be dominant with respect to a T cell proliferative response. A similar broad specificity of the CD4+ T cell response has been reported for MV (Rose *et al.*, 1984). Profound suppression of the proliferative T cell response as well as failure to induce neutralizing antibody was observed in cattle infected with the control capripox vaccine and challenged with the virulent Saudi 1/81 strain indicating development of severe immunosuppression and the probable importance of both humoral immunity and the CD4+ response in recovery from infection (Lund *et al.*, 2000).

## Replicating recombinant vaccines

Successful immunization against experimental infection with RPV has also been achieved using recombinant viruses. Vaccinia and capripox viruses, expressing the envelope glycoproteins, H or F of RPV, have been constructed. All cattle vaccinated with either H or F vaccinia recombinant or combined recombinants produced neutralizing antibodies against rinderpest and were protected against disease when challenged with more than 1000 times the dose of virus (Yilma *et al.*, 1988). More recently a second generation recombinant

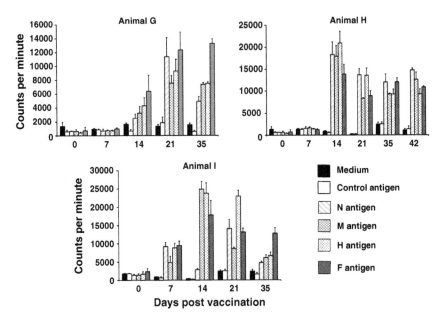

**Figure 10.1**　Proliferative responses of peripheral blood mononuclear cells (PBMC) from RBOK-vaccinated animals to purified RPV N, M, H and F antigens. PBMC were isolated from cattle at the time points indicated after vaccination and subsequent challenge, on day 28 post infection, with the virulent Saudi 1/81 strain of RPV. The proliferative responses of $10^5$ cells to the various rinderpest antigens was determined by measuring [$^3$H] thymidine incorporation. The proliferative responses of PBMC in the medium alone or in the presence of adenovirus derived bacteriophage T7 polymerase antigen are included as controls. Results are expressed as the mean c.p.m. of triplicate cultures. Each value represents the proliferative response obtained with an optimal concentration of the relevant antigen as determined in preliminary studies. (Adapted from Lund *et al.*, 2000)

vaccinia vaccine has been produced which expresses both the RPV H and F genes and produces long-term sterilizing immunity (Verardi *et al.*, 2002). The latter is indicated by the absence of virus from nasal swabs after challenge and failure of animals to mount an anamnestic response. Recombinant vaccinia virus vaccines have also been produced which incorporate the N protein of RPV (Ohishi *et al.*, 1998, 1999). This was initially tested in mice where antibodies to RPV were detected following vaccination (Ohishi *et al.*, 1998). A later study in cattle demonstrated that the recombinant induced both lymphocyte proliferation and cytotoxic T cell responses. However, vaccinated cattle were not protected against challenge with the virulent Saudi 1/81 strain of RPV although there was a delay in onset of disease compared to unvaccinated controls. One of 3 animals challenged with the mild Kenya/eland/96 strain of RPV failed to show signs of disease and the other two had only mild transient fever

(Ohishi *et al.*, 1999). These results suggest that protection again challenge with highly virulent RPV strains may require a CTL response against the viral gly-coproteins as well as the N protein.

Romero *et al.* (1994) constructed a capripox recombinant containing the complete coding sequence of the H protein of the RBOK vaccine strain of RPV under the control of the vaccinia late promoter p11 and inserted into the thymi-dine kinase gene of the KS-1 strain of capripox. This recombinant virus also induced significant levels of neutralizing antibodies and successfully protected against RPV challenge. More recently the H and F proteins have been expressed in cattle, using a disabled human adenovirus vector (Ad 5). These were found to generate low titres of neutralizing antibody to RPV and to fully protect vaccinated animals against virulent RPV challenge in short-term stud-ies to examine duration of immunity (Barrett, unpublished data). It is an impor-tant point to note that all of these recombinant vaccines allow serological differentiation between vaccinated and naturally infected animals, which is of major importance in surveillance of eventual RPV eradication.

## Non-replicating vaccines

Several types of RPV subunit or non-replicating vaccines have been tested. An immune-stimulating complex (ISCOM) incorporating the H protein fully pro-tected three out of four animals against challenge with the fourth showing mild transient clinical signs. However, all animals developed a significant level of antibodies (Kamata *et al.*, 2001). The immunogenicity of proteins pro-duced in insect and plant cell systems has also been investigated. Several stud-ies have been carried out to examine vaccination of mice or cattle with RPV H protein produced in either transgenic tobacco or peanut plants (Khandelwal, *et al.*, 2003a, b). The plant-derived protein was antigenically authentic, as shown by reactivity with H-monospecific and convalescent sera. High titres of antibody were obtained in mice after intraperitoneal inoculation with both plant preparations and these were H-specific and neutralized RPV infection. Leaves of transgenic peanut plants expressing RPV H were also fed to mice and cattle over a 9- or 10-week period. In mice both IgG and IgA antibodies were produced and maintained throughout the study and in cattle a continuing lymphoproliferative response was also demonstrated (Khandelwal *et al.*, 2003b, 2004). These studies indicate the potential for an oral edible vaccine for rinderpest.

In 1993, Bassiri *et al.* reported the construction of a recombinant bac-ulovirus expressing the H and F proteins of RPV and cattle were inoculated with crude extracts from *Spodoptera frugiperda* cells infected with the recom-binant virus. Immunizing mice with F extract alone failed to induce detectable antibody, while H gave an average serum neutralizing (SN) titre of 160. Cattle vaccinated with F or H alone, or a mixture of both antigens, were not protected from challenge with RPV even when the SN titre was greater in cattle than in those vaccinated with recombinant vaccinia virus expressing F. The authors at the time suggested that this lack of protection, in the presence of SN antibody, indicated that live attenuated and recombinant vaccines induce a cell-mediated immune response necessary for protection, which is not generated by subunit or inactivated vaccine virus. However, in later studies this group of workers (Sinnathamby *et al.*, 2001a; Rahman *et al.*, 2003) demonstrated that if cattle or mice are immunized with extracted recombinant baculovirus expressing the H protein on the viral envelope a long-lasting bovine leucocyte antigen (BoLA) class 1 restricted CTL response is induced. The lymphoproliferative response induced by their RPV H plant vaccines (Kandelwal *et al.*, 2003b, 2004) also indicates that a cell-mediated immune response is induced. Therefore it would appear that it is important to have the T cell specific epitopes of H correctly displayed in a non-replicating vaccine in order to generate a protective immune response.

## B and T cell epitopes

To characterize the T cell epitopes of RPV H, Sinnathamby *et al.* (2001b) and Rahman *et al.* (2003) subsequently examined both class II restricted Th (T helper) and class I restricted CTL epitopes of RPV H. In the former study they analysed lymphoproliferative responses of PBLs from cattle to truncated H protein fragments expressed in *E. coli*. One region (aa 113–182) recognized by immune T cells is conserved in the H protein of MV, which was previously shown to contain a dominant Th epitope in the mouse. Synthetic peptides within a region of MV H protein were used to identify a Th epitope located on RPV (aa 123–137) in cattle. A second Th epitope located on the C-terminus of RPV H was mapped to the region corresponding to aa 512. The C-terminal epitope (575–585) was mapped using synthetic peptides corresponding to MV as well as RPV H protein (Sinnathamby *et al.*, 2001a). More recently they employed autologous skin fibroblasts transiently expressing truncated H in a BoLA class I restricted lymphoproliferation assay and found a domain (aa 400–423) which has high homology to the PPRV HN protein and harbours a CTL epitope in both viruses. Subsequently, they identified a BoLA-A11 binding motif (aa 408–416) in the stimulatory domain (Sinnathamby *et al.*, 2004). Autologous cells pulsed with synthetic peptide corresponding to this sequence stimulated CTLs in cattle immunized with recombinant *E. coli* RPV H as well as different breeds of cattle vaccinated with the tissue culture attenuated RPV and PPRV. This group also identified a cytotoxic T cell epitope on recombinant nucleocapsid protein from RPV and PPRV in both Balb/C mice and cattle (Mitra-Kaushik *et al.*, 2001). This 9 amino acid (aa) epitope (RPVN 281–289) was based on a sequence previously shown to be protective for both MV and CDV (Schadeck *et al.*, 1999).

Recently, immunodominant B cell epitopes on RPV H protein have been determined by analysing selected monoclonal antibody-resistant mutants in RPV-infected rabbits (Sugiyama *et al.*, 2002). Six neutralizing epitopes were identified at residues 474, 243, 548 to 551, 597 to 592, 310 to 313 and 383 to 387 from data on the aa substitutions of the H protein of mAb-resistant mutants and the reactivities of mAbs against RPV H. These positions were compared to MV Edmonston and CDV Onderstepoort H proteins. All six epitopes are positioned on the loop of each proposed propeller-like structure of H. The major epitopes were identified as 383–387 and 587–592. The latter is near the C-terminus of RPV H and is located at the same position of MVH which was previously identified from data on reactivity of a synthetic peptide (Makela *et al.*, 1989). Liebert *et al.* (1994) reported that the major antigenic site for MVH is located between residues 368 and 396. A small cysteine cluster region (Cys-381, Cys-386 and Cys-394) of MV was also identified as a linear neutralizing epitope (Ziegler *et al.*, 1996). These two MV epitopes and the RPV 383 to 387 epitope are all located on the β3L23 loop on the top surface of the propeller-like structure. The results suggest that the loop structure β3L23 formed by disulphide bonds between the two β-sheets is a major neutralizing antigenic site in morbilliviruses. Overall study of morbillivirus T and B cell epitopes indicates that many of these are common, as might be expected, and therefore information gained from the study of veterinary viruses such as RPV and CDV in their natural hosts would also apply to MV and would help in the design of subunit or non-replicating recombinant vaccines.

# Immunopathology

## Inflammation

Despite severe depression of both antibody production and the lymphoproliferative response during wild-type RPV infection the occurrence of a local cellular response is indicated from histopathological studies (Wohlsein *et al.*, 1993; Brown and Torres, 1994). Rinderpest is characterized by erosive inflammation of mucous membranes, predominantly of the alimentary tract. Wohlsein *et al.* (1993) reported that in the upper respiratory tract intraepithelial oedema occurs with the sub-epithelial tissue infiltrated by few to moderate numbers of lymphocytes and macrophages in close vicinity to blood and lymphatic capillaries in animals experimentally infected with Saudi 1/81. In the intestines of cattle virus antigen was distributed predominantly in the epithelial cells and histiocytic cells in the lamina propria and was associated with lymphocytic infiltration and necrosis. Ulcerative lesions with infiltration of macrophages and neutrophils were seen and numerous multinucleated giant cells. In the lower digestive tract intraepithelial infiltration of lymphocytes occurred. Slight to moderate infiltration of lymphocytes was also observed in the periportal areas of the liver and single lymphocytes or macrophages were located in interstitial connective tissue of heart and endocrine organs. A few lymphocytes and macrophages were also observed in the eyes and antigen was found in epithelial cells and lymphatic cells in the conjunctival tissue.

These authors also found lymphocytes and macrophages in the meninges although not in brain tissue itself. An early study reported isolation of RPV brain tissue of young cattle experimentally infected with RPV (Bergeon, 1952), although there is no association with central nervous system (CNS) complications with rinderpest in the natural host. These findings raise the possibility that virus could enter the CNS and may be cleared by the immune response or occur too late to be of clinical significance. With canine distemper virus, phocine distemper virus and the cetacean morbilliviruses, as well as more rarely with MV, CNS complications are late sequelae and associated with a marked inflammatory response. The potential neurovirulence and associated inflammatory response of RPV and PPRV has been demonstrated in mice. Imagawa *et al.* (1965) initially demonstrated that the lapinized strain of RPV could be adapted for intracerebral growth in suckling mice. Galbraith *et al.* (2002) subsequently showed that while the virulent Kabete 'O' strain of RPV and its derivative the RBOK vaccine produced no obvious infection, the Saudi 1/81 strain of RPV was neurovirulent for Balb/c and CD1 but not C57 black strains of suckling mice when administered by intracerebral infection. Furthermore the brain areas infected and the immunopathology observed is similar to infection with MV and CDV administered by the same route. Balb/c mice infected with RPV Saudi 181 showed minimal perivascular inflammation, while CD1 mice showed foci of quite pronounced perivascular inflammation throughout the brain (Figure 10.2). Therefore the degree of inflammation with RPV as with MV and CDV in mice

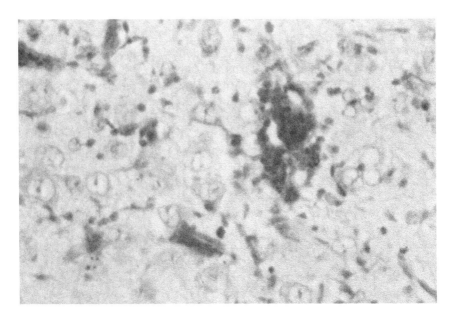

**Figure 10.2** Foci of perivascular inflammation in H&E stained paraformaldehyde-fixed brain section of CD1 mouse infected intracerebrally with RPV Saudi 1/81 (×250)

is related to both the strain of virus and genetic background of the host. While mouse CNS infection is highly artificial, it provides a small animal system where the role of different Saudi 1/81 proteins and immune epitopes in the induction of inflammation could be examined.

## Lymphoid tissue infection

Experimental infections of cattle with the virulent Saudi 1/81 or Kabete 'O' strains of RPV, or rabbits with the lapinized strain of RPV, have shown that the virus has a marked tropism for lymphatic tissues (Chino and Yamanouchi, 1974; Wohlsein *et al.*, 1993; Brown and Torres, 1994). In cattle, viral protein was found to be restricted to B and T cell areas, reticular cells, macrophages and single endothelial cells. This is clearly indicated by lympho-depletion seen in the thymus, Peyer's patches, spleen and pulmonary lymph nodes of infected hosts. In lymphatic organs with marked lymphoid depletion staining was restricted to structures resembling follicular dendritic cells, macrophages and lymphocytes (Wohlsein *et al.*, 1993).

Similar observations were made in rabbits inoculated with lapinized RPV where formation of giant cells and necrotic changes were characteristic with lesions in the lymphoid tissues. Although all the lymphoid tissues were affected by the virus, the mesenteric lymph nodes and the gut-associated lymphoid tissues such as Peyer's patches, caecal tonsils and sacculus rotundus appeared to be attacked by the virus most severely as primary target tissues (Chino *et al.*, 1974). Immunohistochemically virus antigen was localized in the T cell area, CD5+ cells in the rabbit model, at the initial stage of infection but spread to all areas of the lymphoid tissues at the later stages. By flow cytometric analysis, a decrease of the CD4+ and CD5+ subpopulations was observed in the spleen and mesenteric lymph nodes (Okita *et al.*, 1995). The most marked necrosis of lymphoid cells was observed in the spleen and mesenteric lymph nodes, but giant cells were only transiently demonstrated. These necrotic lesions in the intestinal lymphoid tissues in the rabbit model may probably be involved in the manifestation of diarrhoea. In contrast, the superficial lymph nodes, thymus, and spleen showed more marked formation of giant cells at higher degrees and lymphoid necrosis at a relatively lower degree than the other lymphoid tissues. No significant histological changes or virus antigens were detected in the bone marrow. These lymphoid lesions were rapidly repaired and the virus antigen was similarly eliminated within 10 days in spite of their severe nature. Virus antigens tended to persist for several additional days in the mucosal tissues of the intestines (Yamanouchi *et al.*, 1974a). These findings in both cattle and rabbits indicate that RPV affects primarily the lymphoid tissues as the major target, which proceeds to infection of the epithelial tissues.

## Leucocyte infection

To determine which leucocyte sub-types are susceptible to RPV infection, Rossiter *et al.* (1993) infected cloned bovine lymphoblastoid cell lines, transformed by the protozoan parasite *Theileria parva*, with RPV vaccine. The virus grew readily in lymphoid B cells, CD4+ and CD8+ $\alpha/\beta$ T cells and $\gamma/\delta$ T cells resulting in cell death. There did not appear to be a predilection for any particular cell phenotype. *In vitro* experiments also indicated that monocytes and monocyte-derived macrophages serve as targets of productive virus infection, with a higher rate of infection of virulent Saudi virus than that of attenuated RBOK vaccine strain (Nores *et al.*, 1995). It has been shown that RPV like MV and CDV (Tatsuo *et al.*, 2001) and more recently PDV and DMV (Melia and Cosby, unpublished data) use SLAM as an entry receptor on lymphoid cells. SLAM has also been found to be expressed on activated monocytes and dendritic cells. During MV infection SLAM is up-regulated on these cells by the virus and then subsequently down-regulated once the virus has gained cell entry (Kruse *et al.*, 2001; Minagawa *et al.*, 2001). This mechanism is likely to be common to all the morbilliviruses.

## Dendritic cell infection

It was noted by Stolte *et al.* (2002) that there was a close association of RPV antigen with cells of lymphoid follicles morphologically similar to dendritic cells (DC). Recently it has been shown that DC derived from afferent lymph veiled cells (ALVC) are also infected to different degrees by wild-type and vaccine strains of virus (Banyard, Charleston, Barrett and Cosby, unpublished data). It has been reported that a wild-type strain of MV has enhanced uptake and replication in human monocyte derived DC (MoDC) *in vitro*, compared to a vaccine strain. This was found to be associated with strain variations in the H protein and the difference between MV strains was found to be reflected in their ability to infect lymphatic tissue in a cotton rat model (Ohgimoto *et al.*, 2001). RPV infection of DC from ALVC provides a unique opportunity to examine the consequences of morbillivirus infection of lymphoid derived DC compared to MoDC in the natural host. Infection of these cells early in infection would have significant effects on the initial presentation of RPV antigens. This aspect needs further investigation as well as possible differences in infection and replication in particular DC subsets with both wild-type and vaccine strains of RPV.

## Cell death

The mechanism and extent of cell death in lymphatic tissue from cattle infected with the Saudi 1/81, RBT/1 and RGK/1 strains have been examined morphologically by Stolte *et al.* (2002). They used cytological criteria such as cytoplasmic shrinkage and karyorrhexis, with formation of membrane vesicles as well as TUNEL labelling to detect cells undergoing apoptosis, while oncosis (more commonly referred to as necrosis) was recognized by cytoplasmic swelling and karyolysis. The results indicated that cellular disassembly in lymphatic tissues

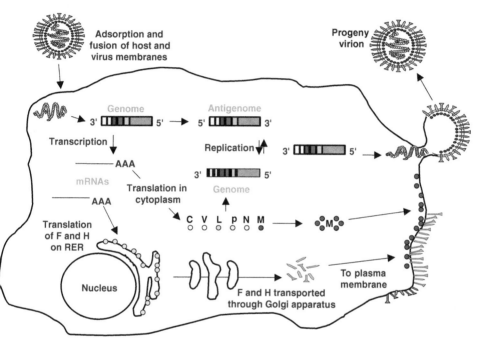

**Plate I** An overview of the life cycle of the paramyxoviruses.

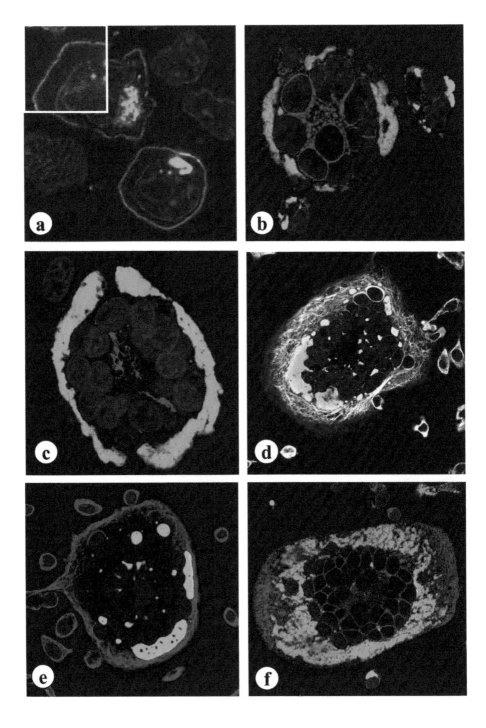

**Plate 2** Infection of B95a cells with GFP-labelled rinderpest virus. The virus causes cell fusion to form large syncytia during infection. Incorporation of the GFP gene within the polymerase protein of the virus enables the virus to be visualized using confocal microscopy as the GFP shows green under UV light. Antibodies are used to stain cellular components and individual images merged to form each panel showing the distribution of the different cellular components, the virus and viral proteins. Nuclei are stained blue in each of the images.

(*a*) Early infection showing the virus (green) localized at the periphery of the cell as a distinct ring around the inside of the plasma membrane. Here, we can also see the viral H protein (red) positioned on the outside of the cell membrane (*inset*).

(*b*) Approximately 48 hours post infection, large cells are observed where the infected cells have fused together to form giant multinucleate syncytia. The viral protein (green) seems to be held in 'lakes' of viral protein whilst the cellular Golgi apparatus (red) has a punctuate appearance and a ubiquitous cytoplasmic distribution.

(*c*) The distribution of the cellular microfilament vimentin (red) during syncytia formation also seems to be affected by syncytia formation. Here it is seen localized to the centre of the cluster of nuclei (blue) whilst again the virus (green) is held in large 'lakes' around the nuclei.

(*d*) The co-localization of viral N protein (red) and the lakes of virus (green) is evident in this image (merged to yellow). However, the presence of viral nucleocapsid protein in the nuclei is also evident. It is understood for several morbilliviruses that the nucleocapsid protein contains a nuclear localization signal although the significance of this in viral infection is unknown. Here the tubulin is present solely at the periphery of the large syncytia, this time visualized in white.

(*e*) The effect of virus infection on tubulin (red) can be quite profound as seen here late on post infection in this huge syncytia. Tubulin seems to be totally excluded from the centre of the giant cell, forced to the periphery of the cell with the nuclei of the fused cells (blue) being crowded into the middle.

(*f*) Late on in infection (96 hours post infection) huge syncytia can be seen containing many tens of nuclei (blue). The virus (green) seems to be distributed around the periphery of the cell while the cellular endoplasmic reticulum has a punctuate appearance and is distributed throughout the cellular cytoplasm.

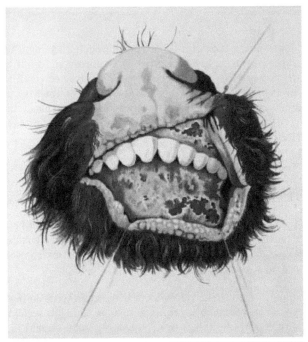

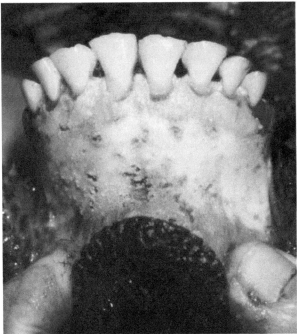

**Plate 3** Rinderpest oral erosion: (*top*) illustration taken from the Third Report of the Commissioners appointed to inquire into the origin and nature etc. of the cattle plague. Printed by George Edward Eyre and William Spottiswoode, London, 1866; (*bottom*) comparison of an animal infected with the highly virulent Saudi/81 strain of rinderpest virus.

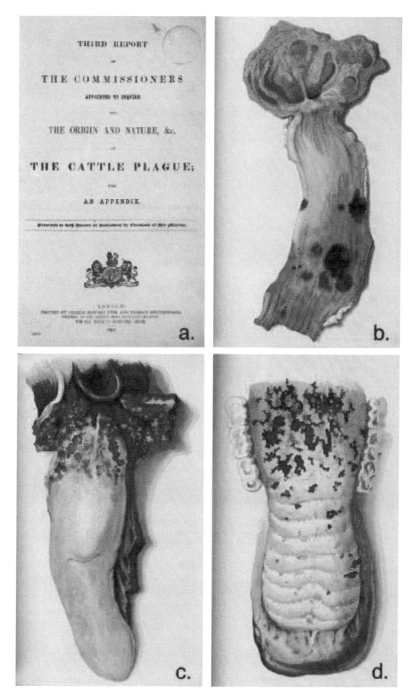

**Plate 4** Illustrations taken from the Third Report of the Commissioners appointed to inquire into the origin and nature etc. of the cattle plague. Printed by George Edward Eyre and William Spottiswoode, London, 1866. (*a*) Title page from the report; (*b*) duodenal lesions; (*c*) tongue lesions; (*d*) lesions on the palate.

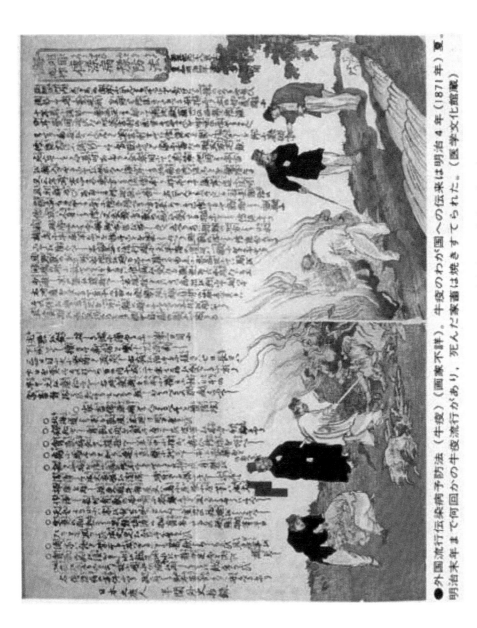

**Plate 5** Nineteenth-century Japanese print showing a pyre of rinderpest infected cattle.

●外国流行伝染病予防法（牛疫）（画家不詳）。牛疫のわが国への伝来は明治4年（1871年）夏、明治末年まで何回かの牛疫流行があり、死んだ家畜は焼きすてられた。（医学文化館蔵）

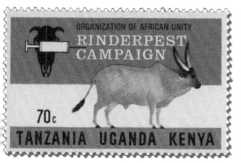
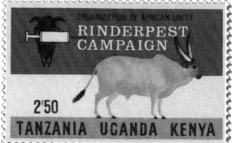
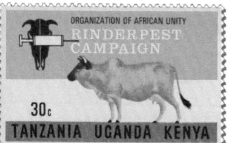
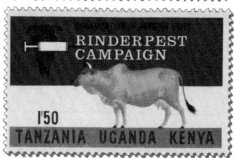
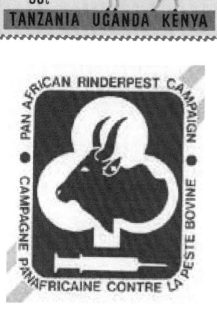
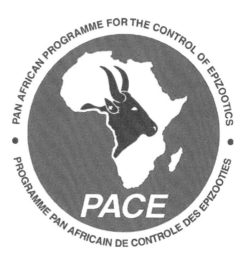

**Plate 6** (*top*) Postage stamps printed to commemorate the 'eradication' of rinderpest from Africa following the JP15 campaign in the 1960s; (*bottom*) emblems for the rinderpest eradication campaigns, PARC and PACE. The PARC emblem incorporated in the clover-leaf outline is the shape of the piece of tissue removed from the ear of a vaccinated animal (or as a brand) allowing observers to determine if the animal has been vaccinated.

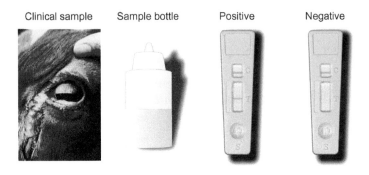

Clinical sample    Sample bottle    Positive    Negative

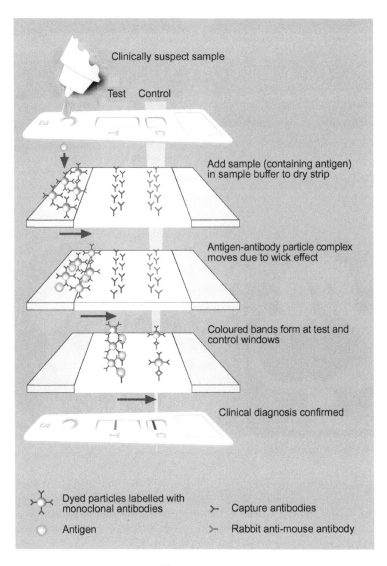

Clinically suspect sample

Test   Control

Add sample (containing antigen) in sample buffer to dry strip

Antigen-antibody particle complex moves due to wick effect

Coloured bands form at test and control windows

Clinical diagnosis confirmed

Dyed particles labelled with monoclonal antibodies

Antigen

Capture antibodies

Rabbit anti-mouse antibody

**Plate 7** Principle of the Clearview™ 'pen-side' test to detect rinderpest antigen.

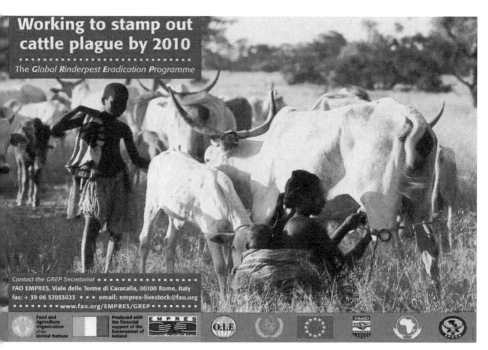

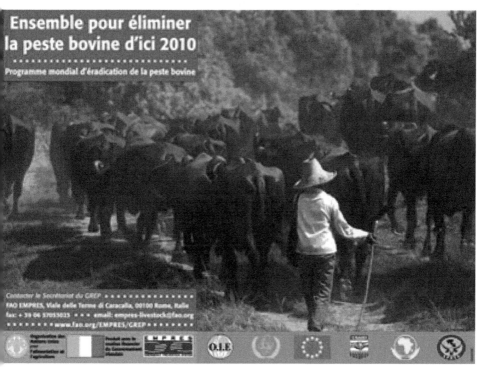

Plate 8  Posters printed by FAO, with funds from international sources, advertising the Global Rinderpest Eradication Programme.

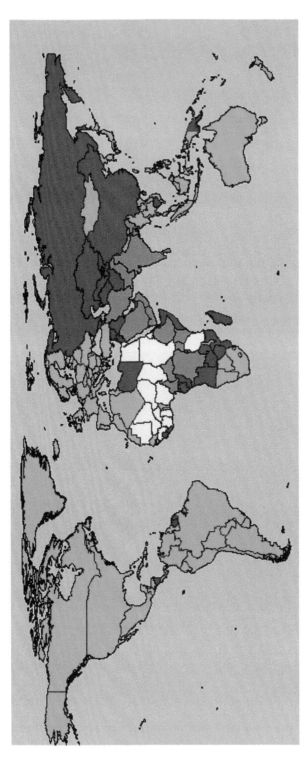

## OIE-Recognized status

■ Free from infection
☐ Free from disease
■ Provisionally free
■ No declaration

The status recognized is zonal for Kenya, Ethiopia, Sudan, Chad and Congo Democratic Republic.

**Plate 9** Accreditation of rinderpest freedom by the OIE Pathway as of August 2005.

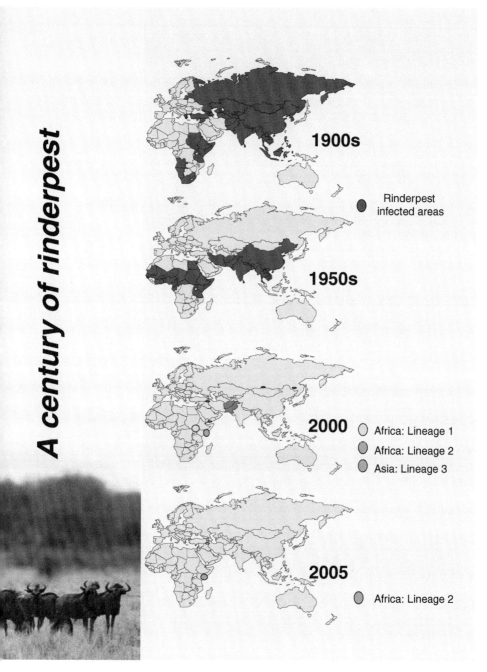

**Plate 10** Endemic areas of rinderpest over the past century.

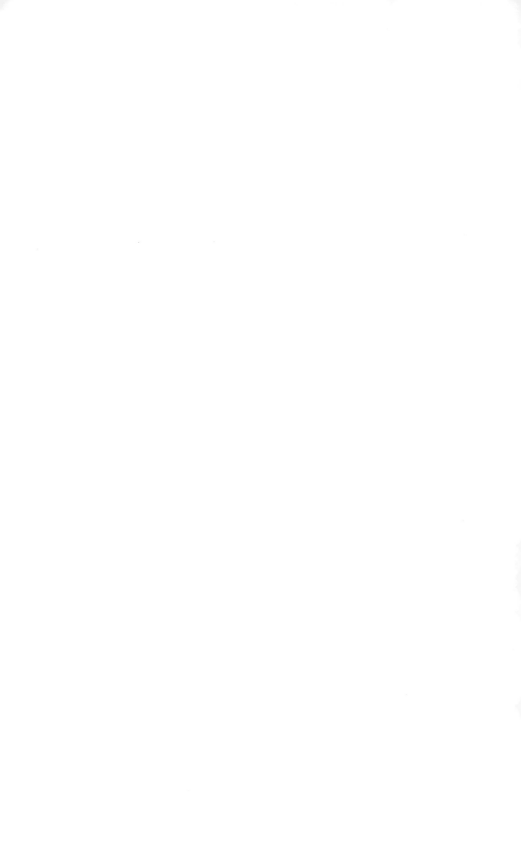

was caused by both apoptosis and oncosis. Cells with DNA strand breaks were observed in follicular and parafollicular areas of lymphatic tissues. A significant correlation was found between the number of TUNEL-positive cells and virus virulence. In cattle infected with the more virulent strains (Saudi 1/81 and RGK/1) the lesions in B and T cell areas were characterized by severe destruction and depletion of lymphocytes and correlated with a high viral load. This is similar to the findings in lymphoid tissues for CDV-infected dogs (Kumagai *et al.*, 2004). However, in the dog study the results suggested that apoptosis also occurs by indirect mechanisms, rather than infection as CDV-antigen negative cells were also found to have DNA strand breaks.

## Autoimmunity

Virus-induced damage of lymphoid cells as demonstrated by lymphoid necrosis and apoptosis causes the release of proteins and nucleic acid from the cell and therefore may not only be related to the immunosuppression but to the development of autoimmunity. Interestingly, MV has been implicated in several autoimmune diseases of humans and although evidence for MV in cases of autoimmunity exists, such as the demonstration of virus-like structures, antigens and nucleic acid in the tissues of patients with autoimmune diseases as well as raised antibody levels to particular viruses or presence of autoimmune antibodies, the link remains controversial. There is, however, no documented evidence for autoimmunity in natural infection of cattle with RPV and, as suggested for CNS infection, development of autoimmunity would be a late sequela of infection which, if it occurs, may go undetected in cattle.

### Autoantibodies

Suggestive evidence for induction of an autoimmune response to RPV was obtained by the comparison of the pathogenicity of the L and LA strains of RPV in rabbits (Fukuda and Yamanouchi, 1981). The L strain which is virulent for rabbits produced marked histological lesions in the lymphoid tissues consisting of both giant-cell formation and necrosis, whereas the LA strain which is less virulent produced only giant-cell formation. Immunosuppression was more profound and prolonged in the L-strain infection than in the LA-strain infection. Although virus-neutralizing antibody developed to a slightly higher titre in LA-strain infection, autoantibodies were detected only in L-strain infection. Rabbits infected with the L strain of RPV provided a unique model of virus-induced autoimmunity, as two types of autoantibodies – antinuclear antibody (ANA) and cold haemagglutinating antibody (HA) – were induced after the virus infection (Fukuda and Yamanouchi, 1976). By indirect immunofluorescence technique using diploid human embryonic lung cells or rabbit kidney cells as targets, ANA of 7S nature which reacts with the nuclei of the cells is demonstrated in all rabbits 2 weeks after the IV inoculation of RPV; the maximum titre reaches up to 1280 or higher 3–4 weeks post inoculation. However, this ANA response is transient and disappears in 6–10 weeks post inoculation. The target antigens of the ANA were shown to be DNA and/or DNA-histone complexes (nucleohistone) (Imaoka *et al.*, 1990).

Cold HA also developed transiently from 1–6 weeks post inoculation. This antibody is of 19S nature and was able to react with rabbit RBC, both autologous and allogeneic cells, at 4 °C but not at 37 °C. Thus it is considered to be the same type of antibody commonly observed in autoimmune haemolytic anaemia which occurs frequently following the infection of mycoplasma pneumonia or infectious mononucleosis. However, no clinical sign of haemolytic anaemia was detected in these rabbits (Fukuda and Yamanouchi, 1976).

## Mechanisms of autoimmunity

The following mechanisms are generally speculated for virus-induced autoimmunity; (i) cross-antigenicity between the virus and self antigens; (ii) modified self antigens in viral envelopes; and (iii) virus-induced disturbance of the immune regulatory system. Some of these mechanisms may occur in RPV infection but have short-lived effects and no significance unless animals recover. Possibly the virus-induced destruction of lymphocytes by RPV and the other morbilliviruses may provide a strong antigenic stimulus consisting of the cellular components released in a large amount from the damaged lymphocytes in the host whose immune functions are disturbed by virus-induced immunosuppression. Development of both ANA and Cold HA antibodies showed a transient pattern in contrast to the persistence of virus-neutralizing antibody. Moreover, formalin-inactivated virus failed to produce the autoantibodies (Imaoka *et al.*, 1990). This indicates that virus infection acts as a trigger of autoantibody production and that cross-antigenicity appears to be unlikely. Recently virulent and avirulent virus strains were cloned from the L strain, and the rescue system of the full genome plasmid of L-virulent strain was developed (Yoneda and Kai, unpublished data). These viruses and recombinant techniques reducing the virulence may give insight into the mechanism of RPV-induced autoimmunity which may follow acute infection and provide a model for MV in humans.

# Immunosuppression

## Secondary infections

Natural or experimental RPV infections of cattle are clearly immunosuppressive, virulent strains inducing severe leucopenia in the affected hosts which, as shown for MV, PPRV and morbillivirus infections in marine mammals, probably results in the development of secondary bacterial infections (Domingo *et al.*, 1995; Griffin and Bellini, 1996; Duignan *et al.*, 1997; Roeder and Obi, 1999). It has been suggested that vaccine strains might also cause transient immunosuppression. An investigation was made into whether vaccination of cattle with tissue culture RPV vaccine would lead to more frequent or more severe infection with trypanosomes in animals grazing in tsetse-infested areas. There was no evidence that vaccinated animals were more likely to acquire trypanosome infections or to show a more severe disease than unvaccinated cattle (Stevenson *et al.*, 1999). However, susceptibility to infection is probably not significantly affected if immunosuppression effects are transient as recently demonstrated for the vaccine and discussed in detail below (Heaney, Cosby and Barrett, unpublished data).

## Mechanisms of immunosuppression

Many mechanisms have been proposed to account for MV-induced immunosuppression, including the inhibition of interferon $\alpha\beta$ production, suppression of the inflammatory response, altered cytokine profiles, direct infection and subsequent destruction of leucocytes, inhibition of immunoglobulin synthesis and cell cycle arrest after direct contact with viral glycoproteins, all aspects of which were recently reviewed by Schneider-Schaulies and references therein (Schneider-Schaulies *et al.*, 2001). Several but not all of these mechanisms have been examined for RPV and other morbilliviruses and will be discussed in the following sections.

## Lymphodepletion

The marked destruction by RPV of the lymphoid tissues in both cattle and rabbits is also observed in the case of measles virus infection, which has the same immunopathological features as RPV infection. More rapid replication of virulent strains of RPV is indicated by the detection of antigens and may give rise to severe lymphodepletion in the thymus, Peyer's patches, spleen and pulmonary lymph nodes (Wohlsein *et al.*, 1993, 1995). The time course of immunosuppression in rabbits closely is correlated with that of severe lymphopenia. Marked destruction of the lymphoid tissues involving both thymus-dependent and thymus-independent areas is induced from 3 days post infection in association with the immunosuppression, and then these lesions are rapidly repaired. Therefore, the destruction of lymphocytes and possibly DC by virulent strains of RPV appears to be a primary mechanism for immunosuppression.

## Inhibition of T and B cell function

While lymphodepletion due to direct virus infection is of obvious importance in immunosuppression by RPV a non-response of leucocytes to mitogens and

unrelated antigens has also been demonstrated. A delayed-type hypersensitivity to tuberculin was an early observation for evidence of immunosuppression by MV (Tamashiro et al., 1987). Similarly a delayed-type skin reaction
to PPD in tuberculin-sensitized rabbits was shown to be completely suppressed for 3–14 days post infection or longer after the RPV infection, and
sensitization to tuberculin was inhibited or delayed by the RPV infection at
the time of immunization with Freund's complete adjuvant. The in vitro
response of peripheral blood lymphocytes to phytohemagglutinin was also
suppressed for 3–28 days post infection, suggesting a suppressive effect on
helper T cells. Failure of cattle infected with virulent strains of RPV to mount
an effective antibody response indicates that B cell as well as T cell function
is impaired. Immunosuppressive effect of RPV L strain in rabbits was shown
in both antibody production as well as cell-mediated immunity (Yamanouchi
et al., 1974a, b). The capacity of rabbits infected with the RPV L strain to
produce antibody to chicken red cells and IgM antibody-forming cells to
sheep red blood cells (SRBC) in the spleen was significantly suppressed for
14 days or longer after virus infection. Both IgM and IgG antibodies in the
serum were similarly suppressed (Penhale and Pow, 1970; Yamanouchi et al.,
1974a, b).

Although MV is rapidly cleared from the host, lymphoproliferative
responses to mitogens and recall antigens are suppressed for up to several
months post infection. Both B and T subsets of leucocytes are affected, but not
the CD4+/CD8+ ratio (Arneborn and Biberfeld, 1983). It has been shown that
MV infection interferes with the differentiation and specialization of lymphocyte functions but does not alter those already established (Fugier-Vivier et al.,
1997). In contrast to the apparent effects of RPV L on CD4+ cells and antibody
in rabbits, production of memory cells was not impaired. Lack of suppression
of memory-cell production, which is relatively independent of T cell-helper
function, may explain why indivi-duals infected with wild-type MV are susceptible to secondary infections but have the ability to clear the MV infection
and retain lifelong immunity. However, vaccination may not be as effective in
this respect as it has been shown recently by Naniche et al. (2004) that there is
a decrease in CD4 T cell memory in subjects who had been vaccinated more
than 21 years previously.

## Contact-mediated inhibition

Although impairment of leucocyte response, following MV and RPV infection,
was recognized, the mechanisms responsible for this have only been investigated in the past few years. An indirect mechanism involving inhibition of non-
infected peripheral leucocytes has now been shown to play a major role. The
method used to demonstrate this for RPV was based on previous studies with
MV. Using a two cell system, Schlender and colleagues showed that small numbers of MV-infected, UV-irradiated, lymphocyte presenter cells (PC) could

inhibit the proliferation of a responder cell (RC) population, either mitogen stimulated naive lymphocytes or human lymphocytic or monocytic cell lines, even after a short contact period (Schlender *et al.*, 1996). More recently Heaney *et al.* (2002) have shown that all members of the morbillivirus genus inhibit the proliferation of a human B lymphoblast cell line (BJAB). Furthermore, they demonstrated that proliferation of freshly isolated, stimulated bovine and caprine PBL is also inhibited by UV-inactivated RPV and PPRV viruses or virus-infected cells (Figure 10.3). As shown for MV (Schlender *et al.*, 1996), the inhibition produced by RPV was specific to cells of lymphoid origin and not a non-specific growth arrest due to contact with other cells such as HeLa and Vero cells.

The inhibitory effect was abolished when the PC and RC populations were physically separated by a semi-permeable membrane, showing that soluble

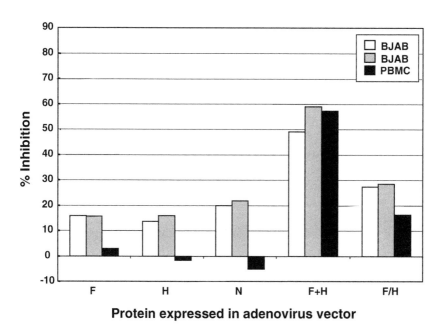

**Protein expressed in adenovirus vector**

**Figure 10.3** Effect of adenovirus recombinants expressing RPV proteins on BJAB cell proliferation. The levels of expression of RPV H and F proteins were determined by FACS analysis using a rabbit anti-RPV hyperimmune serum and FITC conjugated goat anti-rabbit IgG. PC were generated by infecting BJAB cells at MOI of 500 with RPV protein expressing recombinant adenovirus vectors for 48 hours. The recombinant proteins were either expressed alone or co-expressed in pairs, e.g. where H and F were co-expressed in the same cell the designation is F/H. Where a heterologous PC population was generated by mixing equal numbers of cells expressing only one protein the designation is F+H. PC were mixed with uninfected BJAB cells (RC) for 72 hours; then the RC proliferation was determined.

factors do not influence immunosuppression in this model. The data indicate that soluble factors released from PC do not play a role in the proliferation inhibition, but rather direct contact between the two cell populations is required in this *in vitro* system. However, it is possible that soluble factors are released from RC after initial contact with PC and these could also have effects on RC proliferation. Related enveloped RNA viruses, mumps virus (SBL), and SV5 (both Paramyxoviridae) as well as VSV (New Jersey) and FMDV empty capsids did not produce any immunosuppressive effects in this system, indicating that they do not share this mechanism of contact-mediated inhibition with the *Morbillivirus* genus.

The suggestion that RPV vaccination could cause immunosuppression in the host (Jeggo *et al.*, 1987; Stevenson *et al.*, 1999) is unsubstantiated under field conditions. However, Heaney *et al.* (2005) have recently shown, using an *ex vivo* experimental system, based on a proliferation assay, that both wild-type and vaccine strains of RPV can impair the proliferation of host PBMC. In a previous *in vitro* assay little difference could be detected in the proliferation inhibitory effects of wild-type and vaccine strains of RPV (Heaney *et al.*, 2002). This had also previously been found to be the case for MV strains *in vitro* (Schlender *et al.*, 1996). However, in *ex vivo* experiments the extent of the proliferation inhibition is both transient and weak with the vaccine strain, in contrast to either mild or virulent strains of wild-type RPV. Furthermore, the degree of inhibition was found to be directly related to the proportion of infected PBMC during the course of RPV infection, which was highest with virulent strains and lowest in vaccinated animals (Figure 10.4). In a previous study Lund *et al.* (2000) could find no evidence of immune suppression in cattle vaccinated with the RBOK vaccine strain but they did not examine animals in the first few days after infection in contrast to this more recent work.

During the course of acute MV infection, only a proportion of peripheral blood cells have been shown to be infected. This mechanism of inhibition, by direct and transient contact with an infected cell, may account for the widespread non-responsiveness of the immune system when only relatively few cells are infected. As for MV, during the course of RPV infection the majority of circulating PBMC remained virus-free. It was therefore possible to determine their status with regard to contact-mediated inhibition. Heaney, Cosby and Barrett (unpublished data) examined vaccinated cattle with regard to contact-mediated inhibition. Infected cells expressing the RPV H glycoprotein on their surface were removed from the total leucocyte population. The remaining uninfected cells were mitogen-stimulated and compared to cells from an uninfected animal. The stimulation index of the uninfected control animal remained constant over the 12-day test period while, in contrast, the stimulation index of the two experimentally vaccinated animals dropped by over 25%. This indicates that contact-mediated suppression is biologically relevant *in vivo*.

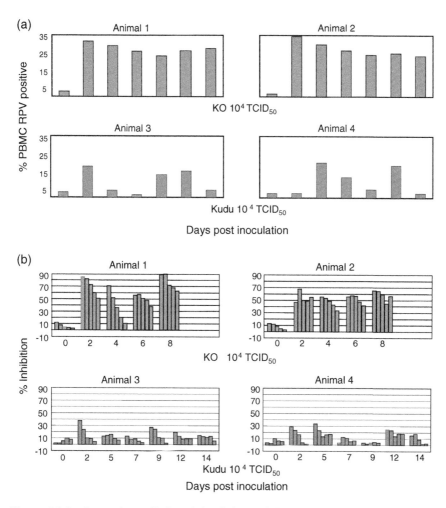

**Figure 10.4** Comparison of infected circulating peripheral blood leucocytes (PBL) with the level of immunosuppression caused by mild and virulent strains of rinderpest virus (unpublished data: Heaney, Cosby and Barrett). (*a*) Percentage of PBL that are infected at different times post inoculation in two cattle infected with virulent (animals 1 & 2) and two with mild (animals 3 & 4) strains of rinderpest virus as measured by FACS analysis. (*b*) Percentage inhibition of proliferation of uninfected PBL by PBL derived from the same animals at the same times post inoculation. Animals 1 & 2 were infected with $10^4$ $TCID_{50}$ of the highly virulent Kabete 'O' (KO) strain of rinderpest. Animals 3 & 4 were infected with $10^4$ $TCID_{50}$ of a mild strain of RPV isolated from a kudu.

## Morbillivirus proteins and immunosuppression

The mechanism of immunosuppression induced by individual morbillivirus proteins has only been investigated in the past few years. Recent studies have determined the importance of the H, N and P genes of RPV in pathogenicity, particularly leucopenia. Recombinant rinderpest viruses were constructed in which the H and P or H, N and P genes of the cattle-derived RBOK vaccine (which is avirulent in rabbits) were replaced with those from the rabbit-adapted RPV-Lv strain, which is highly pathogenic for rabbits (Yoneda *et al.*, 2002, 2004). Rabbits infected with recombinants containing the Lv PH or Lv NPH showed leucopenia, similar to the wild-type lapinized virus. In contrast clinical signs of infection and leucopenia were not observed in animals infected with the the LvH and RBOK viruses. However, both RPV-L and rRPV-lapH induced a marked antibody response in rabbits. Therefore the H protein plays an important role in allowing infection and lymphodepletion to occur in rabbits while the P protein is considered to be a key determinant in cross-species pathogenicity (Yoneda *et al.*, 2004).

Several MV proteins have been reported to play a role in morbillivirus contact-mediated immunosuppression of the host. Schlender *et al.* (1996) showed that interaction of MV glycoproteins F and H with the surface of uninfected peripheral blood leucocytes (PBL) induced immunosuppression *in vitro*. Co-expression of a cleaved form of the F protein and the H proteins of MV on the PC surface was necessary and sufficient to induce the effect, both *in vitro* and in a cotton rat model (Schlender *et al.*, 1996; Niewiesk *et al.*, 1997). Recombinant capripoxvirus and adenovirus vectors expressing RPV proteins have subsequently been used to determine the effect of individual RPV proteins, or combinations of proteins, on the proliferation of the RC population (Heaney *et al.*, 2002). When PC were infected with two adenovirus recombinants, as for MV only the F and H combination of proteins expressed in the same cell showed a significant inhibitory effect on the RC proliferation. When a PC population was generated by mixing equal numbers of cells separately expressing the different proteins, little effect on the RC proliferation was observed. These data indicated that, as for MV, co-expression of both RPV glycoproteins was necessary and sufficient to induce suppression of proliferation.

It has been shown for MV that immune suppression by cell contact inhibition is due to cell cycle arrest, not apoptosis of the RC (Schnorr *et al.*, 1997; Niewiesk *et al.*, 1999). Over 50% of the RC were arrested between $G_0$ and $G_1$ of the cell cycle following co-cultivation with MV-infected PC (Naniche *et al.*, 1999). The remaining lymphocytes did progress through the cell cycle but at a slower rate. When studied at the molecular level it was revealed that the cyclin-dependent kinase (CDK) inhibitor p27[Kip1] protein levels remained high in non-proliferating cell populations (Engelking *et al.*, 1999). Furthermore, there was decreased expression of cyclins D3 and E, which phosphorylate retinoblastoma protein (Rb), allowing entry of cells into the S phase of the cell cycle. Also, the normal upregulation of Rb did not occur (Naniche *et al.*, 1999). It has been reported by Avota *et al.* (2001), that the F and H proteins mediate inhibition of PBL proliferation through Akt kinase as activation of this enzyme was impaired after MV contact both *in vitro* and *in vivo* in a cotton rat model. MV interference with Akt activation is important for immunosuppression, as expression of a catalytically active Akt prevents negative signalling by the MV glycoproteins. This interference with signalling has not been confirmed for the other morbilliviruses but it appears highly likely as the viruses share a common mechanism of inhibition through glycoprotein contact. These workers have also shown for MV that proliferation inhibition is independent of the presence or absence of both known virus binding receptors, SLAM and CD46 (Erlenhoefer *et al.*, 2001). Therefore, the interaction of morbillivirus H and F proteins involves some conformational change that is required to bind the, as yet unidentified, ligand responsible for initiating the process.

Other groups have described immunosuppressive effects of MV nucleocapsid (N) protein. Ravanel *et al.* (1997) demonstrated that MV N protein binds to Fc gamma RII on human and murine B cells and inhibits *in vitro* antibody production. Furthermore, Marie *et al.* demonstrated that this interaction on DC suppresses the inflammatory response *in vivo* in a murine delayed type hypersensitivity model (Marie *et al.*, 2001). More recently, a study by another laboratory reported that the C-terminal fragment of the MV N protein binds to a novel cell surface receptor (NR) and inhibits proliferation of human T cells. They also reported that PPRV N and CDV N bind to both human Fc gamma RIIs and human and murine NR, whereas RPV N only binds to NR (Laine *et al.*, 2003).

Laine *et al.* (2003) reported that MV N protein is released from infected cells following apoptosis and Servet-Delprat *et al.* (2000a) have shown that this also occurs in infected DC. It is likely that N protein is then presented by DC to CD4+ T cells. Both strong cellular and humoral immune responses to N protein are associated with the acute phase of MV infection. In support of the importance of the exogenous pathway and cross-priming, efficient helper CD4+, as well as cytotoxic CD8+ T cell responses against N are generated. It has also been shown that MV-N alone can protect against MV infection in a mouse model system (Niewiesk *et al.*, 1997). Furthermore, N protein binding to Fc gamma RII receptor or possibly the NR receptor on DC may also induce immunosuppression. There are also indications that a feedback mechanism is in place as Servet-Delprat *et al.* (2000b) have reported that inhibition of CD40–CD40L ligand interaction blocks N synthesis in MoDC. Further studies are warranted to dissect these apparently conflicting observations and determine whether findings for MV are common to RPV and the other morbilliviruses.

The P genes of all morbilliviruses give rise to the C and V proteins in addition to P itself. MV V has been shown to inhibit cytokine responses by direct interference with host STAT protein-dependent signalling systems (Palosaari *et al.*, 2003). The interferon-alpha signalling pathway is inhibited through suppression of Jak1 phosphorylation and association of viral accessory proteins, C and V, with interferon-alpha receptor complex (Yokota *et al.*, 2003). Recombinant rinderpest viruses have been constructed in which the expression of these proteins has been suppressed and their growth characteristics in tissue culture have been documented (Baron and Barrett, 2000). However, the effect of these proteins on the immune response remains to be determined.

## Conclusions

Whether an animal recovers from rinderpest infection is probably determined by the balance between virus clearance by immune mechanisms and virus-induced immunosuppression. The immune response during virus clearance and recovery from RPV has not been directly examined in cattle and would require studies with milder wild-type strains where a relatively high survival rate is possible. Furthermore, the extended infection times might allow the possibility of transient or persistent CNS infection or autoimmunity to be investigated. It is also difficult in cattle to distinguish the relative importance of the role of cell-mediated and humoral immunity in either recovery from infection or protection against challenge by vaccination. However, characterization of the inflammatory response in tissues using bovine cell- or cytokine-specific markers, which are now available, should be informative. Also, both the rabbit peripheral infection and mouse CNS infection models provide systems where it is feasible to ablate specific immune functions.

It is apparent that the level of infection in both lymphatic tissues and in PBL is directly correlated with the degree of immunosuppression. Hence highly virulent strains of RPV in addition to causing more direct damage to tissue and leucopenia also infect larger numbers of PBL therefore inducing higher levels of contact-mediated proliferation inhibition. Immunosuppression is a complex and multifaceted process and other mechanisms of suppression need to be studied for morbilliviruses *in vivo*. The RPV cattle virus–host system provides an excellent natural infection system. In the rabbit model it has, already, been demonstrated that RPV affects both T and B cell function but not memory cells. This is an important area for further investigation and may help to explain why during measles virus infection, the response to unrelated antigens can be suppressed on one hand with lifelong immunity to the virus developing on the other.

Studies to date indicate that the role of specific virus proteins in induction of either a protective immune response or immunosuppression is in general the same for both RPV and MV and is probably common for all the morbilliviruses. This similarity can therefore be exploited and leads to the exciting prospect where recombinant RPV can be used in future studies to examine *in vivo* the effects of individual morbillivirus proteins (from both virulent and vaccine strains) on specific immune cell subtypes in the natural host.

## References

Appel, M.J., Shek, W.R. *et al.* (1982) Lymphocyte-mediated immune cytotoxicity in dogs infected with virulent canine distemper virus. *Infect. Immun.* **37** (2), 592–600.
Arneborn, P. and Biberfeld, G. (1983) T-lymphocyte subpopulations in relation to immunosuppression in measles and varicella. *Infect. Immun.* **39** (1), 29–37.

Ata, F.A., al Sumry, H.S. *et al.* (1989) Duration of maternal immunity to peste des petits ruminants. *Vet. Rec.* **124** (22), 590–1.

Avota, E., Avota, A. *et al.* (2001) Disruption of Akt kinase activation is important for immunosuppression induced by measles virus. *Nat. Med.* **7** (6), 725–31.

Baron, M.D. and Barrett, T. (2000) Rinderpest virus lacking the C and V proteins show specific defects in growth and transcription of viral RNAs. *J. Virol.* **74** (6), 2603–11.

Bassiri, M., Ahmad, S. *et al.* (1993) Immunological responses of mice and cattle to baculovirus-expressed F and H-proteins of rinderpest virus – lack of protection in the presence of neutralizing antibody. *J. Virol.* **67**, 1255–61.

Bergeon, P. (1952) Peste bovine: richesse en virus pestique des tissus nerveux et de la moelle osseuse de veaux atteints de peste bovine experimentale. *Bull. Soc. Pathol. Exot.* **12**, 148–52.

Brown, C. and Torres, A. (1994) Distribution of antigen in cattle infected with rinderpest virus. *Vet. Pathol.* **31**, 194–200.

Chino, F. and Yamanouchi, K. (1974) Pathologic changes of the lymphoid system after infections of monkeys with measles virus and of rabbits with rinderpest virus. *Recent Adv. Res.* **14**, 113–29.

Cosby, S.L., Morrison, J. *et al.* (1983) An immunological study of infection of hamsters with large and small plaque canine distemper viruses. *Arch. Virol.* **76** (3), 201–10.

Domingo, M., Vilafranca, M. *et al.* (1995) Evidence for chronic morbillivirus infection in the Mediterranean striped dolphin (*Stenella coeruleoalba*). *Vet. Microbiol.* **44**, 229–39.

Duignan, P.J., Duffy, N. *et al.* (1997) Comparative antibody response in harbour and grey seals naturally infected by a morbillivirus. *Vet. Immunol. Immunopathol.* **55** (4), 341–9.

Engelking, O., Fedorov, L.M. *et al.* (1999) Measles virus-induced immunosuppression in vitro is associated with deregulation of G1 cell cycle control proteins. *J. Gen. Virol.* **80** (Pt 7), 1599–608.

Erlenhoefer, C., Wurzer, W.J. *et al.* (2001) CD150 (SLAM) is a receptor for measles virus but is not involved in viral contact-mediated proliferation inhibition. *J. Virol.* **75** (10), 4499–505.

Fugier-Vivier, I., Servet-Delprat, C. *et al.* (1997) Measles virus suppresses cell-mediated immunity by interfering with the survival and functions of dendritic and T cells. *J. Exp. Med.* **186**, 813–23.

Fukuda, A. and Yamanouchi, K. (1976) Autoimmunity induced in rabbits by rinderpest virus. *Infect. Immun.* **13** (5), 1449–53.

Fukuda, A. and Yamanouchi, K. (1981) Comparison of autoimmunity induction with virulent and attenuated rinderpest virus in rabbits. *Jpn. J. Med. Sci. Biol.* **34** (3), 149–59.

Galbraith, S.E., McQuaid, S. *et al.* (2002) Rinderpest and peste des petits ruminants viruses exhibit neurovirulence in mice. *J. Neurovirol.* **8** (1), 45–52.

Griffin, D. and Bellini, W.J. (1996) Measles virus. In: D.K. and P.H. Fields *et al.*, Fields *Virology*, 3rd edn. New York: Lippincott–Raven.

Heaney, J., Barrett, T. *et al.* (2002) Inhibition of in vitro leukocyte proliferation by morbilliviruses. *J. Virol.* **76** (7), 3579–84.

Heaney, J., Cosby, S.L. and Barrett, T. (2005) Inhibition of host PBMC proliferation *ex vivo* by rinderpest virus. *J. Gen. Virol.*, in press.

Imagawa, D.T. (1965) Propagation of rinderpest virus in suckling mice and its comparison to murine adapted strains of measles and distemper. *Arch. Gesamte Virusforsch.* **17** (2), 203–15.

Imaoka, K., Kanai, Y. *et al.* (1990) Temporary breakdown of immunological tolerance to dsDNA and nucleohistone antigens in rabbits infected with rinderpest virus. *Clin. Exp. Immunol.* **82**, 522–6.

Jeggo, M.H., Wardley, R.C. *et al.* (1987) A reassessment of the dual vaccine against rinderpest and contagious bovine pleuropneumonia. *Vet. Rec.* **120** (6), 131–5.

Kamata, H., Ohishi, K. *et al.* (2001) Rinderpest virus (RPV) ISCOM vaccine induces protection in cattle against virulent RPV challenge. *Vaccine* **19** (25–26), 3355–9.

Khandelwal, A., Renukaradhya, G.J. *et al.* (2004) Systemic and oral immunogenicity of hemagglutinin protein of rinderpest virus expressed by transgenic peanut plants in a mouse model. *Virology* **323**, 284–91.

Khandelwal, A., Sita, G.L. *et al.* (2003a) Expression of hemagglutinin protein of rinderpest virus in transgenic tobacco and immunogenicity of plant-derived protein in a mouse model. *Virology* **308** (2), 207–15.

Khandelwal, A., Sita, G.L. *et al.* (2003b) Oral immunization of cattle with hemagglutinin protein of rinderpest virus expressed in transgenic peanut induces specific immune responses. *Vaccine* **21** (23), 3282–9.

Kobune, F., Chino, F. *et al.* (1976) Studies on recovery mechanism from rinderpest virus infection in rabbits. I. Effect of anti-thymocyte serum and thymectomy. *Jpn. J. Med. Sci. Biol.* **29** (5), 265–75.

Kruse, M., Meinl, E. *et al.* (2001) Signaling lymphocytic activation molecule is expressed on mature CD83+ dendritic cells and is up-regulated by IL-1 beta. *J. Immunol.* **167** (4), 1989–95.

Kumagai, K., Yamaguchi, R. *et al.* (2004) Lymphoid apoptosis in acute canine distemper. *J. Vet. Med. Sci.* **66** (2), 175–81.

Laine, D., Trescol-Biemont, M.C. *et al.* (2003) Measles virus (MV) nucleoprotein binds to a novel cell surface receptor distinct from FcgammaRII via its C-terminal domain: role in MV-induced immunosuppression. *J. Virol.* **77** (21), 11332–46.

Libeau, G., Diallo, A. *et al.* (1992) A competitive ELISA using anti-N monoclonal antibodies for specific detection of rinderpest antibodies in cattle and small ruminants. *Vet. Microbiol.* **31**, 147–60.

Liebert, U.G., Flanagan, S.G. *et al.* (1994) Antigenic determinants of measles virus hemagglutinin associated with neurovirulence. *J. Virol.* **68**, 1486–93.

Lund, B.T., Tiwari, A. *et al.* (2000) Vaccination of cattle with attenuated rinderpest virus stimulates CD4(+) T cell responses with broad viral antigen specificity. *J. Gen. Virol.* **81** (Pt 9), 2137–46.

Makela, M.J., Salmi, A.A. *et al.* (1989) Monoclonal antibodies against measles virus haemagglutinin react with synthetic peptides. *Scand. J. Immunol.* **30** (2), 225–31.

Marie, J.C., Kehren, J. *et al.* (2001) Mechanism of measles virus-induced suppression of inflammatory immune responses. *Immunity* **14** (1), 69–79.

Minagawa, H., Tanaka, K. *et al.* (2001) Induction of the measles virus receptor SLAM (CD150) on monocytes. *J. Gen. Virol.* **82** (Pt 12), 2913–17.

Mitra-Kaushik, S., Nayak, R. *et al.* (2001) Identification of a cytotoxic T-cell epitope on the recombinant nucleocapsid proteins of rinderpest and peste des petits ruminants viruses presented as assembled nucleocapsids. *Virology* **279** (1), 210–20.

Naniche, D., Garenne, M. *et al.* (2004) Decrease in measles virus-specific CD4 T cell memory in vaccinated subjects. *J. Infect. Dis.* **190** (8), 1387–95.

Naniche, D., Reed, S.I. *et al.* (1999) Cell cycle arrest during measles virus infection: a G0-like block leads to suppression of retinoblastoma protein expression. *J. Virol.* **73** (3), 1894–901.

Niewiesk, S., Brinckmann, U. *et al.* (1993) Susceptibility to measles virus-induced encephalitis in mice correlates with impaired antigen presentation to cytotoxic T lymphocytes. *J. Virol.* **67** (1), 75–81.

Niewiesk, S., Eisenhuth, I. *et al.* (1997) Measles virus-induced immune suppression in the cotton rat (*Sigmodon hispidus*) model depends on viral glycoproteins. *J. Virol.* **71**, 7214–19.

Niewiesk, S., Ohnimus, H. *et al.* (1999) Measles virus-induced immunosuppression in cotton rats is associated with cell cycle retardation in uninfected lymphocytes. *J. Gen. Virol.* **80** (Pt 8), 2023–9.

Nores, J.E.R., Anderson, J. *et al.* (1995) Rinderpest virus infection of bovine peripheral blood monocytes. *J. Gen. Virol.* **76** (Pt 11), 2779–91.

Ohgimoto, S., Ohgimoto, K. *et al.* (2001) The haemagglutinin protein is an important determinant of measles virus tropism for dendritic cells in vitro. *J. Gen. Virol.* **82** (Pt 8), 1835–44.

Ohishi, K., Inui, K. *et al.* (1999) Cell-mediated immune responses in cattle vaccinated with a vaccinia recombinant expressing the nucleocapsid (N) protein of rinderpest virus (RPV). *J. Gen. Virol.* **80** (Pt 7), 1627–34.

Ohishi, K., Kamata, H. *et al.* (1998) Construction of recombinant vaccinia virus expressing rinderpest virus nucleocapsid protein and its immunogenicity in mice. *J. Vet. Med. Sci.* **60**, 655–6.

Okita, M., Mori, T. *et al.* (1995) Immunohistochemical studies of lymphoid tissues of rabbits infected with rinderpest virus. *J. Comp. Pathol.* **112**, 41–51.

Palosaari, H., Parisien, J.P. *et al.* (2003) STAT protein interference and suppression of cytokine signal transduction by measles virus V protein. *J. Virol.* **77** (13), 7635–44.

Penhale, W.J. and Pow. I.A. (1970) The immunodepressive effect of rinderpest virus. *Clin. Exp. Immunol.* **6** (4), 627–32.

Permar, S.R., Klumpp, S.A. *et al.* (2004) Limited contribution of humoral immunity to the clearance of measles viremia in rhesus monkeys. *J. Infect. Dis.* **190** (5), 998–1005.

Plowright, W. (1984) The duration of immunity in cattle following inoculation of rinderpest cell-culture vaccine. *J. Hyg.* **92** (3), 285–96.

Provost, A., Maurice, Y. and Borredon, C. (1968) [Rinderpest protection induced in cattle by measles vaccine. Application to calves with passive immunity by maternal antibo-dies.] *Rev. Elev. Méd. Vét. Pays Trop.* **21** (2), 145–64.

Rahman, M.M., Shaila, M.S. *et al.* (2003) Baculovirus display of fusion protein of peste des petits ruminants virus and hemagglutination protein of rinderpest virus and immunogenicity of the displayed proteins in mouse model. *Virology* **317**, 36–49.

Ravanel, K., Castelle, C. *et al.* (1997) Measles virus nucleocapsid protein binds to Fc gamma RII and inhibits human B cell antibody production. *J. Exp. Med.* **186**, 269–78.

Rima, B.K., Cosby, S.L. *et al.* (1990) Humoral immune responses in seals infected by phocine distemper virus. *Res. Vet. Sci.* **49** (1), 114–16.

Rima, B.K., Duffy, N. *et al.* (1991) Correlation between humoral immune responses and presence of virus in the CNS in dogs experimentally infected with canine distemper virus. *Arch. Virol.* **121** (1–4), 1–8.

Roeder, P. and Obi, T. (1999) *Recognising Peste-des-Petits Ruminants: A Field Manual.* FAO Animal Health Manuals No. 5. Rome: FAO.

Romero, C.H., Barrett, T. *et al.* (1994) Recombinant capripoxvirus expressing the hemagglutinin protein gene of rinderpest virus: protection of cattle against rinderpest and lumpy skin disease viruses. *Virology* **204**, 425–9.

Rose, J.W., Bellini, W.J. *et al.* (1984) Human cellular immune response to measles virus polypeptides. *J. Virol.* **49** (3), 988–91.

Rossiter, P.B., Herniman, K.A.J. *et al.* (1993) The growth of cell culture-attenuated rinderpest virus in bovine lymphoblasts with B-cell, CD4+ and CD8+ alpha-beta T-cell and gamma-delta T-cell phenotypes. *J. Gen. Virol.* **74**, 305–9.

Schadeck, E.B., Partidos, C.D. *et al.* (1999) CTL epitopes identified with a defective recombinant adenovirus expressing measles virus nucleoprotein and evaluation of their protective capacity in mice. *Virus Res.* **65** (1), 75–86.

Schlender, J., Schnorr, J.J. *et al.* (1996) Interaction of measles virus glycoproteins with the surface of uninfected peripheral blood lymphocytes induces immunosuppression *in vitro.* *Proc. Natl Acad. Sci. USA* **93**, 13194–9.

Schlereth, B., Buonocore, L. *et al.* (2003) Successful mucosal immunization of cotton rats in the presence of measles virus-specific antibodies depends on degree of attenuation of vaccine vector and virus dose. *J. Gen. Virol.* **84** (Pt 8), 2145–51.

Schneider-Schaulies, S., Niewiesk, S. *et al.* (2001) Measles virus induced immunosuppression: targets and effector mechanisms. *Curr. Mol. Med.* **1** (2), 163–81.

Schnorr, J.J., Seufert, M. *et al.* (1997) Cell cycle arrest rather than apoptosis is associated with measles virus contact-mediated immunosuppression in vitro. *J. Gen. Virol.* **78**, 3217–26.

Servet-Delprat, C., Vidalain, P.O. *et al.* (2000a) Consequences of Fas-mediated human dendritic cell apoptosis induced by measles virus. *J. Virol.* **74** (9), 4387–93.

Servet-Delprat, C., Vidalain, P.O. *et al.* (2000b) Measles virus induces abnormal differentiation of CD40 ligand-activated human dendritic cells. *J. Immunol.* **164** (4), 1753–60.

Sinnathamby, G., Naik, S. *et al.* (2001a) Recombinant hemagglutinin protein of rinderpest virus expressed in insect cells induces humoral and cell mediated immune responses in cattle. *Vaccine* **19** (28–29), 3870–6.

Sinnathamby, G., Nayak, R. *et al.* (2001b) Mapping of T-helper epitopes of Rinderpest virus hemagglutinin protein. *Viral Immunol.* **14** (1), 83–92.

Sinnathamby, G., Seth, S. *et al.* (2004) Cytotoxic T cell epitope in cattle from the attachment glycoproteins of rinderpest and peste des petits ruminants viruses. *Viral Immunol.* **17**, 401–10.

Stevenson, P., Rossiter, P.B. *et al.* (1999) Rinderpest vaccination and the incidence and development of trypanosomosis in cattle. *Trop. Anim. Hlth Prod.* **31** (2), 65–73.

Stolte, M., Haas, L. *et al.* (2002) Induction of apoptotic cellular death in lymphatic tissues of cattle experimentally infected with different strains of rinderpest virus. *J. Comp. Pathol.* **127** (1), 14–21.

Sugiyama, M., Ito, N. *et al.* (2002) Identification of immunodominant neutralizing epitopes on the hemagglutinin protein of rinderpest virus. *J. Virol.* **76** (4), 1691–6.

Tamashiro, V.G., Perez, H.H. *et al.* (1987) Prospective study of the magnitude and duration of changes in tuberculin reactivity during uncomplicated and complicated measles. *Pediatr. Infect. Dis. J.* **6** (5), 451–4.

Tatsuo, H., Ono, N. *et al.* (2001) Morbilliviruses use signaling lymphocyte activation molecules (CD150) as cellular receptors. *J. Virol.* **75** (13), 5842–50.

Verardi, P.H., Aziz, F.H. *et al.* (2002) Long-term sterilizing immunity to rinderpest in cattle vaccinated with a recombinant vaccinia virus expressing high levels of the fusion and hemagglutinin glycoproteins. *J. Virol.* **76** (2), 484–91.

Wohlsein, P., Trautwein, G., Harder, T.C., Liess, B. and Barrett, T. (1993) Comparative aspects of pathogenicity of measles, canine distemper, and rinderpest viruses. *Jpn. J. Med. Sci. Biol.* **33**, 41–66.

Wohlsein, P., Wamwayi, H.M. *et al.* (1995) Pathomorphological and immunohistological findings in cattle experimentally infected with rinderpest virus isolates of different pathogenicity. *Vet. Microbiol.* **44** (2–4), 141–9.

Yamanouchi, K. (1980) Comparative aspects of pathogenicity of measles, canine distemper, and rinderpest viruses. *Jpn. J. Med. Sci. Biol.* **33** (2), 41–66.

Yamanouchi, K., Chino, F. *et al.* (1974a) Pathogenesis of rinderpest virus infection in rabbits. I. Clinical signs, immune response, histological changes, and virus growth patterns. *Infect. Immun.* **9** (2), 199–205.

Yamanouchi, K., Fukuda, A. *et al.* (1974b) Pathogenesis of rinderpest virus infection in rabbits. II. Effect of rinderpest virus on the immune functions of rabbits. *Infect. Immun.* **9** (2), 206–11.

Yilma, T., Hsu, D. *et al.* (1988) Protection of cattle against rinderpest with vaccinia virus recombinants expressing the HA or F gene. *Science* **242** (4881), 1058–61.

Yokota, S., Saito, H. *et al.* (2003) Measles virus suppresses interferon-alpha signaling pathway: suppression of Jak1 phosphorylation and association of viral accessory proteins, C and V, with interferon-alpha receptor complex. *Virology* **306** (1), 135–46.

Yoneda, M., Bandyopadhyay, S.K. *et al.* (2002) Rinderpest virus H protein: role in determining host range in rabbits. *J. Gen. Virol.* **83** (Pt 6), 1457–63.

Yoneda, M., Miura, R. *et al.* (2004) Rinderpest virus phosphoprotein gene is a major determinant of species-specific pathogenicity. *J. Virol.* **78**, 6676–81.

Ziegler, D., Fournier, P. *et al.* (1996) Protection against measles virus encephalitis by monoclonal antibodies binding to a cystine loop domain of the H protein mimicked by peptides which are not recognized by maternal antibodies. *J. Gen. Virol.* **77** (Pt 10), 2479–89.

# History of vaccines and vaccination

# 11

## WILLIAM P. TAYLOR,* PETER L. ROEDER† AND MARK M. RWEYEMAMU‡

*Littlehampton, Sussex, United Kingdom
†Food and Agriculture Organization, Animal Health Service, Animal Production and Health Division, Rome, Italy
‡Woking, Surrey, UK

## Introduction

Having defined rinderpest as an entity, the first half of the history of man's acquaintance with this ruinous condition was devoted to attempts to cure sick animals. Retrospectively, the well-researched history of this period provides much that will interest the student of veterinary medicine (Spinage, 2003). Drawing on the discovery in Russia by Semmer (1893) that serum taken from a recovered animal had protective powers, the second half as it were, begins with the final realization that the disease could be in fact be cured by the use of immune serum or repulsed by inducing a protective immunity in uninfected animals. The subsequent development of rinderpest vaccines paved the way for numerous attempts to modify the epidemiology of the virus by creating livestock populations so heavily immune that they could no longer support the presence of the virus. Of course, with understanding, other means of preventing the spread of the virus became available, such as either the destruction or quarantining of infected animals and the control of the movement of in-contacts. However, when weighed against the cultural inappropriateness of heavily policed control methods in those parts of the world still supporting endemic rinderpest in the twentieth century, the impetus to develop and improve methods of vaccinating livestock against rinderpest became the engine driving rinderpest control.

Early in the development of rinderpest vaccines came the realization that if live virus was used to immunize the host, a lifelong immunity could be

ISBN-13: 978-0-12-88385-1
ISBN-10: 0-12-88385-6

induced. This attribute allowed individual herds to be protected indefinitely using an initial vaccination campaign and annual follow-up vaccination of young replacement stock. If undertaken on a wide enough scale, the individual farmer's herd became the national herd at which point it became clear that if vaccine could eliminate rinderpest from a national herd, it could do the same job at the international level. It was then only a question of time before eradication became the compelling issue relating to rinderpest. Hopefully, history will judge that we have now moved far beyond control and, with the elimination of two of the three field lineages (see Chapter 6), are well on the way to achieving global eradication.

Companion papers describe the genesis of the Global Rinderpest Eradication Programme and its impact on the fate of the virus. This contribution attempts to describe the development of rinderpest vaccines and the history of their use within the on-going, global assault on rinderpest.

## Immune serum and serum-simultaneous vaccination

Ten years after its commencement, in 1897 the great African rinderpest epizootic finally spread from the Transvaal to Cape Colony. Ahead of this event, in October 1896, a team comprised of Arnold Theiler, Transvaal Government Veterinarian, and Herbert Watkins-Pitchford, Chief Veterinary Surgeon, Natal, had already begun work in Transvaal studying immune serum as a curative method, the simultaneous inoculation of virus and immune serum as a prophylactic method and the preparation of hyperimmune serum in goats. In early 1897 Dr Theiler's efforts were subsumed into another team led by Drs Bordet and Danysz, brought in from the Pasteur Institute, Paris; this team reported its results in June 1897 (Mack, 1970; Vogel and Heyne, 1996; Spinage, 2003). The technique involved the use of serum alone or in combination with infective blood given before or after the serum treatment. They had, however, demonstrated the protective effects of immune serum leading to the development of the so-called French Method.

In the midst of the search for a preventive method, Robert Koch arrived in Cape Town – at the beginning of December, 1896 – and began work at Kimberley with a team of local staff comprised of Drs George Turner (Medical Officer of Health, Cape Colony, and Alexander Edington (Director of the Bacteriological Institute, Grahamstown). In February, 1897, Koch reported that bile from an infected ox was (generally) non-infective and (behaving in a manner analogous to an inactivated rinderpest vaccine) could produce immunity to rinderpest – after which he immediately left for India on a different mission. However, in the same report Koch indicated that convalescent serum gave a short-term passive protection but a mixture of immune serum and virulent

224 Rinderpest and Peste des Petits Ruminants

blood produced an active immunity. In 1898, Turner and Koch's chosen replacement, Wilhelm Kolle, confirmed the value of the serum–virus simultaneous method which, until the later development of inactivated vaccines, was the most effective way of immunizing cattle against rinderpest and a method widely used in both Africa and India.

Writing from India, Pool and Doyle (1922) pointed out that there was little to distinguish the serum-simultaneous method from the use of serum alone as the animals passively protected with serum were in any case mixed with infected animals and would themselves be infected by the live virus. In India the serum-only method had been in use for the past 20 years but now a switch to the serum-simultaneous method was taking place. Apparently an earlier attempt to introduce the serum-simultaneous method in Madras had resulted in high mortality, which brought the method into disrepute but now, 10 years later, imported stock in Military Dairy Farms were being vaccinated by this method. Its future was seen in the elimination of outbreaks where the administration of live virus would present no danger, the virus already being present. Accordingly, it was seen as the method *par excellence* for a country such as India. Nevertheless, Pantulu (1934) indicated that the serum-only method continued in use in the Madras Presidency until 1929 and although serum-simultaneous inoculations were commenced in 1919–20, as late as 1928–29 only 8336 animals had been vaccinated by this means. By the end of 1931–32 however, just over half a million animals had been immunized by the simultaneous method.

According to Pool and Doyle (1922), following the spread of rinderpest to Egypt in 1903, the immune serum method was used from 1904 to 1912 but with unsatisfactory results. In 1912, following an unfavourable review, this method was replaced by the serum-simultaneous method. Over the following eight years nearly half a million vaccinations were carried out and a high level of control was achieved.

In a set of standard operating procedures for the serum-simultaneous method issued by Dr J.T. Edwards, Director of the Imperial (later Indian) Veterinary Research Institute at Mukteswar in northern India (Edwards, 1927/28), it is pointed out that the only difference between a natural attack of the virus and the process of active immunization by the serum-simultaneous method was that, in the former instance, a fatal outcome was often seen but, in the latter, the severity of the attack is artificially controlled. If the operation were correctly undertaken the animal should not show any outward sign of bodily disturbance but emerge with a lifelong immunity to rinderpest. The method was not recommended for young weak calves or cows in advanced pregnancy. It was also pointed out that inoculated animals were potentially infectious and should be physically separated from non-inoculated animals. Much effort was devoted to estimating the potency of the serum and computing the amount to be used on various breeds of imported and native cattle and buffaloes. A further consideration was the short shelf-life of the virulent blood, which was as brief as nine days in warm weather; however, the main drawback to the serum-simultaneous method seems to have been the danger that the virus inoculum, drawn from a reacting ox, could contain piroplasms capable of infecting the recipient animal.

Based on the impact of draconian legislation (calling for the immediate slaughter of infected animals) as early as 1908 rinderpest had been eliminated from European Russia, although persisting in Transcaucasia and Kazakhstan (Laktionov, 1967). However, having already discovered the protective property of blood, serum and milk from recovered animals, the Russians went on to discover, develop and apply the serum-simultaneous method. Laktionov does not discuss the impact, if any, of contemporary events in southern Africa but does state that the discovery was confirmed by 'a committee of authoritative scientists'. Subsequently, stations to combat rinderpest were set up in Chita, Zuryabad and Tabakhmel. While it was imperfect and led to the creation of virus carriers which spread the infection, it was far more effective than anything that had gone before and by 1928, in the space of 2–3 years, the serum-simultaneous method had eradicated rinderpest from the whole of Russia.

## Inactivated rinderpest vaccines

In the 1920s a number of workers succeeded in immunizing cattle with inactivated preparations of infected bovine tissues (spleen, tonsils, lymph nodes) using toluol, eucalyptol, formalin or chloroform. Thereafter the pulp was either issued as a wet preparation, or oven dried and issued as a powder. In India, the pioneering results showing protection following two inoculations with glycerine-inactivated rinderpest (Kakizaki, 1918), could not be reproduced and inactivated vaccines were never explored. Nevertheless, inactivated vaccines were developed and Daubney (1953a) praised their advent for the relief they gave from the costly and laborious serum-virus simultaneous method.

According to Scott (1987), rinderpest was first eradicated from Iran in 1931 using a formalin-inactivated vaccine, while a formalin and saponin preparation was used when the virus reinvaded in 1949. Inactivated vaccines helped to eradicate rinderpest from the Philippines and Thailand before the Second World War. In the Philippines, a variety of vaccination techniques made little headway (Koch's glycerinated bile, serum alone, serum-simultaneous), the turning point being the development of a phenol-glycerine inactivated vaccine (Boynton, 1928). In Sri Lanka, a hitherto intractable rinderpest problem was solved in 1934 through the importation of formalized inactivated rinderpest vaccine from East Africa. In 1939 an outbreak spread from Manchuria to Russia (Primorsky Kray) and when the use of hyperimmune serum and strict quarantine failed to suppress the outbreak the inclusion of a formol-inactivated vaccine in the arsenal led to its elimination within five months (Laktionov, 1967).

During the Second World War, and before the advent of cell cultures, 100 000 doses of inactivated rinderpest vaccine were produced at Grosse Isle, Canada for the contingent protection of American and Canadian cattle (Shope, 1949).

Twenty percent (w/v) suspensions of infected bovine tissues were successfully inactivated using 0.75% cent chloroform or 1 in 1000 formalin; cattle could be immunized with a 20 ml dose of either preparation. However, based on the inordinate requirement for bovine virus donors, it was decided to experiment with a strain of the virus (Kabete O) adapted to growth in embryonated eggs. Although the virus was present, the resulting inactivated vaccine was a failure and it was concluded that the large-scale production of an inactivated vaccine was both impractical and excessively expensive.

Even so inactivated vaccines were still in use in several African and Asian countries as late as 1963 (Vittoz, 1963). Later modifications were the use of either aluminium hydroxide or saponin as adjuvants.

While attempts to produce inactivated vaccines from attenuated strains adapted to eggs, goats or rabbits failed (see Scott, 1964 for details), a preparation made from low passage cell culture vaccine succeeded but was never exploited. Scott highlighted safety as the great advantage of inactivated vaccines but a short immunity as a disadvantage. This could be as low as 6 months following a single inoculation or up to 2 years, depending on the adjuvant employed. In addition, a risk associated with the declining immunity was that rinderpest could make an inapparent entry into a group of vaccinated animals spreading slowly but steadily, until finally the majority of the group contracted a severe infection. A case in point was the introduction of rinderpest into Malta in 1947 by cattle that had been given inactivated vaccine in the Sudan (Daubney, 1953a). In contemporary terms, however, a short but effective immunity can be seen as a desirable characteristic, permitting the early resumption of serosurveillance for the presence of wild virus following an attempted suppression of the virus by the use of vaccine.

## Goat-attenuated rinderpest vaccines

The history of goat vaccine, the first of several live attenuated rinderpest vaccines, is divided between India and Africa. Whereas the attenuation of Kabete O in Kenya (see below) came about as a result of an elective decision to develop and standardize a goat-attenuated vaccine, in India the earlier introduction of an attenuated goat-adapted rinderpest strain as a vaccine for cattle was a much less organized affair. To a large extent the ultimate success originated from the studies of Edwards at Mukteswar. Although Edwards was perhaps initially unaware of the studies by Schein (1926) in Indo-China in which Schein described serial passage in goats resulting in attenuation for cattle, he would have been aware of Koch's early belief in the possibility of attenuating rinderpest by passage in goats.

At any rate, in an independent study begun in 1926, Edwards undertook to try to 'fix' a strain of rinderpest (Hill Bull virus, which is to India what the Kabete O strain is to Kenya) in goats. Following an initial introduction into a goat fetus, it was possible to continue a passage series in adult goats using viraemic blood derived from the dam. With passage, the virus became increasingly virulent for goats, resulting in a fatal infection in the majority of instances. Over the following two years Edwards maintained two passage series, one in goats alone and the other alternating between goats and bulls. Without mentioning the passage levels, in his 1928 address to the Central Provinces Veterinary Association (Edwards, 1930), he stated that 'during the past few months, the virus has shown a very striking attenuation in virulence for cattle [i.e. no mortality], and this attenuation is seen equally clearly with both the "direct" and "alternate" strains'. That said, the viruses still produced pyrexia, mouth lesions and diarrhoea in Hill Bulls.

In undertaking this adaptation Edwards was in fact looking for a solution to a problem associated with the serum-simultaneous method in which virulent rinderpest virus of bovine origin was normally employed. Although an inoculation of immune serum promoted recovery from the resulting rinderpest infection, a complicating factor was the simultaneous inoculation of bovine piroplasms and a severe illness. Edwards admitted that the attenuation of rinderpest by passage in goats was a fortuitous result as his primary intention had been to develop a piroplasm-free inoculum. In his 1928 address he asserts that the immunodepressive effect of the rinderpest component led to the reactivation of latent piroplasms within the host, but in his later review (Edwards, 1949) he was more clearly indicating the dangers of introducing piroplasms with the use of a virulent bovine inoculum. In any case following the observed attenuation by passage in goats, it was decided (*circa* 1928) to issue goat virulent blood instead of bovine virulent blood. It was expected that this would lead to the more widespread adoption of the serum-simultaneous method and a wider improvement of livestock health.

In any discussion of goat vaccines, it is important to appreciate the existence of variable levels of innate resistance to rinderpest seen among different races and breeds of cattle. In general it is accepted that breeds of *Bos indicus* are considerably more resistant than breeds of *Bos taurus*. We have recently learnt (N.P.S. Karki, personal communication) that, in contrast to the plains cattle of India which are *Bos indicus*, Himalayan hill cattle (i.e. Hill Bulls), which have always been regarded as having a higher (but puzzling) degree of innate susceptibility to rinderpest, are *Bos taurus*. Accordingly, in 1928, plains cattle were inoculated with goat virus alone and they survived with less impairment to their health than had been the case with Hill Bulls (although they did develop pyrexia).

Edwards was greatly concerned with the need to introduce a modified live virus within a 'Jennerian' system of vaccination and although he departed from India without being able to see the results of his rinderpest attenuation exploited in that way, it did eventually happen. Already in 1928 there seems to have been a move towards the use of goat-adapted rinderpest within the serum-simultaneous method and from 1931 onwards it was increasingly used in northern and southern India as a vaccine in its own right.

Working in Madras, southern India, Saunders and Ayyar (1936) sought to verify the attenuating effect of the serial passage of rinderpest virus in goats. Over a series of 150 passages, each of which was inoculated into a buffalo, the mortality rate over the first 100 passages was around 50 per cent but during the next 50 passages it fell to 24 per cent. According to Krishnamurti (1945), cited by Daubney (1949), the attenuated Madras strain at its 400th goat passage level, when combined with the standard Mukteswar strain to give a virus known as Madras No.2 and then passaged a further 225 times, still produced a mortality rate of around 17% in calves.

The goat-adapted vaccine was widely used in South Asia for the protection of cattle and more resistant breeds of buffalo. It was used in the successful eradication of rinderpest from Thailand after the Second World War (where it could only be used in cattle as it was lethal in buffaloes). It was introduced into Myanmar in 1935, the strain coming from Madras. After the war a replacement strain was supplied from the Veterinary Research Institute, Izatnagar, and finally, in 1966 a strain was imported from Cairo (presumably a sub-strain of Kabete O) which was said to be more attenuated than either of the Indian introductions (Thet Swe, 1991). Goat vaccine was still used to vaccinate cattle and buffaloes in Bangladesh and Myanmar in 1990.

In India two strains of the virus were available at Mukteswar in 1952 – a line that had been maintained by direct goat passage for many years and a second line that had been similarly maintained except for out-passages in Hill Bulls every two or three months. Daubney (1953b), examining proposals for the launching of an all-India rinderpest eradication programme, recommended the adoption of a standard product using the direct line. Standardized goat-adapted virus went in to regular manufacture at Mukteswar in 1953 and continued until 1973 (Y.P. Nanda, personal communication). It was subsequently made at Izatnagar, the main campus of the Indian Veterinary Research Institute and in biological production units at state level where it continued to be used for many years being only gradually replaced by tissue culture vaccine.

In 1936 or so, the Mukteswar goat virus was made available in Kenya, where it was tested in grade and zebu cattle; at 16 and 18 per cent respectively, the mortality rates were deemed to be unacceptably high. Accordingly, between 1937 and 1945 Daubney and Hudson mirrored the work undertaken in India and Indo-China but with the Kabete O strain of rinderpest virus, a highly virulent strain isolated in 1911 and subsequently maintained in the laboratory by needle-passage in cattle (MacOwen, 1955). After 50 passages in goats the virus still killed all experimental cattle in 7–9 days. Between the 69th and 80th passages, animals still died but took longer to do so (12–16 days) and at the 85th passage the first recovery occurred. Between the 85th and 150th passage, 15 of 17 (92.3%) experimental animals survived (Daubney, 1949). Clinically, the pathogenicity of the virus also changed and so after 80 passages the only universal sign was a pyrexia of 4–5 days although this could still be accompanied by serous ocular discharge, nasal discharge and diarrhoea in some but not all animals. Necrotic mouth lesions were not seen after the 100th passage.

By the time the virus had been passaged 250 times it was considered sufficiently attenuated to be used on zebu cattle (*Bos indicus*), although it was still
capable of causing 2% mortality among healthy stock. At between 250 and 400
passages there may have been some slight further attenuation, but even so the
virus still provoked a pyrexia in 95% of zebu vaccinates and was still too virulent for use on European (*Bos taurus*) stock. Nevertheless, at this point it was
introduced for the vaccination of zebu cattle and referred to as KAG (variously
Kenya/Kabete Attenuated Goat).

When first used in Nigeria in 1941, it was too virulent unless given with
immune serum but it was possible to further attenuate it during local production. Unfortunately this sub-line was lost but in 1945 a replacement virus was
sent from Kabete and a fresh passage series was undertaken. Subsequently,
after between 13 and 26 passages in Nigeria (the exact passage level seems to
be unknown), the virus was sent to Egypt, where it was regarded as apprecia-
bly milder than the virus being used in Kenya. Following a further 25 passages
in the Abbassia laboratories in Cairo, vaccine production began there in 1947.
Crawford (1947) pointed out

> a very curious feature of the history of the development of this method of immu-
> nisation is that in most cases when introduced into a new territory, very severe
> reactions with considerable (cattle) mortality followed its use. This was the case in
> Nigeria just as had been the case when Edwards' virus was introduced into Kenya.

Daubney on the other hand, writing in 1949, felt that there was an element of
subjectivity about the variable residual virulence of this virus.

In cattle KAG was expected to provoke a temperature reaction in nearly all
susceptible zebu. An absence of such reactions led to a suspicion that poor
quality vaccine had been used. In Nigerian vaccine camps it was normally
expected that animals would remain in the camp until the third day, when they
would all react and lie down. On the following day they would all stand up
again and the camp would be disbanded. The virus was generally regarded as
non-transmissible between cattle.

Daubney spoke of the reinfection of Egypt in April 1945 through cattle
imported from Anglo-Egyptian Sudan, indicating that by the end of 1945 the
infection was widely disseminated throughout upper and Lower Egypt. Twenty-
one months later, with the outbreak still raging, desiccated goat vaccine was
introduced as a method of mass immunization and six months after that the epidemic had been eradicated. By 1948, some 15 million head of cattle across
East, West, Central and North Africa had been vaccinated with goat virus vaccine (Daubney, 1949).

This vaccine was considered to be cheap and efficacious. The immunity to
rinderpest it produced is long-lived – up to 14 years was reported by Brown and
Raschid (1958), who found neutralizing antibodies in unchallenged cattle living on the island of Pemba, off the East African coast. The only associated
problem was the need for low temperature conservation and the difficulty of

supplying this in the field. However, the keeping quality was improved by desiccation and storage under vacuum.

## Rabbit-attenuated rinderpest vaccine

Brotherston (1957) reflected that through the loss of the rabbit colony at Mukteswar (in which he was attempting to passage rinderpest), providence had pushed Edwards towards the development of a goat-attenuated vaccine in India, where it was most needed, while the shortage of goats in Japan and Korea had forced Nakamura to use rabbits leading to the subsequent development of a vaccine better suited to the more susceptible Asiatic livestock breeds.

Although the attenuation of rinderpest for calves had been demonstrated by passage in rabbits by Cèbe and Perrin (1935), by adapting the virulent Fusan strain to rabbits by intravenous injection, Nakamura et al. (1938) were credited with demonstrating the use of rabbits as a substrate for the growth of the virus (Nakamura III). Apparently the adapted virus was intended for use in serum-simultaneous vaccination attempts on ultra susceptible breeds of cattle (Nakamura et al., 1943). Appreciation of Nakamura's work (in the West) was delayed by the Second World War and because the trials were undertaken in Korea and the results published in Japanese journals.

A slight temperature elevation was reported in the initial passages, becoming more marked as adaptation proceeded and after the first few passages pathognomonic lesions could be observed in the abdomen of infected rabbits. Peyer's patches appeared swollen and to be composed of greyish-white nodules due to necrosis of the germinal centres which began 48 hours after infection. Similar lesions were present in the appendix and sacculus rotundus along with swelling of the mesenteric lymph nodes. The Nakamura virus was carried to very high passage levels. After 150 passages it caused a high mortality rate in Korean cattle, and even at the 325th passage level it still caused occasional deaths in these hypersusceptible animals. In Indian and Mongolian cattle respectively, the 160th and 350th passage of the virus caused only slight reactions. In 1941 the rabbit passaged virus was distributed in Mongolia where, unsupported by serum, it was used safely and effectively on calves (Isogai, 1944). In the 20 or so years between its introduction and the later development of tissue culture rinderpest vaccine (see below), lapinized vaccine was widely used in Africa and Asia, generally in conjunction with goat vaccine but on breeds of cattle with levels of innate resistance unsuited to that variant.

Having been used in north China during the Second World War, it was acquired and used by the Chinese National Research Bureau of Animal Industry in 1945 but the results only became known when they were subsequently presented in Nairobi (Cheng and Fischman, 1949); at passage 630 it had been used for the preparation of a vaccine which caused only mild reactions in cattle and buffaloes. Thereafter, the Food and Agriculture Organization of the

United Nations (FAO) disseminated this vaccine to a number of countries including Egypt, Thailand, India, Kenya, Pakistan and Ethiopia.

Lapinized rinderpest virus is readily adaptable to a number of additional hosts including goats, sheep, and calves but not chick embryos. In Thailand, where rabbits were virtually unobtainable, Hudson and Wongsonsarn (1950) developed a reactor vaccine using Asiatic pigs which is credited with the eradication of rinderpest from that country (Scott, 1964).

In China many different breeds of cattle, buffaloes and yaks showed differing susceptibilities to the effects of rinderpest. Mongolian cattle were most resistant, with mortality rates of 50–70%. Yellow cattle and buffaloes (swamp) experienced death rates of 80% or more while Korean cattle and yaks suffered virtually 100% mortality.

From about 1950 Chinese workers at the Harbin Veterinary Institute attempted to develop a more satisfactory live attenuated vaccine because the Nakamura III vaccine was difficult to produce in the amounts needed, one rabbit being sufficient to produce only 600 doses. Starting from the 400th rabbit passage level the virus was adapted to goats to give an effective reactor vaccine giving good protection and being generally safe to use. However, both lapinized as well as the lapinized/caprinized vaccines gave very severe reactions with nervous signs in yaks. Passage in goats was continued up to 200 passages but was still unsuitable for Korean cattle and yaks. The virus was then passaged another 150 times in sheep to produce a vaccine made from lymph nodes and spleen which was safe and efficacious in all species and breeds, even yaks and Korean cattle. In yaks the duration of vaccine immunity was tested to exceed 5 years. This vaccine was used for the final eradication thrust in China (Academician Shen Rong-xian, former Director of Harbin Veterinary Research Institute, China, personal communication).

## Egg-attenuated rinderpest vaccine

An attenuated avianized rinderpest vaccine was developed at Grosse Isle, Canada, during the Second World War using the Kabete O strain (Shope et al., 1946). Daubney (1947), with reference to the larger number of highly susceptible breeds for which the vaccine was suitable, thought that it possessed a flexibility that the goat-adapted strains lacked. In 1946 the seed virus was introduced to East Africa and China by veterinarians working under the United Nations Relief and Rehabilitation Administration (UNRRA). In addition, a number of lots of the Grosse Isle vaccine were inoculated into small numbers of calves of Chinese Yellow Cattle, which developed a pyrexia of over 40 °C but then resisted challenge. In China a further 200 000 doses were apparently successfully inoculated in the field but ultimately the Grosse Isle strain was lost in both regions (Scott, 1964).

Having failed to establish the Grosse Isle virus in routine production in China, the UNRRA team then attempted unsuccessfully to adapt two virulent local strains (Lanchow and Szechwan) and one from Cairo (Cheng *et al.*, 1949). Then Dr K.V.L. Kesteven of UNRRA visited the Kenyan government veterinary research laboratory at Kabete, near Nairobi, and returned with two samples of their chorio-allantoic membrane (CAM)-passaged virus, presumably Kabete O – K66 and L66. One of these, L66, was CAM-passaged twice (L66p$_2$), then passaged twice in calves, four more times on 10-day-old CAMs and thereafter used to initiate a yolk sac passage series. After 16 passages by this route the virus was sufficiently attenuated to be used as a vaccine. In addition, Kabete O itself was adapted to the CAM and after 48 passages, had become partially attenuated. A second Kabete O variant was CAM passaged 17 times and then adapted to yolk sac passage (without attenuation).

One feature of avianized rinderpest which was particularly highly regarded was that, by varying the passage level, different degrees of attenuation could be produced. It could be attenuated to the point where there was no pyrexia associated with its replication in the host. On the other hand, it appeared possible to passage the virus to a point where it no longer protected. In late 1948 the United Nations teams withdrew from the mainland and, as outlined above, the vaccine subsequently used to prosecute the fight against rinderpest in China was derived from the Nakamura III lapinized virus.

In Egypt, attempts to adapt the Kabete O virus to eggs met with little success. At Kabete itself, a line of virus was attenuated after 33 membrane passages and a small number of yolk sac passages. After 25 yolk sac passages there was no reaction in cattle and they were solidly immune to challenge. Avianized vaccine produced at Grosse Isle was used in Kenya and Somalia and conferred an immunity to challenge. The duration of immunity was felt to be long-lasting.

The impetus for the development of an avianized strain of the virus was the inability to attenuate lapinized rinderpest to a point of safety for Korean and Japanese cattle. Starting with the Nakamura III virus at its 763rd rabbit passage and after using a brief alternating passage series on the CAM and then rabbits, the virus could be established and passaged in chick embryos by the intravenous inoculation of the spleen. After 246 such passages it only caused mild reactions in Japanese black cattle (Nakamura and Miyamoto, 1953). This virus was subsequently back-passaged in rabbits (lapinized–avianized–lapinized) and used to vaccinate Korean and Vietnamese cattle (Scott, 1964).

## Tissue culture rinderpest vaccines

With the advent of cell culture techniques and a realization of the research advantages that these could offer, it was natural that workers should attempt to adapt existing attenuated laboratory strains of rinderpest to this exciting new medium. According to Johnson (1962a), Wilde tried in 1956 but could not detect the growth of goat- or rabbit-adapted strains in chick embryo fibroblasts.

Then in 1959 Johnson himself attempted to grow goat-, rabbit- and egg-attenuated strains in homologous cells and in bovine kidney (BK) cells but again without success. Plowright and Ferris (1959a) similarly failed to demonstrate growth of the goat- and rabbit-attenuated viruses in homologous cells or in BK cells or in cells from bovine embryonic kidneys. However, using the virulent Kabete O virus, these authors reported a breakthrough. During the first four passages on established BK monolayers they were able to demonstrate growth without cytopathic effect. Thereafter, using cells infected in suspension and allowed to form monolayers, cytopathic effects became readily apparent. Infected cells were seen to react by becoming either rounded or stellate or by being recruited into multinucleate syncytia. In the penultimate section of their introductory remarks the authors quietly stated that they had, incidentally, furnished another attenuated strain suitable for the immunization of cattle!

In a companion publication, Plowright and Ferris (1959b) described the results obtained by continuing to passage the Kabete O virus in BK cells. Compared with the parent strain, the virulence for cattle actually increased over the first ten passages as manifested by an increased mortality rate (rising from 60 to 100%) and shorter average survival time post-infection (falling from 9 to 3 days). In addition, necrotic mouth lesions were now apparent – their absence being an unusual but constant feature of the parent, needle-passaged strain. In other respects too, this per-acute strain differed from normal virulent strains. In the small intestine, an organ often spared by virulent strains, it caused diffuse epithelial necrosis and massive haemorrhages together with oedema and haemorrhage of the lymph nodes of the head and neck. It had also become readily transmissible by contact. By the 16th passage however, the virulence had returned to a level equivalent to that of the parent virus. The ability to cause mouth lesions, diarrhoea or death of the host also diminished after the 16th passages and from the 21st passage level onwards only temperature reactions remained frequent. Finally, no temperature reactions were observed with virus at the 70th, 90th or 122nd BK cell passages (Plowright, 1962).

As had already been established, naturally attenuated variants of rinderpest could arise in the field (Robson *et al.*, 1959) while in the laboratory Kabete O had already been attenuated by passage in eggs and goats, showing that a variety of different selection pressures can promote the emergence of rinderpest sub-populations with this characteristic. Accordingly, it may be supposed that the process of attenuation described by Plowright represented the overgrowth of either one, or a succession of avirulent variants at the expense of the more virulent sub-populations present in the original virus pool. That variants with differing levels of virulence might exist in the same virus pool was suggested by the rapid selection by terminal dilution of an avirulent virus from a parent Kabete O pool which, after 22 BK passages, still caused pyrexia (De Boer and Barber, 1964).

In Africa in the early 1960s, goat-attenuated virus was given to indigenous animals and the relatively more attenuated lapinized vaccine was used on high grade and hypersusceptible non-humped West African breeds of cattle.

However, as Johnson (1962b) pointed out, caprinized rinderpest vaccine was capable of causing severe reactions in cattle and associated weight loss. Moreover the reactions in cattle less than one year old prevented its use in that age group and consequently this generation of animals were commonly implicated in rinderpest outbreaks. Lapinized virus too was capable of causing reactions in hypersusceptible West African short-horned cattle, especially in the rainy season, and was seemingly fragile in the field. It was therefore easy to understand the rapidity and finality with which Plowright's tissue culture adaptation of Kabete O replaced its predecessors.

In the ensuing years considerable effort was put into fully characterizing what became known as tissue culture rinderpest vaccine (TCRV). In contrast to the earlier vaccines, the potency of which could only be estimated in laboratory animals, the potency of TCRV could obviously be estimated easily and very cheaply in cell cultures. The question then was, how did the tissue culture potency relate to the immunizing potency in cattle? A number of authors have been involved in trials both in cattle and in small ruminants aimed at determining this correlation (Plowright, 1962; Johnson, 1962b; Bansal and Joshi, 1974, Taylor and Best, 1977). By undertaking parallel titrations in animals and cell cultures, infected as freshly trypsinized cell suspensions, an approximation to a 1:1 relationship was generally obtained. However, Bansal et al. (1974a) using virus at the 104th BK passage level, compared median cell culture infectivity with 100% immunizing potency and reported differences of between 10- and 100-fold. In a subsequent report with TCRV grown in lamb kidney cultures, a 10-fold difference was observed between the median end points in cell cultures and cattle (Bansal et al., 1980). Overall, irrespective of the cell titration system employed, no one would disagree with Plowright's conclusion that it was no longer necessary to test the immunizing potency of TCRV by cattle inoculation.

Field trials in East Africa showed that TCRV of the 90th and 91st passages was safe for use in heavily pregnant cows, in high grade dairy calves of Jersey breeding, in yearling grades of Ayrshire, Hereford or Friesian breeding and in yearling East African zebus (Plowright, 1962). Trials in West Africa showed that TCRV of the 66–70th passages was safe to use on White Fulani cattle but still induced mild hyperthermia in non-humped hypersusceptible cattle of the Ndama, Ketetu and Muturu breeds; these trials were undertaken in the wet season when adverse reactions were normally most severe. Although some 85% of inoculated animals sustained a mild pyrexia, none of them suffered weight losses while control animals given lapinized virus did (Johnson, 1962b). In India, Bansal et al. (1974b) demonstrated the safety of TCRV for hill cattle but recorded mild pyrexia in Red Dane and Brown Swiss. This group did not record any adverse reactions when TCRV made in LK cells was inoculated into Red Sindhi, Gir or Hariana cattle or into Murrah buffaloes (Bansal et al., 1980). TCRV was found to be safe to use on Himalayan yaks in Pakistan (Roland Geiger and Manzoor Hussain, personal communication) and in Nepal (Dr G.N. Gongal, personal communication).

Johnson (1962b) stated that in White Fulani cattle, neutralizing antibodies first appeared between 7 and 17 days after vaccination and that the higher the dose inoculated, the earlier this response was detected. He also quoted unpublished results by Johnson and Macleod (1962) making parallel estimations of the responses of cattle to TCRV, to goat vaccine, to lapinized vaccine and to avianized vaccine. Antibodies were formed at approximately the same rates against the first three vaccines but more slowly against the avianized virus. Although no neutralizing antibodies were evident, cattle inoculated with TCRV had already developed a resistance to challenge after four days. Plowright (1962) showed that in animals receiving small doses of TCRV, the development of neutralizing antibodies was still incomplete 3 weeks after inoculation. Similar results were reported by Bansal et al. (1980).

Plowright (1962) showed that Kabete O virus at the 41st passage level, back-passaged four times in cattle, produced thermal reactions in the recipients but no contact transmission. By the 90th passage, seven serial back-passages failed to induce any reversion to virulence or a capacity for contact transmission. Similar results were obtained by Johnson (1962b) and Bansal et al. (1974b). Although TCRV multiplies in the lymphoid system of the vaccinated host its failure to transmit correlates with its inability to replicate in the nasal or alimentary mucosae of the vaccinated ox (Taylor and Plowright, 1965). Plowright's final conclusion (Plowright, 1972) was that TCRV is safe and immunogenic for cattle of all breeds and ages and of either sex.

Plowright and Ferris (1961) correlated the presence of neutralizing antibodies in cattle with resistance to challenge and subsequent workers have looked at the duration of immunity to TCRV as indicated either by resistance to challenge or by the presence of neutralizing antibodies. A detailed examination of the duration of immunity of East African cattle began in 1960 and was reported by Plowright and Taylor (1967), Rweyemamu et al. (1974) and, finally, by Plowright (1984). Grade dairy animals or improved zebus were vaccinated at between 8 and 13 months of age, maintained in rinderpest-free environments, bled at 6-month intervals and individually deleted from the experiment following challenge with virulent rinderpest virus. Antibody levels declined between 12 and 18 months but then remained stable for 3 or more years. Otherwise, any traces of maternal antibody at the time of vaccination were seen to influence the level of neutralizing antibody produced, though not the ability to withstand parenteral challenge. However, it was clear that if the level of neutralizing antibody were low, then a limited post-exposure viraemia could ensue although no adverse clinical reaction occurred. One such animal apparently transmitted infection to a contact control without itself showing any reaction. Otherwise this experiment showed that East African zebus were capable of withstanding either parenteral or contact challenge with virulent rinderpest at intervals up to and including 11 years and at the same time they neither circulated the virus, discharged it in their nasal secretions nor infected in-contact animals. Comparable results were obtained with high grade animals challenged at intervals between 6 and 10 years after vaccination. Serologically, the majority of individuals showed no increase in antibody titre following challenge, although delayed non-anamnestic increases were occasionally seen. It was, and still is, concluded that a long-lived immunity results from a single subcutaneous inoculation of a fully rinderpest-susceptible animal. Bansal and Joshi (1979) recorded resistance to virulent challenge at 8.3 years following a single vaccination.

Contradictory evidence relating to the duration of immunity was reported by Provost *et al.* (1969a), who showed that by the end of 24 months, challenge virus could replicate in the nasal passage of vaccinated cattle and by 36 months challenged animals would die of rinderpest. However, given that extremely long immunities seem to be characteristic of attenuated rinderpest vaccines (Bansal *et al.*, 1971), the weight of evidence suggests that TCRV can be expected to produce an enduring resistance to challenge. However, the observation of Provost *et al.* (1969a) had a profound effect on national vaccination policies in West Africa in the aftermath of JP15 (see Chapter 13). In Nigeria for instance, the recommended policy of only vaccinating replacement stock was modified in favour of the considerably more expensive option of attempting to keep the whole of the national herd in a constant state of annual revaccination. Undoubtedly, such national policy decisions were also influenced by the desire to incorporate contagious bovine pleuropneumonia (CBPP) control into rinderpest control programmes by administering a combined vaccine (Provost *et al.*, 1969b), which generated an immunity to CBPP lasting only months.

In a further series of experiments undertaken at Muguga, the stability of TCRV was examined, both after lyophilization and after reconstitution after lyophilization (Plowright *et al.*, 1970, 1971). It was convincingly demonstrated that after lyophilization in a cryoprotectant solution containing sucrose and lactalbumin hydrolysate the vaccine had a prolonged stability at either $-20\,°C$ or $+4\,°C$. Degradation constants ($\log_{10}$ median cell culture infectious doses [$CCID_{50}$] per day) derived from the reported results were between 0.00286 and 0.00324 at $20–22\,°C$, between 0.0111 and 0.0178 at $37\,°C$ and at around 0.0878 at $56\,°C$. After reconstitution in saline to field working strength the degradation constants ($CCID_{50}$ per hour) were found to be 0.0108 at $4\,°C$, 0.0184 at $25\,°C$ and 0.0356 at $37\,°C$ respectively. Similar results were obtained by Bansal *et al.* (1980). Dilution in distilled water at between 4 and $37\,°C$ caused immediate temperature-dependent losses of 50–90% of the virus present (Plowright *et al.*, 1970, 1971).

Before the introduction of shelf freeze-dryers, rinderpest vaccine was dried in a two-stage process involving primary drying with a centrifugal dryer (12 hours) followed by secondary drying over phosphorus pentoxide for 36 hours; the product was contained in all-glass ampoules sealed under vacuum. As shown by Johnson (1962a), unless well stabilized, over 99% of the virus could be lost during the drying process. With the advent of shelf freeze-dryers, vaccine was dried in rubber-stoppered glass vials and primary and secondary drying were both carried out in the same machine. Primary drying is considered to be the period during which sublimation is taking place, and ends when the product temperature reaches ambient temperature; secondary drying continues for a further period of between 33 and 50% as long again. In the mid-1980s the Institute for Animal Health, Pirbright, recommended a primary drying run with an initial product temperature of $-40\,°C$, raised to ambient temperature over the next 16–18 hours to be followed by a secondary drying run of 20–24 hours (total time 40–48 hours) and completed by hydraulic stoppering and capping (Leslie Rowe, personal communication). The residual moisture level of this product was not routinely estimated. Expected release titres should have been of the order of $10^{5.5}$ CCID$_{50}$ per ml and release for use within a cold chain.

In order to achieve a distribution system independent of a cold chain, Mariner *et al.* (1990) attempted to develop a more thermostable variant of TCRV. This problem was approached by taking the standard Kabete O strain grown them Vero cells to harvest titres sometimes exceeding $10^{7.0}$ CCID$_{50}$, mixing them with a variety of freeze-drying stabilizers and subjecting them to a variety of freeze-drying cycles. Lactalbumin-sucrose was established as the best cryoprotectant. The most effective primary drying cycle used vacuum regulation (100–130 mTorr) and consisted of 16 hours with the shelf temperature at $-30\,°C$, rising to $0\,°C$ over 8 hours and held at that temperature for a further 18 hours. During the secondary drying cycle the shelf temperature was raised to $25\,°C$ over a 6-hour period and held at that temperature for the following 18 hours, after which it was raised to $35\,°C$ over 2 hours and held at that temperature for the next 4 hours. During this secondary drying, the maximum possible vacuum (20–30 mTorr) was applied.

Post drying, a two stage degradation curve was established, a rapid initial decay followed by a gradual linear component with a boundary at around seven days post drying. Degradation constants were determined using this second degradation component. Following the above routine the product was characterized by a small infectivity loss during drying, a very low level of residual moisture (*c.* 1%) and a very low degradation constant (0.0057 CCID$_{50}$ per day at $37\,°C$). Vaccine made according to this method is generally referred to as Thermovax and is used in the field without cold chain support. In order that the vaccine can lose 90% of its content during 30 days' field exposure at high ambient temperatures and still contain a cattle field dose of $10^{2.5}$ CCID$_{50}$ per ml on reconstitution, the release titre should be at least $10^{5.7}$ CCID$_{50}$ per ml. In addition the product titre should be at least $10^{4.7}$ CCID$_{50}$ per ml determined following an abbreviated stability test consisting of 14 days' storage at $45\,°C$ and a residual moisture level of 1–1.5%. Under field conditions the vaccine may be removed from the cold chain on one occasion, and should then be destroyed if not used within 30 days. Under the Pan-African Rinderpest Campaign (PARC) programme, a joint Institut d'Elevage et de Médecine Vétérinaire des Pays Tropicaux and Tufts University School of Veterinary Medicine project succeeded in transferring the technology for the manufacture of Thermovax to a small number of African vaccine manufacturers. Historically speaking, the 38th BK passage of Kabete O yielded a virus with similar properties (16b-1009) which was, for a time, used for the manufacture and refrigeration-free distribution of rinderpest vaccine from the Farcha Laboratory in Chad (Provost and Borredon, 1972).

According to its development criteria, Thermovax was intended for use within alternative vaccination programmes (delivery without the use of capitalized resources such as cold chains, vehicles and large teams) and community-based vaccination programmes (trained pastoralists travelling with their herds and offering vaccination and treatment to their immediate communities). It has been used within alternative vaccination programmes in Sudan, Somalia, Uganda and Ethiopia. During an assessment of a community-based vaccination programme with Thermovax in the north of Cameroon, it was found that 86% of vaccinated cattle were protected.

In 1963, and following the development of Plowright's TCRV, Russian workers adapted the Nakamura III virus to grow in calf kidney cells, intending to use it as a vaccine in place of their inactivated vaccine (Laktionov, 1967). It was removed from manufacture in the 1970s because of adverse reactions. In Japan, the AKO line of lapinized–avianized Nakamura III virus was grown on Vero cells to produce a strategic stock-pile suitable for use in Japanese cattle (Sonoda, 1983). Similarly, a strategic reserve of the Chinese lapinized–caprinized–ovinized vaccine is produced currently in lamb kidney cell culture.

In 1961 a virulent rinderpest strain was isolated in Kabul and maintained through 37 cattle passages. It was subsequently attenuated by 70 passages in primary calf kidney cells and introduced as a vaccine in 1978. The attenuation was carried out by Ivanushinkov at the Research Agricultural Institute in Kazakhstan where, until 1989, the vaccine was also produced but in 1992 production was moved to the Pakrov Biopreparation plant near Moscow. The vaccine was intended for routine use in the border immune belt between the USSR and neighbouring countries and to repulse introductions of rinderpest if needed. Known as K37/70, denoting attenuation by 37 passages in cattle followed by 70 passages in primary calf kidney cell cultures from the original Kabul strain, the vaccine, extensively tested during appraisal and widely used subsequently, is regarded as safe for use in cattle and yaks. Unfortunately in three, perhaps four instances, outbreaks of clinical rinderpest have been observed in areas where this vaccine had been recently administered (Georgia, 1989–90; Tuva and Chitta, 1991–93; Amur, 1998). Not unexpectedly, a comparison of the F gene nucleotide sequence (bases 840 to 1161) shows that K37/70 and the Kabul strain differ by only the base at position 885. Additionally, comparing K37/70 vaccine virus with the virulent virus isolated from the Amur outbreak, the viruses are virtually identical and the substitution at position 885 is still present, suggesting a unique relationship between the two viruses (Sergei Starov and Pavel Ayanot, personal communication). On the other hand, the Amur virus has a further base change at position 1147 leading to the suggestion that K37/70 can, and has, reverted to virulence and regained the ability to transmit among cattle on more than one occasion and that virulence can be regained very rapidly, not requiring the accumulation of a large number of point mutations.

## Combined rinderpest vaccines

Macadam (1964) showed that cattle could be satisfactorily immunized simultaneously with both rinderpest and anthrax/blackquarter vaccines provided that the TCRV and bacterial preparations were separately reconstituted.

The results of the simultaneous vaccination of cattle with TCRV and foot-and-mouth (FMD) vaccine are mentioned in three reports. Kathuria *et al.* (1976) vaccinated calves with TCRV and mono- or polyvalent inactivated FMD vaccine simultaneously at different sites. All animals receiving monovalent FMD and TCRV, and 66% of animals receiving polyvalent FMD and TCRV vaccines reacted to challenge with FMD virus; controls not receiving rinderpest vaccine did not. Compared with controls, FMD virus neutralizing antibody levels were lower in animals receiving both vaccines. The preliminary conclusion from this trial was that simultaneous vaccination against rinderpest and FMD might not be possible. Ten years later Hedger *et al.* (1986) showed that the serological response in Omani cattle receiving TCRV and inactivated trivalent FMD vaccine at separate sites did not differ from the satisfactory levels in controls receiving only one vaccine. Finally, Guillemin *et al.* (1987) showed that animals receiving both vaccines at separate sites developed satisfactory antibody levels to both valencies and were protected against challenge.

At a time when both rinderpest and contagious bovine pleuropneumonia (CBPP) were endemic in Nigeria, field officers took to reconstituting TCRV in broth culture CBPP vaccine. Macadam *et al.* (1964) showed that this procedure was only acceptable if the ox serum used in the manufacture of broth vaccine was from rinderpest-susceptible animals – which were in short supply. In Chad, Provost *et al.* (1969b) developed a mixed freeze-dried vaccine with a streptomycin-resistant mutant of the $KH_3J$ strain of CBPP and TCRV made at the 36th BK passage level. From 1970 the $KH_3J$ strain was often replaced with the more immunogenic strain $T_1SR$ and the Kabete O rinderpest valency was sometimes replaced by one of its thermostable clones, 16b-1009. Whatever its formulation, the combined vaccine, known as Bisec, was widely used in West, Central and East Africa.

## Recombinant vaccines and differentiation between vaccine and wild virus infection

As the world is progressively cleared of rinderpest, control activity is progressively being focused away from mass vaccination and seromonitoring onto verification of rinderpest freedom whilst attempting to disclose and eliminate residual reservoirs of infection. Serosurveillance is an essential tool to achieve this yet, whilst of generally satisfactory performance in terms of specificity and sensitivity, the currently available conventional assays are compromised by being unable to differentiate between wild infection and vaccination. Thus, serosurveillance is impossible in the face of ongoing vaccination and for several years after vaccination has ceased. Clearly a marked vaccine with a differentiating test is needed and would be of great benefit. Development of recombinant vaccines has been described by several groups of scientists (Yilma *et al.*, 1988; Yamanouchi *et al.*, 1993; Romero *et al.*, 1994) using vaccinia or capripox vectors expressing the fusion (F) and haemagglutinin (H) proteins of rinderpest virus, either alone or in combination, and these have been shown to be highly efficacious (Ohishi *et al.*, 2000; Verardi *et al.*, 2002). Combined with a differentiating serological test in the form of an ELISA based on a baculovirus-expressed rinderpest N protein, a vaccinia recombinant vaccine expressing F and H rinderpest proteins would appear to have considerable potential (Yilma *et al.*, 2003). Unfortunately the N-based ELISA has shown performance characteristics rendering it unsuitable as an OIE-prescribed test (OIE, 2004) and to date none of the recombinant vaccines has been licensed for general use. An alternative approach has been to explore the production of positively marked vaccines by inserting genes for the expression of jellyfish green fluorescent protein and influenza A haemagglutinin into the Kabete vaccine strain of rinderpest virus (Walsh *et al.*, 2000). The haemagglutinin-marked vaccine retained immunogenicity and with its companion indirect ELISA to detect the strong haemagglutinin antibody response appeared to have potential for field use. Whether or not this vaccine will find practical use remains unclear given that antibodies to influenza A virus are widespread in cattle (Crawshaw and Brown, 1999). At present the most attractive candidate as a marked vaccine is the heterologous PPR vaccine (Diallo *et al.*, 1989) as it is known that PPR virus induces good protection against rinderpest in cattle (Dardiri *et al.*, 1976). Discriminatory monoclonal antibody-based ELISA antibody assay systems are available (Anderson *et al.*, 1991; Anderson and McKay, 1994). However, the use of this vaccine has yet to gain broad support despite the clear advantages it would offer for focal vaccination to eliminate reservoirs of rinderpest infection in the Somali pastoral ecosystem whilst allowing serosurveillance to continue. Another approach that is being pursued is the potential to use transgenic plants as vaccine delivery systems. Preliminary experimental work with these vaccines is promising but it remains to be demonstrate if they can protect target species. If so, it would constitute a major advance for the control of PPR, even if it is too late for rinderpest (see Chapter 12).

## The salient features of different rinderpest vaccines

The salient features of the different rinderpest vaccines discussed may be summarized as in Table 11.1.

In the respective developmental phases, much was made of the duration of immunity attributable to the different rinderpest vaccines as this property was of considerable value when it was expected that a vaccinated animal might be exposed to infection at any time in its life. Similarly, within buffer zones an enduring immunity is a useful attribute. On the other hand, it is not a terribly important character where rinderpest eradication is being attempted. To break a transmission chain it is the campaign manager's ability to saturate the population with vaccine and achieve a temporary but very high prevalence of resistant animals (an immunosterilized population; Taylor *et al.*, 2002a) that produces the desired result, and this result does not depend on the ability of the

**Table 11.1** Features of different rinderpest vaccines

| Vaccine | Attributes |
|---|---|
| Inactivated | Safe |
| | Short duration of immunity |
| Serum-simultaneous | Inherent degree of danger in its use – could recreate frank rinderpest or transmit piroplasms if bovine tissues are used |
| | Lifelong immunity |
| | Useful but not ideal for the immunization of large numbers of livestock |
| Rabbit-attenuated | Safer than goat-attenuated but could cause adverse reactions in highly susceptible breeds |
| | Supplies constrained by access to rabbits |
| | Lifelong immunity |
| Egg-attenuated | Virulence could be modified continuously |
| | Long immunity (debatable) |
| Goat-attenuated | Relatively safe but not sufficiently attenuated for use on highly susceptible breeds |
| | Did not transmit piroplasms |
| | Could be produced on large scale therefore relatively cheap |
| | Difficult to standardize to modern requirements |
| | Lifelong immunity |
| Tissue culture-attenuated Kabete O | Robust |
| | Highly immunogenic with lifelong immunity |
| | Cheap |
| | Ease of manufacture |
| | Lifelong immunity |
| | Safest of all |
| Poxvirus recombinant vaccines | Robust |
| | Highly immunogenic |
| | Cheap |
| | No possibility of reverting to virulence to re-establish rinderpest |
| | Ease of manufacture |
| | Safety questions not fully resolved |
| | May be used as marker vaccines |

virus to generate a long-lived immunity. The following chapter will describe the evolution of this sentiment.

# References

Anderson, J. and McKay, J.A. (1994) The detection of antibodies against peste des petits ruminants virus in cattle, sheep and goats and the possible implications to rinderpest control programmes. *Epidemiol. Infect.* **112**, 225–31.

Anderson, J., McKay, J.A. and Butcher, R.N. (1991) The use of monoclonal antibodies in competitive Elisa for the detection of antibodies to rinderpest and peste des petits ruminants viruses. In: *Seromonitoring of Rinderpest throughout Africa: Phase One.* Proceedings of the Final Research Coordination Meeting of the IAEA Rinderpest Control Projects, Côte d'Ivoire, 19–23 November 1990. IAEA-TECDOC-623, pp. 43–53.

Bansal, R.P. and Joshi, R.C. (1974) Studies on use of tissue culture rinderpest vaccine among sheep and goats. *Indian Vet. J.* **51**, 631–4.

Bansal, R.P. and Joshi, R.C. (1979) Immunogenicity of tissue-culture rinderpest vaccine. *Indian J. Anim. Sci.* **49**, 260–5.

Bansal, R.P., Chawla, S.K., Sharma, S.D. and Menon, M.S. (1971) Studies on duration of immunity conferred by attenuated rinderpest vaccines. *Indian J. Anim. Sci.* **41**, 18–26.

Bansal, R.P., Chawla, S.K., Joshi, R.C. and Shukla, D.C. (1974a) Use of attenuated rinderpest tissue culture vaccine in cattle. *Indian J. Anim. Sci.* **44**, 441–6.

Bansal, R.P., Chawla, S.K., Joshi, R.C. and Shukla, D.C. (1974b) Studies on attenuated rinderpest vaccine of tissue culture origin. *Ind. J. Anim. Sci.* **44**, 520–4.

Bansal, R.P., Joshi, R.C. and Kumar, S. (1980) Studies with tissue culture adapted strain of rinderpest virus in lamb kidney cell cultures. *Bull. Off. Int. Epizoot.* **92**, 37–46.

Boynton, W.H. (1928) Rinderpest, with special reference to its control by a new method of prophylactic treatment. *Philipp. J. Sci.* **36**, 1–35.

Brotherston, J.G. (1957) Rinderpest: some notes on control by modified virus vaccines. II. Lapinised virus. *Vet. Rev. Annot.* **3**, 45–56.

Brown, R.D. and Raschid, A. (1958) The duration of immunity following vaccination with caprinised virus in the field. Annual Report, East African Veterinary Research Organisation, 1956–57, p. 21.

Cèbe, J. and Perrin, J. (1935) *Bull. Econ. Indoch.* **38**, 795 (abstracted in *Vet. Bull.* **6**, 744, 1936).

Cheng, S.C. and Fischman, H.R. (1949) Lapinised rinderpest virus. In: K.V.L. Kesteven (ed.), *Rinderpest Vaccines: Their Production and Use in the Field.* FAO Agricultural Studies No. 8. Washington: FAO.

Cheng, S.C., Chow, T.C. and Fischman, H.R. (1949) Avianised rinderpest vaccine in China. In: K.V.L. Kesteven (ed.), *Rinderpest Vaccines: Their Production and Use in the Field.* FAO Agricultural Studies No. 8. Washington: FAO.

Crawford, M. (1947) The immunology and epidemiology of some virus diseases. *Vet. Rec.* **59**, 537–42.

Crawshaw, T.R. and Brown, I. (1999) Bovine influenza. *Vet. Rec.* **145**, 556–7.

Dardiri, A.H., De Boer, C.J. and Hamdy, F.M. (1976) Response of American goats and cattle to peste des petits ruminants. In: Proceedings of the 19th Annual Meeting of the American Association of Veterinary Laboratory Diagnosticians, pp. 337–44.

Daubney, R. (1947) Recent developments in rinderpest control. *Bull. OIE* **26**, 36–45.

Daubney, R. (1949) Goat-adapted virus. In: K.V.L. Kesteven (ed.), *Rinderpest Vaccines: Their Production and Use in the Field*. FAO Agricultural Studies No. 8. Washington: FAO.

Daubney, R. (1953a) Rinderpest vaccination. *Bull. Epizoot. Dis. Afr.* **1**, 12–18.

Daubney, R. (1953b) *Report to the Government of India on Rinderpest Control*. Rome: FAO, Rome.

De Boer, C.J. and Barber, T.L. (1964) Segregation of an avirulent variant of rinderpest virus by the terminal dilution technique in tissue culture. *J. Immunol.* **92**, 902–7.

Diallo, A., Taylor, W.P., Lefèvre, P.C. and Provost, A. (1989) Atténuation d'une souche de virus de peste des petits ruminants: candidat pour un vaccin homologue vivant. *Rev. Elev. Méd. Vét. Pays Trop.* **42**, 311–19.

Edwards, J.T. (1927/28) *Active Immunisation of Cattle by Means of the 'Serum Simultaneous' or 'Serum-virus' Method*, 3rd edn. Mukteswar publications.

Edwards, J.T. (1930) The problem of rinderpest in India. *Imp. Inst. Ag. Res. Pusa Bull.* **199**, 1–16.

Edwards, J.T. (1949) The uses and limitations of the caprinised virus in the control of rinderpest (cattle plague) among British and Near-Eastern cattle. *Br. Vet. J.* **105**, 209–53.

Guillemin, F., Mosienyane, M., Richard, T. and Mannathoko, M. (1987) Immune response and challenge of cattle vaccinated simultaneously against rinderpest and foot-and-mouth disease. *Rev. Elev. Med. Vet. Pays Trop.* **40**, 225–9.

Hedger, R.S., Taylor, W.P., Barnett, I.T.R., Riek, R. and Harpham, D. (1986) Simultaneous vaccination of cattle against foot-and-mouth disease and rinderpest. *Trop. Anim. Hlth Prod.* **18**, 21–5.

Hudson, J .R. and Wongsonsarn, C. (1950) The utilisation of pigs for the production of lapinised rinderpest vaccine. *Br. Vet. J.* **106**, 453–72.

Isogai, S. (1944) On the rabbit virus inoculation as an active immunization method against rinderpest for Mongolian cattle. *Jpn. J. Vet. Sci.* **6**, 388–90 (Biological Abstracts 26 1147–52).

Johnson, R.H. (1962a) Rinderpest in tissue culture. I: Methods for virus production. *Br. Vet. J.* **118**, 107–16.

Johnson, R.H. (1962b) Rinderpest in tissue culture. III: Use of the attenuated strain as a vaccine for cattle. *Br. Vet. J.* **118**, 141–50.

Kakizaki, C. (1918) Study on the glycerinated rinderpest vaccine. *Kitasato Arch. Exp. Med.* **2**, 59–66.

Kathuria, B.K., Uppal, P.K. and Kumar, S. (1976) Studies on simultaneous vaccination of cattle against rinderpest and foot and mouth disease. *Indian Vet. J.* **53**, 571–6.

Krishnamurti, R. (1945) A comparative study of rinderpest Bull-Goat-Virus, with a brief survey of the work done with rinderpest goat virus in Madras. *Indian J. Vet. Sci. Anim. Husb. Calcutta* **15**, 247–52.

Laktionov, A.M. (1967) Borba s chumoi krupnogo rogatogo skota. *Trudy Vsesoyuznogo Inst. Eks. Vet.* **34**, 302–11.

Macadam, I. (1964) The response of zebu cattle to tissue culture rinderpest vaccine mixed in (1) blackquarter vaccine and (2) anthrax spore vaccine. *Bull. Epizoot. Dis. Afr.* **12**, 401–3.

Macadam, I., Ezebuiro, E.O. and Oreffo, V.O.C. (1964) The response of zebu cattle to mixed contagious bovine pleuro-pneumonia and tissue culture rinderpest vaccines. *Bull. Epizoot. Dis. Afr.* **12**, 237–40.

Mack, R. (1970) The great African cattle plague epidemic of the 1890s. *Trop. Anim. Hlth Prod.* **2**, 210–19.

MacOwen, K.D.S. (1955) Origin of Kabete 'O' strain of rinderpest. *Annv. Rep. Vet. Ser. Dept. Kenya*, p. 29.

Mariner, J.C., House, J.A., Sollod, A.E., Stem, C., van den Ende, M.C. and Mebus, C.A. (1990) Comparison of the effect of various chemical stabilisers and lyophilisation cycles on the thermostability of a Vero cell-adapted rinderpest vaccine. *Vet. Microbiol.* **21**, 195–209.

Nakamura, J. and Miyamoto, T. (1953) Avianization of lapinised rinderpest virus. *Am. J. Vet. Res.* **14**, 307–17.

Nakamura, J., Fukusho, K. and Kuroda, S. (1943) Rinderpest: laboratory experiments on immunisation of Chosen cattle by simultaneous inoculation with immune serum and rabbit virus. *Jpn. J. Vet. Sci.* **5**, 455–77 (abstracted in *Vet. Bull.* **22** (1944), 186–7).

Nakamura, J., Wagatuma, S. and Fukusho, K. (1938) On the experimental infection with rinderpest virus in rabbits. I. Some fundamental experiments. *J. Jpn. Soc. Vet. Sci.* **17**, 185–204 (abstracted in *Vet. Bull.* **17** (1939), 536).

Ohishi, K., Inui, K., Barrett, T. and Yamanouchi, K. (2000) Long-term protective immunity to rinderpest in cattle following a single vaccination with a recombinant vaccinia virus expressing the virus haemagglutinin protein. *J. Gen. Virol.* **81**, 1439–46.

OIE (2004) Rinderpest, Ch 2.1.4 in: *Manual of Diagnostic Tests and Vaccines for Terrestrial Animals*, 5th edn. Paris: OIE, pp. 142–52.

Pantulu, C.S. (1934) *Report of the Special Rinderpest Officer, Madras Presidency*. Madras: Government Press, pp. 1–54.

Plowright, W. (1962) The application of monolayer tissue culture techniques in rinderpest research. II. The use of attenuated culture virus as a vaccine for cattle. *Bull. Off. Int. Epizoot.* **57**, 253–76.

Plowright, W. (1972) The production and use of rinderpest cell culture vaccine in developing countries. *World Anim. Rev.* **1**, 14–18.

Plowright, W. (1984) The duration of immunity in cattle following inoculation of rinderpest cell culture vaccine. *J. Hyg. (Camb.)* **92**, 285–96.

Plowright, W. and Ferris, R.D. (1959a) Studies with rinderpest virus in tissue culture. I. Growth and cytopathogenicity. *J. Comp. Pathol.* **69**, 152–72.

Plowright, W. and Ferris, R.D. (1959b) Studies with rinderpest virus in tissue culture. II. Pathogenicity for cattle of culture-passaged virus. *J. Comp. Pathol.* **69**, 173–84.

Plowright, W. and Ferris, R.D. (1961) Studies with rinderpest virus in cell culture. III. The stability of cultured virus and its use in virus neutralisation tests. *Arch. Gesamte Virusforsch.* **11**, 516–33.

Plowright, W. and Taylor, W.P. (1967) Long-term studies of the immunity in East African cattle following inoculation with rinderpest culture vaccine. *Res. Vet. Sci.* **8**, 118–28.

Plowright, W., Herniman, K.A.J. and Rampton, C.S. (1971) Studies with rinderpest culture vaccine. IV. Stability of the reconstituted product. *Res. Vet. Sci.* **123**, 40–6.

Plowright, W., Rampton, C.S., Taylor, W.P. and Herniman, K.A.J. (1970) Studies on rinderpest culture vaccine. III. Stability of the lyophilised product. *Res. Vet. Sci.* **11**, 71–81.

Pool, W.A. and Doyle, T.M. (1922) Studies in rinderpest. *Memoirs of the Department of Agriculture in India. Veterinary Series, Vol III*. Pusa: Agriculture Research Institute, pp. 122–35.

Provost, A. and Borredon, C. (1972) Un vaccin mixte antibovipestique-antipéripneumonique lyophilisé utilisable, sur le terrain, sans réfrigeration. I. Sélection de virions bovipestiques à inactivation thermique retardée. *Rev. Elev. Méd. Vét. Pays Trop.* **25**, 507–20.

Provost, A., Borredon, C. and Queval, R. (1969b) Recherches immunologiques sur la péripneumonie. XI. Un vaccin vivant mixte antibovipestique antipéripneumonique inoculé en un seul temps. Conception – production – controles. *Bull. Off. Int. Epizoot.* **72**, 166–203.

Provost, A., Maurice, Y. and Borredon, C. (1969a) Comportement clinique et immunologique, lors de contamination bovipestique, de bovins vaccinés depuis plusieurs années contre la peste bovine avec des vaccins de cultures cellulaires. *Rev. Elev. Méd. Vét. Pays Trop.* **22**, 453–64.

Robson, J., Arnold, R.M., Plowright, W. and Scott, G.R. (1959) The isolation from an eland of a strain of rinderpest virus attenuated for cattle. *Bull. Epizoot. Dis. Afr.* **7**, 97–102.

Romero, C.H., Barrett, T., Chamberlain, R.W., Kitching, R.P., Fleming, M. and Black, D.N. (1994) Recombinant capripox expressing the haemagglutinin protein gene of rinderpest: protection of cattle against rinderpest and lumpy skin disease. *Virology* **204**, 425–9.

Rweyemamu, M.M., Reid, H.W. and Okuna, N. (1974) Observations on the behaviour of rinderpest virus in immune animals challenged intranasally. *Bull. Epizoot. Dis. Afr.* **22**, 1–9.

Saunders, P.T. and Ayyar, K.K. (1936) An experimental study of rinderpest virus in goats in a series of 150 direct passages. *Indian J. Vet. Sci.* **6**, 1–86.

Schein, H. (1926) *Bull. Soc. Path. Exot.* **19**, 915.

Scott, G.R. (1964) Rinderpest. *Adv. Vet. Sci.* **9**, 113–224.

Scott, G.R. (1987) Review of Rinderpest campaigns in the past (global). FAO Expert Consultation on the Global Strategy for Control and Eradication of Rinderpest. Rome: FAO.

Semmer E. (1893) Rinderpest-infektion und Immunisierung und Schutzimpfung gegen Rinderpest. *Berl. Tierärztl. Wochenschr.* **23**, 590–1.

Shope, R.E. (1949) Inactivated virus vaccine. In: K.V.L. Kesteven (ed.), *Rinderpest Vaccines: Their Production and Use in the Field.* FAO Agricultural Studies No. 8. Washington: FAO.

Shope, R.E., Griffith, H.J. and Jenkins, D.L. (1946) The cultivation of rinderpest virus in developing hen's egg. *Am. J. Vet. Res.* **7** (Part II), 135–41.

Sonoda, A. (1983) Production of rinderpest tissue culture live vaccine. *Jpn. Agr. Res. Q.* **17**, 191–8.

Spinage, C.A. (2003) *Cattle Plague: A History.* New York: Kluwer Academic/Plenum Publishers.

Taylor, W.P. and Best, J.R. (1977) Simultaneous titrations of tissue culture rinderpest vaccine in goats and cell cultures. *Trop. Anim. Hlth Prod.* **9**, 189–90.

Taylor, W.P. and Plowright, W. (1965) Studies on the pathogenesis of rinderpest in experimental cattle. III. Proliferation of an attenuated strain in various tissues following subcutaneous inoculation. *J. Hyg. (Camb.)* **63**, 263–75.

Taylor, W.P., Roeder, P.L., Rweyemamu, M.M., Melewas, J.N., Majuva, P., Kimaro, R.T., Mollel, J.N., Mtei, B.J., Wambura, P., Anderson, J., Rossiter, P.B., Kock, R., Melengeya, T. and Van den Ende, R. (2002a) The control of rinderpest in Tanzania between 1997 and 1998. *Trop. Anim. Hlth Prod.* **34**, 471–87.

Thet Swe (1991) Rinderpest Eradication in Myanmar in South Asia Rinderpest eradication Campaign. Proceedings of the Regional Expert Consultation on Rinderpest eradication in South Asia. Bangkok, June 1990.

Verardi, P.H., Fatema, H.A., Ahmad, S., Jones, L.A., Beyene, B., Ngotho, R.N., Wamwayi, H.M., Yesus, M.B., Egziabher, B.G. and Yilma, T.D. (2002) Long-term sterilizing immunity to rinderpest in cattle vaccinated with a recombinant vaccinia virus expressing high levels of the fusion and haemagglutinin glycoproteins. *J. Virol.* **76**, 484–91.

Vittoz, R. (1963) Report of the Director on the Scientific and Technical Activities of the Office International des Epizooties from May 1962 to May 1963. Paris: OIE.

Vogel, S.W. and Heyne, H. (1996) Rinderpest in South Africa – 100 years ago. *J. S. Afr. Vet. Assoc.* **67**, 164–70.

Walsh, E.P., Baron, M.D., Rennie, L., Monahan, P., Anderson, J. and Barrett, T. (2000) Recombinant rinderpest vaccines expressing membrane anchored proteins as genetic markers: evidence for exclusion of marker protein from the virus envelope. *J. Virol.* **74**, 10165–75.

Yamanouchi, K., Inui, K., Sugimoto, M., Asano, K., Nishimaki, F., Kitching, R.P., Takamatsu, H. and Barrett, T. (1993) Immunisation of cattle with a recombinant vaccinia vector expressing the haemagglutinin gene of rinderpest virus. *Vet. Rec.* **132**, 152–6.

Yilma, T., Aziz, F., Ahmad, S., Jones, L., Ngotho, R., Wamwayi, H., Beyene, B., Yesus, M., Egziabher, B., Diop, M., Sarr, J. and Verardi, P. (2003) Inexpensive vaccines and rapid diagnostic kits tailor-made for the global eradication of rinderpest, and technology transfer to Africa and Asia. *Afr. Asia Dev. Biol. (Basel)* **114**, 99–111.

Yilma, T., Hsu, D., Jones, L., Owens, S., Mebus, C., Yamakana, M. and Dale, B. (1988) Protection of cattle against rinderpest with vaccinia virus recombinants expressing the HA and F genes. *Science* **242**, 1058–61.

# New generation vaccines against rinderpest and peste des petits ruminants

# 12

## THOMAS BARRETT* AND KAZUYA YAMANOUCHI†

*Institute for Animal Health, Pirbright Laboratory, Surrey, UK
†Nippon Institute for Biological Science, Tokyo, Japan

## Introduction

The history of rinderpest vaccine development is comprehensively described in Chapter 11, but it was not until a safe, cheap, effective and easy to administer vaccine became available that eradication of rinderpest globally could be considered a feasible proposition. The search for such a vaccine culminated in the Tissue Culture Rinderpest Vaccine (TCRV) produced by Plowright and Ferris in Kenya in the late 1950s (Plowright and Ferris, 1962). This vaccine has been widely used in many parts of the world for more than forty years and is responsible for the success of the global rinderpest eradication programme. Without such a safe and effective vaccine we could not have reached the point where rinderpest has ceased to be a major animal disease threat and is on the verge of extinction. In most respects the TCRV is an ideal vaccine, giving solid lifelong protection following a single inoculation. However, the vaccine is perceived to have two weaknesses; first, thermolability and secondly the response in vaccinated animals is identical to that produced by natural infection in recovered animals. As the TCRV is mostly required for use under hot and arid conditions it required the establishment of an effective cold chain to deliver the vaccine to the field, which is inconvenient and costly. However, the absolute necessity for a cold chain has since been largely overcome by improved freeze-drying techniques (Mariner et al., 1990; see also Chapter 13). This has enabled the TCRV (Thermovax) to be kept for reasonably long periods at temperatures as high as

ISBN-13: 978-0-12-88385-1
ISBN-10: 0-12-88385-6

37 °C while freeze-dried. Once reconstituted in a high salt solution, however, it must be administered to cattle within 2 hours. Although a cold chain may not be entirely necessary, it can be justified on two counts: first to ensure the vaccine is regarded as something important and cared for in a responsible manner and secondly to ensure no deterioration after release from the manufacturer. At the current stage of the eradication campaign, where vaccination is only used to contain outbreaks of disease, thermolability, therefore, is not a major issue but the inability to distinguish vaccinated animals from those naturally infected with the virus is a serious problem since if TCRV is used, serological surveys can be confused if vaccinated animals are moved into disease-free areas, and that makes it more difficult to be sure that the wild-type virus is not still circulating and masked by vaccination. It was not until the advent of recombinant DNA technology that new generation rinderpest vaccines could be made which could solve the problems of thermolability and the inability to identify vaccinated animals.

# The first recombinant vaccines

Recombinant DNA technology has been widely used to produce new vaccines for many diseases, including rinderpest (Yamanouchi et al., 1998) and thermolability was the main reason used to justify the development of the recombinant rinderpest vaccines. The first to be produced were vaccinia recombinants, so-called vectored vaccines, which used the DNA genome of an established vaccine strain of vaccinia (the vector) as the backbone for the insertion of foreign genes coding for immunogenic proteins from the desired pathogen. Vaccination with the recombinant then induces a protective immune response to the disease concerned. Vaccinia virus is very suitable for genetic manipulation, as it has a large DNA genome with many non-essential genes which can be removed and replaced by the desired antigen (Mackett et al., 1982). The first and most successful vaccine product of this type was the vaccinia/rabies recombinant vaccine, which is now widely used in Europe and the USA to control rabies (Brochier et al., 1991; Pastoret and Brochier, 1996). This can withstand the extremes of temperature found under field conditions. The first vaccinia recombinant vaccines for rinderpest were developed in the late 1980s and these used the two surface glycoprotein genes of the virus, the fusion (F) and haemagglutinin (H) protein genes, as the immunizing antigens (Yilma et al., 1988; Barrett et al., 1989).

These were based on the WR strain of the virus but this was not considered sufficiently attenuated to be suitable for licensing in the absence of smallpox in the human population. In addition, this vaccinia strain produced severe lesions at the site of inoculation in animals (Belsham et al., 1989). An expert committee convened by OIE in 1989 to consider guidelines for the use of these vaccines recommended the use of safer strains of vaccinia which have been shown to be sufficiently attenuated in authoritative trials. A rinderpest recombinant based on the LC16mO strain was tested in cattle in Britain (Yamanouchi *et al.*, 1993) and the Wyeth strain in the USA (Giavedoni *et al.*, 1991). Subsequently the duration of immunity in African (Verardi *et al.*, 2002) and European cattle (Inui *et al.*, 1995) was shown to be reasonably long-lasting, certainly sufficient to control an outbreak situation.

Another poxvirus vector, capripox virus (the agent of sheep and goat pox) has also been used to produce a recombinant rinderpest vaccine. Using the established capripox vaccine as a vector it is possible to protect cattle against two diseases, rinderpest and lumpy skin disease, the latter being caused by a close relative of sheep and goat pox (Romero *et al.*, 1993, 1994a, 1994b; Ngichabe *et al.*, 1997). Similar long-term trials showed that protection using the capripox recombinant is reasonably long-lasting (at least three years), although a disadvantage is that pre-existing antibodies to LSDV interfere with the vaccine take (Ngichabe *et al.*, 2002). Due to the strong antigenic relationships within the *Morbillivirus* genus (see Chapter 3), goats can also be protected from peste des petits ruminants virus using the vectored rinderpest vaccines despite the fact that no anti-peste des petits ruminants antibody responses were detectable (Jones *et al.*, 1993; Romero *et al.*, 1995). More recently the capripox vector has been used to develop a homologous recombinant vaccine for peste des petits ruminants virus (Berhe *et al.*, 2002). This acts as a dual vaccine which also protects sheep and goats from infection with capripox virus.

The vaccinia and capripox recombinant vaccines can also act as effective marker vaccines for rinderpest and peste des petits ruminants as their serological signature lacks responses to the nucleocapsid (N) proteins of the viruses. The N proteins are highly antigenic and specific tests have been developed to distinguish these two closely related viruses in ELISAs specific for the N protein (Libeau *et al.*, 1995) and they can be used to identify recombinant vaccinated animals as well as vaccinated animals that subsequently become infected. Specific ELISAs are also available to detect the serological response to H proteins of the two viruses (Anderson *et al.*, 1996; see also Chapter 8). Controversy over the release of genetically manipulated organisms has hampered the licensing of these vaccines for field use and they are all still at the experimental stage.

## Reverse genetics and vaccine development

Advances in biotechnology over the past 10 years have revolutionized our approach to new vaccine design for viruses such as rinderpest which have single-stranded negative sense RNA genomes (ssnRNA viruses). Reverse genetics systems, the process whereby the genomes of RNA viruses can be genetically altered through a DNA copy and live virus rescued from the altered

DNA, have been developed for this group of viruses. This technology allows their genomes to be genetically modified (Conzelmann and Schnell, 1994). The rinderpest vaccine virus genome can also be manipulated using reverse genetics (Figure 12.1), allowing site-specific mutagenesis of the rinderpest virus vaccine genome (Baron and Barrett, 1997, 2000). This enables an alternative approach to the production of marker vaccines, i.e., by altering their genomes, either by adding marker genes (making a positively marked vaccine) or by deleting an antigenic component (making a negatively marked vaccine).

The first problem encountered when adding marker genes is where to insert these extra genes. Unlike DNA viruses, the genomes of non-segmented negative strand RNA viruses are very economical in their coding capacity (see Chapter 3). Their genomes have a single transcription promoter located at the 3' end and the closer a gene is to this promoter the more the mRNA will be produced and, consequently, the more protein (Whelan *et al.*, 2004). The gradient in mRNA transcription results in abundant transcripts for the 3' proximal genes and low numbers of transcripts from the promoter distal genes. The virus proteins with genes closest to the promoter, the N and phospho (P) proteins, are

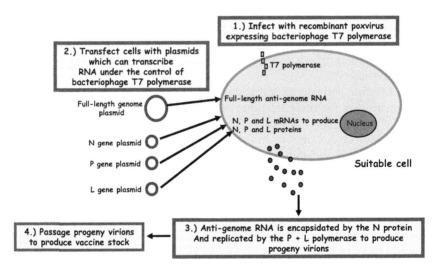

**Figure 12.1**   Reverse genetics technology for RNA viruses. This diagram outlines the protocol to rescue a negative sense single strand RNA virus from a cDNA copy of the genome. The cells to be used for rescue are grown to 70% confluence and are infected with a recombinant poxvirus expressing the bacteriophage T7 polymerase. One hour later they are transfected with a plasmid containing the full-length genome copy along with three other plasmids containing the genes for the N, P and L proteins which are required to encapsidate and replicate the RNA copy of the virus genome transcribed from the full-length plasmid. Transcription of RNA from all four plasmids is under the control of the bacteriophage T7 promoter. After 4–5 days virus cytopathic effects are seen in the transfected cells and the rescued virus can then be amplified for further characterization.

produced most abundantly in infected cells and, as would be expected, are required in large amounts for efficient replication. Disrupting the ratios of these two proteins might adversely affect virus growth and so it was decided to insert the marker gene between the P gene and the matrix (M) protein gene, the next in the genome sequence of morbilliviruses. Versions of the TCRV were produced where the green fluorescent protein (GFP) gene was expressed in different ways (cytoplasmic, secreted, membrane anchored) to see which would produce the best serological response to the marker protein (see Figure 12.2). All were highly effective in protecting animals from challenge with virulent rinderpest virus; however, a consistent and measurable antibody response to the GFP protein was only achieved in the recombinant vaccine where the GFP was anchored on the cell membrane (rRPV-AncGFP) (Walsh *et al.*, 2000a, b).

Another potential marker protein which has been incorporated as a marker into the TCRV is the influenza A haemagglutinin (HA) protein. This vaccine (rRPV-InsHA) produced a strong antibody response to the influenza HA marker protein in all animals vaccinated. This recombinant showed that it is also possible using this technology to produce dual vaccines to protect against two diseases (Walsh *et al.*, 2000b). The GFP and HA vaccines are both 'positively marked' and can be used to determine the effectiveness of a vaccination programme and the level of vaccine cover achieved in vaccinated herds, but they do not allow the identification of vaccinated animals that have subsequently become infected by wild-type virus. This may not be a problem as the parent TCRV is thought to give long-lasting sterilizing immunity; however, ideally a negatively marked vaccine, where some antigenic component has been deleted, is required. The missing component of the vaccine will only be detected in a vaccinated animal if it subsequently becomes infected. Negative marker DNA vaccines have been used for some time, for example the marker vaccine for Aujeszky's disease, which has a non-essential glycoprotein gene deleted (Oirschot *et al.*, 1990). Vaccinated animals lack a response to the missing protein and so can be distinguished from naturally infected animals and vaccinated animals that subsequently become infected with wild-type virus. However, the tight constraints imposed by an RNA genome means that no such 'luxury' antigenic gene is available for deletion in ssnRNA viruses.

## Chimeric marker vaccines

Since there are no genes that can be removed or replaced by foreign marker genes in ssnRNA viruses, another approach had to be taken to make negative marker vaccines for rinderpest and peste des petits ruminants viruses. The solution was to make chimeric viruses with genes for immunogenic proteins derived from the related virus. For example, the H and F glycoprotein genes of the rinderpest vaccine were substituted by the corresponding genes from peste des petits ruminants virus resulting in a recombinant marker vaccine for the latter

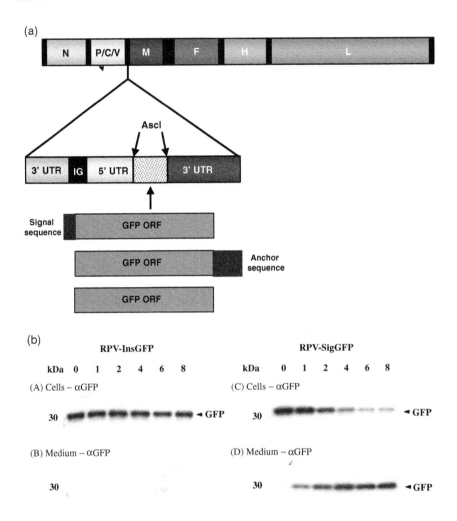

**Figure 12.2** Insertion of the green fluorescent protein (GFP) into the rinderpest virus genome. (*a*) This diagram shows the gene order on the rinderpest virus genome and the position where the GFP was inserted, either as a simple gene or one manipulated to express the GFP as a secreted protein. The signal sequence is required to allow translation of the protein on the rough endoplasmic reticulum and direct the protein to the surface for excretion into the medium. (*b*) The production of normal GFP is shown in frames (A) and (B) while that of the secreted GFP is shown in frames (C) and (D). It can be seen that the intracellular concentration of the normal form remains constant (A) and no GFP appears in the medium (B). In contrast with the secreted form the intracellular concentration decreases as the extracellular concentration increases. (Data from Walsh *et al.*, 2000a)

(Das *et al.*, 2000). Virus-specific ELISAs can then be used to identify which serological responses are present in any serum sample from vaccinated small ruminants, being positive in the RP N ELISA and positive in the PPR H ELISA.

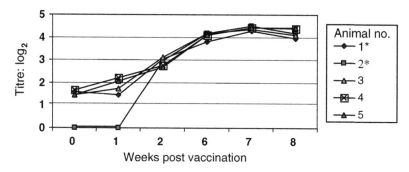

**Figure 12.3** Virus neutralizing antibodies induced on vaccination of cattle with the chimeric rRPV-PPRN virus. Animals 1 and 2 were vaccinated with the normal TCRV and animals 3, 4 and 5 with rRPV-PPRN. Titres are expressed as $\log_2$ values.

The N protein genes can also be swapped to produce a negative marker vaccine. A rinderpest chimeric vaccine (rRPV-PPRN), where the N protein gene is derived from peste des petits ruminants virus while all other vaccine components are from the TCRV, has been produced and would be a suitable negatively marked vaccine for rinderpest (Parida *et al.*, 2004). The rescued virus grew to as high a titre as the parental TCRV and induced a similar VNT response (Figure 12.3). Again, animals vaccinated with this chimeric vaccine can be distinguished from naturally infected ones using two available ELISAs mentioned above. Vaccinated animals become positive in the PPRV-specific N test and remain negative in the RPV-specific N test. The opposite is true in the case of H protein-specific antibodies. Vaccinated animals that subsequently become infected with wild-type virus would become double-positive for the N protein antibodies of both viruses.

Another very promising approach to marker vaccine development, and one that has been used to produce a marker vaccine for Newcastle disease virus, is to delete a highly antigenic, but non-essential, epitope and develop tests specifically designed to detect responses to the resulting serological response to the new vaccine. These researchers identified a highly antigenic epitope in the N protein of the virus and replaced it with a foreign sequence, in this case a B-cell epitope from mouse hepatitis virus (Mebatsion *et al.*, 2002). Vaccinated mice lacked a response to the deleted N protein epitope and developed a strong response to the mouse hepatitis virus epitope. This is now an active field of research to produce rinderpest and peste des petits ruminants marker vaccines.

## Alternative approaches

Before the TCRV was developed attempts were made to use inactivated (e.g. formalin-inactivated) forms of the virus as vaccines but they were not very successful in protecting cattle from rinderpest or any other host susceptible to viruses in the *Morbillivirus* genus. They produce only a short-term protective response (Appel *et al.*, 1984) and, in the case of measles virus, inactivated vaccines increased the pathology of disease when children were subsequently exposed to the wild-type virus. Baculovirus-expressed rinderpest F and H protein antigens have been used to produce so-called subunit vaccines (Yamanouchi *et al.*, 1998). However, a complete failure to protect cattle from rinderpest was seen when these recombinants expressing the H and fusion (F) proteins of rinderpest were used to vaccinate cattle, although they induced a strong neutralizing antibody response (Bassiri *et al.*, 1993). The nature of the antibodies produced in response to vaccination with inactivated antigens is therefore crucial for inducing protection since hyperimmune serum can give short-term protection, as can inactivated whole virus (see Chapter 10). In contrast, when a baculovirus-expressed H protein was incorporated into ISCOMs, which are known to stimulate a cell-mediated response with subunit vaccines (deVries *et al.*, 1988; Ennis *et al.*, 1999), a good level of protection was achieved (Kamata *et al.*, 2001). Similarly, when recombinant baculovirus particles expressed the rinderpest H protein, where the antigens on the virus envelope, the protein induced protective antibodies (Sinnathamby *et al.*, 2004). Therefore it appears that the appropriate type of antibody response and an effective cellular immune response are major factors in the protective response induced by morbillivirus vaccines (see Chapter 10).

The prospect of producing effective edible vaccines against rinderpest and peste des petits ruminants is very attractive. Although still at an early stage of development, several studies have been carried out to examine vaccination of mice and cattle with RPV-H protein produced in either transgenic tobacco or peanut plants. The plant-derived protein was antigenically authentic as shown by reactivity with H-monospecific and convalescent sera. High titres of antibody were obtained in mice after intraperitoneal inoculation with both plant preparations and these were H-specific and neutralized RPV infection. Leaves of transgenic peanut plants expressing RPV-H were also fed to mice and cattle over a 9- or 10-week period. In mice both IgG and IgA antibodies were produced and maintained throughout the study and in cattle a continuing lymphoproliferative response was also demonstrated (Khandelwal *et al.*, 2003, 2004). These studies indicate the potential for an oral edible vaccine for rinderpest and PPR.

## Companion diagnostic tests

Marker vaccines are only useful if suitable tests (companion diagnostic tests) are available to monitor the vaccination levels and to follow the spatial course of the infection. The OIE, at its General Session held in May 2003, adopted a resolution to provide a much broader recognition of diagnostic tests as fit for a specified purpose, not just for international trade. It is expected that in the near future the OIE will abandon the test prescribed/alternative classification for important transboundary diseases (List A diseases) and replace it with a classification based on fitness for purpose. So, in future, all animal diagnostic tests will be validated according to fitness for a specified use. New tests will have to be independently validated with respect to variables such as specificity, sensitivity, repeatability and reproducibility. Tests for new recombinant TCRV marker vaccines (e.g. epitope deletions/insertions) will need to be developed and validated independently and the nature of these tests will depend on the type of marker vaccine used and whether it is a positive or negative marker vaccine.

## Safety of recombinant vaccines

An important consideration when developing genetically modified virus vaccines is safety. One of the major concerns with using vaccinia-based recombinants is the risk to vaccinators, particularly in Africa where the number of people immunosuppressed due to HIV infections is high.

In the case of the vaccines produced by reverse genetics, the possibility that the marker proteins could be incorporated into the virus envelope and thus alter the tropism, and possibly the pathogenicity, of the vaccine produced, was also considered. Therefore, in the case of the flu HA-marker vaccine, a receptor site mutant version of the influenza HA protein gene was used in which the receptor binding domain of the HA was mutated to severely reduce its binding efficiency. In addition, viruses have mechanisms to exclude the incorporation of foreign proteins into their envelopes and immunoprecipitation studies using antibodies to the GFP and HA marker proteins failed to precipitate the recombinant vaccine viruses, indicating that the marker protein is excluded from the virus envelopes. Later immunoelectron microscopic studies confirmed that budded virus envelopes were free of the marker influenza HA protein (Walsh *et al.*, 2000b) (Figure 12.4). Whether or not this vaccine will find practical use remains unclear given that antibodies to influenza A virus are widespread in cattle (Crawshaw and Brown, 1999); however, influenza HA genes are very mutable and it is unlikely that a current HA strain would cross-react with the X31 laboratory strain used to generate rRPV-InsHA.

## Prospects for the use of recombinant vaccines in the field

The next phase will be to test the new RPV marker vaccines in a larger number of cattle, in particular African breeds of cattle, to determine the average level of antibody response to the marker antigens, to validate the companion diagnostic tests and to establish the minimum vaccine dose that will give solid protection along with an acceptable marker antibody response in vaccinated animals. Extensive safety trials would need to be conducted before these vaccines are licensed for field use.

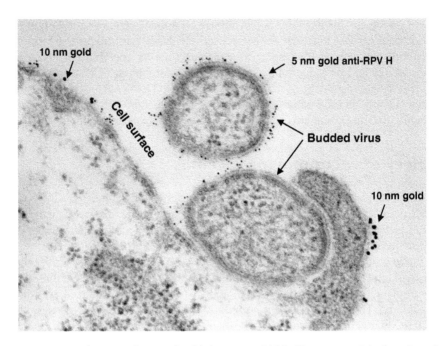

**Figure 12.4** Electron micrograph with immunogold labelling to reveal the location of the rinderpest virus H proteins (5 nm particles) and the influenza HA proteins (10 nm gold particles). (Adapted from Walsh *et al.*, 2000b)

In the final stages of the rinderpest eradication campaign, where very limited use of vaccines to control outbreaks will be sanctioned, it would be a great advantage to be able to identify vaccinated cattle serologically. However, even if rinderpest is eradicated before any of these marker vaccines is approved for use, all this effort will not have been in vain since the knowledge gained can be usefully channelled into producing a safe and effective marker vaccine for peste des petits ruminants virus and other morbillivirus diseases. Epidemics of peste des petits ruminants virus can severely affect the rural economies of many developing countries, particularly in West Africa and South Asia and the poorer farmers, who depend more on small ruminants for their livelihoods, suffer disproportionately. The control and possible elimination of peste des petits ruminants is now a target for the FAO.

The new reverse genetics technology for manipulating morbillivirus genomes, in addition to its practical usefulness in allowing the development of marker vaccines, also enables us to investigate, on a rational scientific basis, the molecular determinants of virulence and attenuation in this virus group (Nagai, 1999). The molecular basis of attenuation of the TCRV has been shown to be due to the accumulation of a number of separate mutations in the N, P, F and L genes, none of which is itself so sufficiently debilitating that there is strong selective pressure in favour of the revertant (Baron *et al.*, 2005). Powerful attenuating mutations were also found to arise in the promoter regions of the virus (Banyard *et al.*, 2005). This research gives valuable insights when assessing the safety of both existing and new vaccines that may yet be produced for other morbilliviruses.

# References

Anderson, J., Barrett, T. and Scott, G.R. (1996) *Manual on the Diagnosis of Rinderpest,* 2nd edn. Rome: FAO.
Appel, M.J., Shek, W.R., Shesberadaran, H. and Norrby, E. (1984). Measles virus and inactivated canine distemper virus induce incomplete immunity to canine distemper. *Arch. Virol.* **82** (1–2), 73–82
Banyard, A., Baron, M.D. and Barrett, T (2005) A role for virus promoters in determining the pathogenesis of rinderpest virus in cattle. *J. Gen. Virol.* **86** (Pt 4), 1083–92.
Baron, M.D., Banyard, A., Parida, S. and Barrett, T. (2005) The Plowright vaccine strain of rinderpest virus has attenuating mutations in most genes. *J. Gen. Virol.* **86** (Pt 4), 1093–101.
Baron, M.D. and Barrett, T. (1997) Rescue of recombinant rinderpest virus from cloned cDNA. *J. Virol.* **71**, 1265–71.
Baron, M.D. and Barrett, T. (2000) Rinderpest viruses lacking the C and V proteins show specific defects in growth and transcription of viral RNAs. *J. Virol.* **74** (6), 2603–11.
Barrett, T., Belsham, G.J., Shaila, M.S. and Evans, S.A. (1989) Immunisation with a vaccinia recombinant expressing the F protein protects rabbits from challenge with a lethal dose of rinderpest virus. *Virology* **170**, 11–18.
Bassiri, M., Ahmad, S., Giavedoni, L., Jones, L., Saliki, J.T., Mebus, C. and Yilma, T. (1993) Immunological responses of mice and cattle to baculovirus-expressed F and H proteins of rinderpest virus: lack of protection in the presence of neutralizing antibody. *J. Virol.* **67** (3),1255–61.
Belsham, G.J., Anderson, E.C., Murray, P.K., Anderson, J. and Barrett, T. (1989) The immune response and protection of cattle and pigs generated by a vaccinia virus recombinant expressing the F protein of rinderpest virus. *Vet. Rec.* **124**, 655–8.
Berhe, G., Minet, C., Le Goff, C., Barrett, T., Ngangnou, A., Grillet, C. Libeau, G., Fleming, M., Black, D.N. and Diallo, A. (2002). Development of a dual recombinant vaccine to protect small ruminants against peste des petits ruminants and capripox infections. *J. Virol.* **77**, 1571–7.
Brochier, B., Kieny, M.P., Costy, F., Coppens, P., Bauduin, B., Lecocq, J.P., Languet, B., Chappuis, G., Desmettre, P., Afiademanyo, K. *et al.* (1991). Large-scale eradication of rabies using recombinant vaccinia-rabies vaccine. *Nature* **354** (6354), 520–2.
Conzelmann, K.K. and Schnell, M. (1994) Rescue of synthetic genome analogs of rabies virus by plasmid-encoded DNA. *J. Virol.* **68**, 713–19.
Crawshaw, T.R. and Brown, I. (1999) Bovine influenza. *Vet. Rec.* **145**, 556–7.
Das, S.C., Baron, M.D. and Barrett. T. (2000) Recovery and characterisation of a chimeric rinderpest virus with the glycoproteins of peste des petits ruminants virus: Homologous F and H proteins are required for virus viability. *J. Virol.* **74**, 9039–47.
deVries, P., van Binnendijk, R.S., van der Marel, P., van Wezel, A.L., Voorma, H.O., Sundquist, B., Uytdehaag, F.G. and Osterhaus, A.D. (1988) Measles virus fusion protein presented in an immune-stimulating complex (iscom) induces haemolysis-inhibiting and

fusion-inhibiting antibodies, virus-specific T cells and protection in mice. *J. Gen. Virol.* **69**, 549–59.

Ennis, F.A., Cruz, J., Jameson, J., Klein, M., Burt, D. and Thipphawong, J. (1999) Augmentation of human influenza A virus specific cytotoxic T lymphocyte memory by influenza vaccine and adjuvanted carriers (ISCOMS). *Virology* **259** (2), 256–61.

Giavedoni, L., Jones, L., Mebus, C. and Yilma, T. (1991) A vaccinia virus double recombinantn expressing the F and H genes of rinderpest virus protects cattle against rinderpest and causes no pock lesions. *Proc. Natl Acad. Sci. USA* **88**, 8011–15.

Inui, K., Barrett, T., Kitching, R.P. and Yamanouchi, K. (1995) Long term immunity in cattle vaccinated with a recombinant rinderpest vaccine. *Vet. Rec.* **137**, 669–70.

Jones, L., Giavedoni, L., Saliki, J.T., Brown, C., Mebus, C. and Yilma, T. (1993) Protection of goats against peste des petits ruminants virus with a vaccinia double recombinant expressing the F and H genes of rinderpest virus. *Vaccine* **11**, 961–4.

Kamata, H., Ohishi, K., Hulskotte, E., Osterhaus, A.D.M.E., Inui, K., Yamanouchi, K. and Barrett, T. (2001) Rinderpest virus (RPV) ISCOM vaccine induces protection in cattle against virulent RPV challenge. *Vaccine* **19**, 3355–9.

Khandelwal, A., Lakshmi Sita, G. and Shaila, M.S. (2003) Oral immunization of cattle with hemagglutinin protein of rinderpest virus expressed in transgenic peanut induces specific immune responses. *Vaccine* **21**, 3282–9.

Khandelwal, A., Renukaradhya, G.J., Rajasekhar, M., Sita, G.L. and Shaila, M.S. (2004) Systemic and oral immunogenicity of hemagglutinin protein of rinderpest virus expressed by transgenic peanut plants in a mouse model. *Virology* **323**, 284–91.

Libeau, G., Perhaud, C., Lancelot, R., Colas, F., Guerre, L., Bishop, D.H.L. and Diallo, A. (1995). Development of a competitive ELISA for detecting antibodies to the peste des petits ruminants virus using a recombinant nucleoprotein. *Res. Vet. Sci.* **58**, 50–5.

Mackett, M., Smith, G.L. and Moss, B. (1982) Vaccinia virus: a selectable eukaryotic cloning and expression vector. *Proc. Natl Acad. Sci. USA* **79**, 7415–19.

Mariner, J.C., House, J.A., Sollod, A.E., Stem, C., van den Ende, M.C. and Mebus, C.A. (1990) Comparison of the effect of various chemical stabilisers and lyophilisation cycles on the thermostability of a Vero cell-adapted rinderpest vaccine. *Vet. Microbiol.* **21**, 195–209.

Mebatsion, T., Koolen, M.J., de Vaan L.T. *et al.* (2002) Newcastle disease virus (NDV) marker vaccine: an immunodominant epitope on the nucleoprotein gene of NDV can be deleted or replaced by a foreign epitope. *J. Virol.* **76**, 10138–46.

Nagai, Y. (1999) Paramyxovirus replication and pathogenesis: reverse genetics transforms understanding. *Rev. Med. Virol.* **9**, 83–99.

Ngichabe, C.K., Wamwayi, H.M., Barrett, T., Ndungu, E.K., Black, D.N. and Bostock, C.J. (1997) Trial of a capripoxvirus-rinderpest recombinant vaccine in African cattle. *Epidemiol. Infect.* **118**, 63–70.

Ngichabe, C.K., Wamwayi, H.M., Ndungu1, E.K., Mirangil, P.K., Bostock, C.J., Black, D.N. and Barrett, T. (2002) Long-term immunity in African cattle vaccinated with a recombinant capripox-rinderpest virus vaccine. *Epidemiol. Infect.* **128**, 343–9.

Oirschot, J.T., van Terpstra C., Moormann, R.J.M., Berns, A.J. and Gielkens, A.L.J. (1990) Safety of an Aujeszky's disease vaccine based on deletion mutant strain 783 which does not express thymidine kinase and glycoprotein 1. *Vet. Rec.* **127**, 443–6.

Parida, S., Walsh, E.P., Anderson, J., Baron, M.D. and Barrett, T. (2004) Development of marker vaccines for rinderpest virus using reverse genetics technology. In: *Applications of Gene Based Technologies for Improving Animal Production and Health in Developing Countries.* New York: Kluwer Academic/Plenum.

Pastoret, P.P. and Brochier, B. (1996). The development and use of a vaccinia-rabies recombinant oral vaccine for the control of wildlife rabies; a link between Jenner and Pasteur. *Epidemiol. Infect.* **116**, 235–40.

Plowright, W. and Ferris, R.D. (1962) Studies with rinderpest virus in tissue culture. The use of attenuated culture virus as a vaccine for cattle. *Res. Vet. Sci.* **3**, 172–82.

Plowright, W. and Taylor, W.P. (1967) Long-term studies of the immunity in East African cattle following inoculation with rinderpest culture vaccine. *Res. Vet. Sci.* **8**, 118–28.

Romero, C.H., Barrett, T., Chamberlain, R.W., Kitching, R.P., Fleming, M. and Black, D.N. (1994a) Recombinant capripoxvirus expressing the haemagglutinin protein gene of rinderpest virus: protection of cattle against rinderpest and lumpy skin disease. *Virology* **204**, 425–9.

Romero, C.H., Barrett, T., Evans, S.A., Kitching, R.P., Gershon, P.D. and Black, D.N. (1993) A single vaccine for the protection of cattle against rinderpest and lumpy skin disease. *Vaccine* **11**, 737–42.

Romero, C.H., Barrett, T., Kitching, R.P., Bostock, C.J. and Black, D.N. (1995) Protection of goats against peste des petits ruminants with recombinant capripoxviruses expressing the fusion and haemagglutinin protein genes of rinderpest virus. *Vaccine* **13**, 36–40.

Romero, C.H., Barrett, T., Kitching, R.P., Carn, V.M. and Black, D.N. (1994b) Protection of cattle against rinderpest and lumpy skin disease with a recombinant capripoxvirus expressing the fusion protein gene of rinderpest virus. *Vet. Rec.* **135**, 152–4.

Sinnathamby, G. (2004). Cytotoxic T cell epitope in cattle from the attachment glycoproteins of rinderpest and peste des petits ruminants viruses. *Viral Immunol.* **17** (3), 401–10.

Verardi, P.H., Aziz, F.H., Ahmad, S., Jones, L.A., Beyene, B., Ngotho, R.N., Wamwayi, H.M., Yesus, M.G., Egziabher, B.G. and Yilma, T.D. (2002) Long-term sterilizing immunity to rinderpest in cattle vaccinated with a recombinant vaccinia virus expressing high levels of the fusion and haemagglutinin glycoproteins. *J. Virol.* **76**, 484–91.

Walsh, E.P., Baron, M.D., Rennie, L., Anderson, J. and Barrett, T. (2000a) Development of a genetically marked recombinant rinderpest vaccine expressing green fluorescent protein. *J. Gen. Virol.* **81**, 709–18.

Walsh, E.P., Baron, M.D., Rennie, L., Monahan, P., Anderson J. and Barrett, T. (2000b) Recombinant rinderpest vaccines expressing membrane anchored proteins as genetic markers: evidence for exclusion of marker protein from the virus envelope. *J. Virol.* **74**, 10165–75.

Whelan, S.P.J., Barr, J.N. and Wertz, G. (2004) Transcription and replication of nonsegmented negative-strand RNA viruses. In: Y. Kawaoka (ed.), *Biology of Negative Strand RNA Viruses: The Power of Reverse Genetics.* New York: Springer.

Yamanouchi, K., Barrett, T. and Kai, C. (1998) New approaches to the development of virus vaccines for veterinary use. *Rev. Sci. Tech. OIE* **17**, 641–53.

Yamanouchi, K., Inui, K., Sugimoto, M., Asano, K., Nishimaki, F., Kitching, R.P., Takamatsu, H. and Barrett, T. (1993) Immunisation of cattle with a recombinant vaccinia vector expressing the haemagglutinin gene of rinderpest virus. *Vet. Rec.* **132**, 152–6.

Yilma, T., Hsu, D., Jones, L., Owens, S., Mebus, C., Yamakana, M and Dale, B. (1988) Protection of cattle against rinderpest with vaccinia virus recombinants expressing HA and F genes. *Science* **242**, 1058–61.

# Use of rinderpest vaccine in international programmes for the control and eradication of rinderpest

# 13

**WILLIAM P. TAYLOR,\* PETER L. ROEDER† AND MARK M. RWEYEMAMU‡**

*\*Littlehampton, Sussex, UK*
*†Food and Agriculture Organization, Animal Health Service, Animal Production and Health Division, Rome, Italy*
*‡Woking, Surrey, UK*

## The dawn of control through vaccination

Writing in 1928, J.T. Edwards drew a distinction between countries in which the imposition of livestock standstill orders was an accepted means of controlling livestock disease, and endemically infected countries where such methods were impracticable, 'or even quite impossible' (Edwards, 1930). As far as rinderpest was concerned however, he did believe that there were ways forward. At that time it was possible to passively protect cattle at the scene of an outbreak with convalescent serum, which protected for about 10 days, or using the serum-simultaneous method, which provided a long-lived active immunity and a way of forestalling the infection altogether.

Although he felt that the day of eradication was far distant, employing the serum-simultaneous method, he proposed a strategy based on the creation of either belts or a wide scattering of immune animals to 'effectively reduce the transmission chain and thus bring about a commensurate diminution in the virulence of the infection for the cattle population generally'. These remarks suggest that, while prepared to dream of eradicating rinderpest from India,

ISBN-13: 978-0-12-88385-1
ISBN-10: 0-12-88385-6

Edwards was also prepared to accept attempts to reduce the incidence level as the more pragmatic way forward. He also envisaged the need for a live attenuated vaccine as an essential additional tool. In 1931 a number of Indian states (e.g. Mysore, Bengal, Central Province) came to discover that the Edwards' Mukteswar caprinized virus could be used on plains cattle without the simultaneous administration of immune serum and that the virus could be used in the face of an outbreak to develop an 'interference'. By 1934 it was possible to issue the virus in the form of desiccated spleen powder.

By 1936 all aspects of a 'new system' of rinderpest control, i.e. through the use of a live attenuated vaccine, were in place but the unfortunate truth was that subsequent progress towards eradication made little headway. Edwards illustrated this point using figures taken from the Punjab, where the introduction of the goat vaccine was made gradually and in quantities that seem minute in relation to the 16 million cattle population. In 1936–37 some 169000 animals were inoculated but the following year this rose to 805035. In fact immune serum continued to be used in outbreak situations and in 1937–38 rinderpest still accounted for 52% of the total mortality among cattle. In 1938–39, 17241 cattle died of rinderpest so that although a cheap and efficient prophylactic had become available, there was little evidence of its ability to make any permanent inroad on the level of virus transmission. The responsibility for this state of affairs was placed on the incessant movement of diseased and suspected animals purchased by dealers (Edwards, 1949).

In Burma (now Myanmar) on the other hand, by steadily adding to the immunized proportion of the livestock population, itself only 3.75 million strong, it was possible to detect profound effects on the epidemiology of the disease. These results led Edwards to propose a rule for the suppression of rinderpest (Edwards, 1949). He suggested that when dealing with cattle with the intention of creating a threshold above which rinderpest could not retain its footing, it was necessary to create and maintain within the population a proportion of permanently (and solidly) immune animals amounting to not less than 60% of the total population.

In the course of his discussions, Edwards clearly pinned his hopes on the use of live attenuated rinderpest vaccine as the means of controlling rinderpest in India. He understood that rinderpest might be eliminated by the use of a rinderpest-induced immunity in two totally different ways. The ideal method would be to immunize the entire target population within a very short period of time – in which case the durability of the immunization was not as important as the intensity of the coverage. The more practical scenario, based on the Burmese experience, was to profit from the lifelong immunity associated with live rinderpest vaccines and 'bank' each year's campaign results until the balance was sufficiently large to bring the virus under a beneficial level of control. These deliberations place Edwards firmly at the head of the movement to eliminate rinderpest from India. By the time this was finally achieved some 50 years later, both methods had been tried, with pulsed intensified vaccination providing the final thrust.

Turning to Africa and the contemporary situation and the availability of attenuated egg, goat and rabbit strains of rinderpest, Daubney (1953) wrote

> whenever a determined effort at mass vaccination with one of these living vaccines has been made, the impact of the campaign upon the incidence of the disease has been dramatic. In Tanganyika huge tracts of territory were freed from infection in the early 1940s; in Egypt, a mass-immunisation campaign cleared the country of rinderpest in the short space of eight months. Given sufficient will to succeed and sufficiently wholehearted inter-territorial co-operation, the task of eradicating rinderpest from Africa is well within our compass and should not take too many years.

Holding Daubney's theme, the present section discusses two enormous and successful vaccination-oriented rinderpest eradication programmes, one in Africa and one in India. Jointly and severally these programmes have had a major impact on the distribution of the virus and have made major contributions towards its eradication. The first discussion takes up the role of vaccines and vaccination in the elimination of rinderpest from West Africa and the subsequent realization that, once the vaccination campaigns have been completed, a process to replace follow-up vaccination must be set in place. The second, in India, demonstrates how a newly agreed international accreditation process to replace follow-up vaccination with disease surveillance might be integrated within a refocused, time-bound and ultimately successful rinderpest eradication programme.

# The joint campaign against rinderpest (JP15)

In the 1940s and 1950s, although the time of the great African rinderpest epizootic had long since passed, the disease continued to rage in Africa in a disquieting way, checked only by the strenuous and repetitive efforts of veterinary services across the East African and sub-Sahelian regions of the continent. Neither control nor eradication seemed possible, one reason being the compartmentalization that existed between the veterinary services concerned (Lepissier, 1971). Nevertheless, there was a growing awareness that increasing supplies of freeze-dried, attenuated goat-adapted vaccine provided a tool for the improved control, or even attempts at eradication. Thus, the first resolution of the African Rinderpest Conference of 1948 stated that 'it is the considered opinion of the Conference that in spite of any agricultural, sociological or administrative repercussions, control of rinderpest with a view to its complete eradication is desirable and necessary in the interests of Africa as a whole'. The Conference further resolved that 'rinderpest can be eradicated from Africa with the biological immunizing agents already at our disposal' and, in recognizing the need for international collaboration, recommended the establishment of an African Rinderpest Organization comprised of the African Information Bureau on Rinderpest (quickly to become the Inter-African Bureau of Epizootic Diseases).

In 1961, the Commission for Technical Cooperation in Africa South of the Sahara (CCTA) met in Kano, northern Nigeria, and decided to initiate a programme of joint action against rinderpest. Eventually running to six phases, taking in both West and East Africa, and later described as 'the biggest animal disease operation of its kind ever undertaken', the first phase was a more modest affair. It aimed at demonstrating the effectiveness of coordinated disease control in reducing the incidence of rinderpest in the 8 million cattle living in the Lake Chad Basin area of Cameroon, Chad, Niger and Nigeria. Administratively, this operation was designated as Phase I of JP15. Subsequent phases were administered by the Scientific, Technical and Research Commission (STRC) of the OAU.

H.E. Lepissier, the International Coordinator of Phases I–III, distinguished between sanitary prophylaxis (basic zoo-sanitary measures such as slaughter of sick animals, segregation of contacts and movement controls within an infected area) and medical prophylaxis (mass vaccination/immunization). He considered that in West and Central Africa countries where extensive livestock keeping was practised, the route to eradication lay through a two-stage process with medical prophylaxis leading to a high degree of control and sanitary prophylaxis eliminating the last vestiges of infection. These principles were built into JP15 and from the outset the first objective was to be the use of a programme of mass immunization of cattle as the means of breaking the virus' endemic hold on the population. The second objective was to move to the progressive introduction of zoo-sanitary measures as the ultimate means of eradicating the virus (Lepissier, 1971). Pending the success of sanitary prophylaxis and to prevent any recrudescence in the number of outbreaks, an annual vaccination programme in young stock would be retained. Vaccine then, was not seen as the only key to achieving the eradication of rinderpest; however, the Final Report of the Central and West African Phases of JP15 includes a discussion in relation to conservatory measures which foresaw the emergence of further problems, but offered no solution.

The characteristics required of a rinderpest vaccine for use in an extensive livestock husbandry system, and which both the goat and cell culture attenuated vaccines satisfied, were:

- to rapidly induce a durable and reliable immunity
- to be easy to use in the field
- to give no, or only a slight, post vaccinal reaction
- to be cheap.

Based on these criteria, the action plan for Phase I, and all subsequent West African phases, called for the vaccination of all eligible cattle (young calves were not included) with live attenuated rinderpest vaccine during each of three successive dry seasons. The launching of Phase I in the dry season of 1962–63 marked the start of both international cooperation and international coordination in rinderpest eradication in Africa. The estimated vaccine requirements were 7 650 000 doses, which were produced at the Farcha Laboratory in Chad and the Vom Laboratory in Nigeria; the Coordinator was appointed to ensure the synchronization of the individual national campaigns. In August 1962, before Phase I had even begun, a meeting in Bamako, Mali, agreed to extend the programme westwards to cover all the rinderpest-affected areas of West Africa, to which end, two further phases were chalked out (Table 13.1).

Two live attenuated vaccines were extensively used in JP15. In Kano it had been decided that only goat vaccine would be used. However, this vaccine produced some untoward reaction whereas TCRV, already under experimentation at Vom, did not. In Bathurst, Gambia, in 1964, TCRV was officially endorsed for use on the hypersensitive cattle breeds of the West African Coastal Region, hitherto immunized with lapinized vaccine. In fact TCRV had already replaced goat vaccine as the only vaccine in use in Nigeria and production of TCRV began in Bamako, Farcha and Dakar in 1965. In the course of the three phases 50.6 million doses of goat vaccine were supplied, compared to 43.75 doses of TCRV. In terms of gross vaccine output, Dakar produced nearly 56 million doses while Vom, Farcha and Bamako produced 25, 23 and 21 million doses, respectively.

Rowe (1966) showed that after one round of vaccination the proportion of immune bovines stood at just over 70%, rising to 90% after two rounds and remaining at this level after three rounds. By examining the reduction in the number of rinderpest outbreaks in the regions participating in Phase I, the effectiveness of these high immunity levels is easily appreciated, the more so when it is considered that national vaccination had gone on in the preceding years. The results are summarized in Table 13.2. By and large most of the vaccination work was completed in the first 6 months of each dry season and the abrupt creation of very high levels of immunity that this produced was undoubtedly an important element in the almost immediate end of enzootic infection. This was especially clear in Nigeria.

**Table 13.1** Countries participating in the JP15, Phases I–III

| Phase | Timetable | Participating countries |
|---|---|---|
| I | 1962–65 | The Lake Chad basin area of part of Cameroon, Chad and Niger, and Sokoto, Zaria, Plateau and Niger Provinces of Nigeria |
| II | 1964–67 | Benin (former Dahomey), Ghana, Côte d'Ivoire, Mali, Niger, Nigeria, Togo, Burkina Faso (former Upper Volta) |
| III | 1966–69 | Mali, Gambia, Mauretania, Senegal, Sierra Leone, eastern Chad, Guinea, Liberia |

**Table 13.2**  The ability of high inputs of rinderpest vaccine to reduce the numbers of rinderpest outbreaks in endemically infected Phase I cattle populations

| Country | Average number of outbreaks per annum over the previous 10 years[a] | Results of dry season vaccination by years | | | | | |
|---|---|---|---|---|---|---|---|
| | | 1962–63 | | 1963–64 | | 1964–65 | |
| | | Proportion of herd vaccinated | No. of recorded outbreaks | Proportion of herd vaccinated | No. of recorded outbreaks | Proportion of herd vaccinated | No. of recorded outbreaks |
| C'roon | 148 | 97.6 | 0 | 108.0 | 2 | 98.9 | 0 |
| Niger | 196 | 91.3 | 47 | 90.2 | 18 | 106.9 | 4 |
| Nigeria | 375 | 86.2 | 91 | 105.3 | 2 | 111.1 | 2 |
| Chad | 250 | 92.2 | 37 | 100.3 | 6 | 99.2 | 4 |

[a]In vaccinated zone.
*Source:* Data from Lepissier, 1971

**Table 13.3**  Phase II rinderpest outbreaks reported in countries and regions of countries vaccinated for three seasons, starting October 1964

| Country\Year | 1964 | 1965 | 1966 | 1967 |
|---|---|---|---|---|
| Mali – region | 102 | 41 | 19 | 4 |
| Niger | 60 | 1 | 2 | 1 |
| Burkina Faso | 32 | 21 | 1 | 0 |

*Source:* Data from Lepissier, 1971

**Table 13.4**  Phase III rinderpest outbreaks reported in countries and regions of countries vaccinated for three seasons starting October 1966

| Country | 1964 | 1965 | 1966 | 1967 | 1968 | 1969 |
|---|---|---|---|---|---|---|
| Mali – region | 60 | 26 | 1 | 0 | 0 | 0 |
| Mauritania | 91 | 60 | 82 | 24 | 12 | 4 |
| Senegal | 110 | 13 | 27 | 33 | 69 | 16 |
| Eastern Chad | 0 | 7 | 12 | 17 | 4 | 2 |

*Source:* Data from Lepissier, 1971

Continuing to generate highly immune cattle populations throughout Phases II and III, JP15 succeeded in bringing rinderpest to a very low incidence level across the whole of West Africa (Tables 13.3 and 13.4). Over the period 1962–69, approximately 100 million doses were used in the furtherance of JP15 and in West Africa, some even considered that rinderpest in Africa had been consigned to history and several countries even produced a series of postage stamps to commemorate the occasion (Plate 6).

At the conclusion of the phase of intensive vaccination endeavour, conservation measures were devolved to National Veterinary Authorities who had in any case implemented the project up to that point, albeit it with international finance and coordination. The difference was that now, the follow-up work was set against departmental budgets and international coordination was at an end. The results were predictably variable. Nigeria was faithful to the JP15 objectives and duly continued with follow-up vaccination, adjusted to take into account Provost's results concerning longevity of protection (see Chapter 11). Surveillance activities were also well carried out and when, in 1973, an infected herd entered Nigeria across the Cameroon border having already been tracked by the Cameroon authorities (Alain Provost, personal communication) it was followed as far as the border village of Mubi where it was sampled, detained and vaccinated. The samples received at Vom were positive by the agar-gel immuno-diffusion test. Although this was the last record of rinderpest in Nigeria in the immediate post-JP15 era, annual vaccination campaigns were not discontinued.

Whereas JP15 itself was frequently criticized in Africa for its insistence on three rounds of mass vaccination when a lesser number might have sufficed, this was not the crux of the matter. Rather it was the absence of a coordinating authority (a role for which the Organization of African Unity's Inter-African Bureau of Animal Health had been proposed) with a responsibility for ensuring, first, that sanitary prophylaxis took over where medical prophylaxis ended and later, when this had succeeded, for advising against continued vaccination. In Nigeria in 1978 there was no clear understanding of how long conservatory measures should continue nor what to do next. Neither was it understood that the virus persisted in Mauritania and that a contingency plan was needed to prevent it re-entering the country, even though the cattle population was known to be growing increasingly susceptible (Taylor and Ojeh, 1981). As we all know now, and as was known locally at the time, a focus of endemic infection remained in the Mauritania/Mali pastoral system, from which reinfection of a number of West African countries took place in the late 1970s, unravelling most of the benefits of JP15.

Who was to blame for the recrudescence of rinderpest across West Africa? Ultimately international leadership that had failed to recognize that mass vaccination was only the beginning of the eradication, and that an accreditation process was also required. Knowing that a fresh attempt to eliminate rinderpest from Africa was under way, in 1989 the OIE met and devised its Rinderpest Pathway (see Chapter 15). The thrust of this important meeting was to understand that follow-up programmes rendered participating countries vulnerable either to the re-establishment of enzootic infection with a virus of reduced virulence or to reinvasion from an infected neighbour. To encourage countries to end their vaccination programmes and in fact place their reliance on sanitary prophylaxis, the meeting attempted to devise an exit strategy based on the successful conclusion of vaccination and a demonstration that the virus had actually stopped circulating. By promoting the so-called Rinderpest Pathway, the OIE has developed a supra-national review system to accredit and protect the rinderpest-free status claimed by its member states.

## Fifty-year struggle to eliminate rinderpest from India: 1954–2004

The Indian Civil Veterinary Department was established in 1891, partly as a recommendation of the India Cattle Plague Commission of 1868. Thus the seeds of rinderpest control were sown at an early date and certainly resonated throughout the writings of Edwards. However, Datta (1954) indicates that it took another 20 or so years before an eradication plan was first articulated – one that envisaged the immunization of 320 million head of cattle, buffaloes, sheep and goats over a 5–10-year period.

In his 1953 report to the Government of India, R.L. Daubney, representing FAO, was asked to advise which vaccine should be used in such a scheme. He found that the Nakamura III strain of lapinized rinderpest vaccine was available at the 1178th direct passage level and this virus was being inoculated into goats to give a lapinized-goat-reactor vaccine. Unfortunately the viral content in first passage goat spleens was too low to provide a practicable vaccine and the concept was shelved. Goat-adapted rinderpest, line W, had been maintained at Mukteswar by direct passage in goats for many years. As a stable characteristic, this virus produced no more than a mild, delayed pyrexia (103 °F/39.4 °C) in the highly susceptible hill cattle. Another passage series of this virus, line Y, was out-passaged in Hill Bulls every 2 or 3 months and, even though there were no data indicating differing levels of virulence, some states used line W and some used line Y. After a series of trials Daubney recommended that the Mukteswar W line of goat-adapted virus was suitable for the great bulk of animals in India.

By 1954 India had gained sufficient confidence in its attenuated goat vaccine as well as in the strength of the veterinary services, to embark on a publicly financed, vaccine-based campaign for rinderpest eradication – the National Rinderpest Eradication Programme (Khera, 1979). Following the success of a small pilot programme (recommended by Daubney) involving 18 districts in a contiguous area of Andhra Pradesh, Karnataka and Maharashtra, the full programme began in 1956–57, running through to 1989. The programme was entirely self-sufficient – no external donors were involved – and aimed at systematically vaccinating 80% of adult cattle and buffaloes in an initial period of 5 years. This would be succeeded by a follow-up period lasting until the disease was eliminated. In this follow-up period the remaining 20% of adult animals plus the annual calf crop (itself estimated at around 20% of the adult population) would be vaccinated.

The decision to exclude sheep and goats from the programme was probably sound. In 1954, PPR was not a recognized pathogen of small ruminants in India – although it may well have been present (Taylor et al., 2002b), as would have been sporadic outbreaks of small ruminant rinderpest contracted by contact with infected cattle. Much later, a number of veterinarians in south India implicated small ruminants in the transmission of rinderpest from village to village but, with respect, were still failing to differentiate between rinderpest and PPR.

Each state undertook its own vaccination programme and up and down the country the success of the initial phase varied considerably. In the northern state of Uttar Pradesh for example (Table 13.5) the main campaign lasted for 8 years (1956–64) and follow-up measures for at least another 20 years. In fact, apart from a reduced vaccination input in 1964–65, it is hard to see a reduced level of vaccination in the follow-up phase. Nonetheless, within 8 years of starting, a notional 80% of the bovine population of Uttar Pradesh had been vaccinated and the incidence level of outbreaks had fallen dramatically – from over a thousand in the first year of the campaign, to a single-figure level by the seventh. In fact, as judged by the low number of yearly outbreaks after 1962, there can be little doubt that the endemic status of rinderpest in Uttar Pradesh had been changed irrevocably. Interestingly, this was probably accomplished without ever achieving particularly high immunity rates as even after 8 years of work, the coverage was only 84% without allowing for failed immunizations or the bovine population turnover. In fact it is quite probable that vaccination rates of between 50 and 60% were the best that had been achieved (the endemicity-breaking level suggested previously by Edwards), yet the outbreak incidence rate plummeted.

After 1962 the epidemiology of the virus appears to have been totally changed. Sporadic outbreaks continued to be reported but the low incidence level suggested the existence of a non-endemic situation, probably because villages no longer sold infected animals to one another. Trade with other states was still there however, causing localized outbreaks by the introduction of infected animals into urban dairies. In Uttar Pradesh then, the follow-up programme was able to prevent a return to endemicity but, by failing to address the residual problem by sanitary prophylaxis, was unable to achieve a rinderpest-free status.

Unfortunately, the follow-up programme was not always able to prevent the re-establishment of endemicity. In the southern state of Andhra Pradesh (Table 13.6), mass vaccination began in 1956, the vaccination rate in the first phase exceeding the nominal bovine population and spectacularly, the rinderpest outbreaks was reduced to zero. However, from the start of the follow-up campaigns in 1961, when the uptake of vaccine fell sharply (as anticipated by the programme), outbreaks were again apparent. Even though escalating quantities of vaccine were subsequently administered, over the next 23 years the outbreak incidence rate remained intractably high. Arguably these outbreaks represented a constant re-introduction of infection from neighbouring states but given the parallel declining incidence of endemically infected states elsewhere in the country, this explanation seems untenable. Realistically, it appears that the virus remained endemic within the village population of Andhra Pradesh throughout this period – a suggestion perhaps supported by the low number of animals involved in the individual outbreaks. This suggests that in spite of an enormous

**Table 13.5**  The results of vaccination against rinderpest between 1956 and 1984 in the Indian state of Uttar Pradesh

| Phase and Year[a] | Outbreaks | Deaths/cases/mean cases per outbreak | Vaccinations undertaken (millions) | Notional bovine population vaccinated (%)[b] |
|---|---|---|---|---|
| *Main* | | | | |
| 1956–57 | 1123 | 10532/19702/17.5 | 5.71 | 14 |
| 1957–58 | 1541 | 10060/18679/12.1 | 1.49 | 18 |
| 1958–59 | 1828 | 11285/24998/13.7 | 2.05 | 23 |
| 1959–60 | 229 | 1378/2957/12.9 | 4.25 | 34 |
| 1960–61 | 70 | 507/1012/14.5 | 2.28 | 39 |
| 1961–62 | 56 | 674/1237/22.1 | 3.52 | 48 |
| 1962–63 | 9 | 68/133/14.8 | 6.56 | 65 |
| 1963–64 | 12 | 63/118/9.8 | 7.56 | 84 |
| *Follow-up* | | | | |
| 1964–65 | 31 | 405/645/20.8 | 2.21 | 89 |
| 1965–66 | 4 | 51/198/49.5 | 4.17 | 100 |
| 1966–67 | 25 | 676/1135/45.4 | 4.18 | 110 |
| 1967–68 | 11 | 131/231/21.0 | 4.18 | 120 |
| 1968–69 | 0 | | 4.85 | 133 |
| 1969–70 | 25 | 555/1128/45.1 | 5.59 | 146 |
| 1970–71 | 5 | 78/149/29.8 | 8.72 | 168 |
| 1971–72 | 0 | | 8.56 | 190 |
| 1972–73 | 1 | 91/100/100.0 | 8.74 | 212 |
| 1973–74 | 2 | 4/21/10.5 | 8.35 | 232 |
| 1974–75 | 2 | 18/38/19.0 | 8.55 | 254 |
| 1975–76 | 1 | 4/15/15.0 | 5.42 | 267 |
| 1976–77 | 4 | 67/210/52.5 | 3.35 | 276 |
| 1977–78 | 0 | | 4.09 | 286 |
| 1978–79 | 2 | 511/889/444.5 | 4.44 | 297 |
| 1979–80 | 3 | 52/243/81.0 | 7.01 | 315 |
| 1980–81 | 0 | | 7.22 | 333 |
| 1981–82 | 1 | 12/206/206.0 | 7.00 | 367 |
| 1982–83 | 0 | | 6.70 | 384 |
| 1983–84 | 1 | 42/563/563.0 | 6.42 | 400 |

Total vaccinations: 153.17 millions

[a]Dates are quoted by fiscal year.
[b]Based on a constant population estimation of 40 million bovines.

follow-up effort, the bovine population remained sufficiently susceptible to continually support the virus, pointing to either poor distribution or poor quality of the vaccine. Unfortunately seromonitoring was not employed as a management tool for investigating the problem.

Across India as a whole, reducing endemic rinderpest with mass vaccination succeeded but required an inordinately long time to do so. In Table 13.7 it can

**Table 13.6**   The results of vaccination against rinderpest between 1956 and 1984 in the Indian state of Andhra Pradesh

| Phase and year[a] | Outbreaks | Deaths/cases/mean cases per outbreak | Vaccinations undertaken (millions) | Notional bovine population vaccinated (%)[b] |
|---|---|---|---|---|
| *Main* | | | | |
| 1955–56 | No data | | 3.11 | 16 |
| 1956–57 | 44 | 251/281/6.4 | 3.74 | 34 |
| 1957–58 | 128 | 985/1895/14.8 | 2.74 | 48 |
| 1958–59 | 53 | 745/1018/19.2 | 3.31 | 64 |
| 1959–60 | 1 | 4/8/8 | 4.46 | 87 |
| 1960–61 | 0 | | 5.98 | 117 |
| *Follow-up* | | | | |
| 1961–62 | 11 | 339/582/52.9 | 1.40 | 124 |
| 1962–63 | 4 | 40/140/35.0 | 0.93 | 128 |
| 1963–64 | 8 | 578/1050/131.3 | 3.26 | 145 |
| 1964–65 | 85 | 1254/3096/36.4 | 4.55 | 167 |
| 1965–66 | 18 | 215/401/22.3 | 2.45 | 180 |
| 1966–67 | 45 | 461/692/15.4 | 2.23 | 191 |
| 1967–68 | 59 | 475/973/16.5 | 2.05 | 202 |
| 1968–69 | 49 | 294/849/17.3 | 2.73 | 215 |
| 1969–70 | 96 | 896/1876/19.5 | 2.90 | 229 |
| 1970–71 | 79 | 527/1569/19.9 | 2.72 | 243 |
| 1971–72 | 9 | 52/124/13.8 | 3.65 | 261 |
| 1972–73 | 10 | 123/291/29.1 | 3.22 | 277 |
| 1973–74 | 9 | 421/761/84.6 | 3.16 | 293 |
| 1974–75 | 39 | 254/917/23.5 | 3.57 | 311 |
| 1975–76 | 12 | 71/185/15.4 | 7.22 | 347 |
| 1976–77 | 25 | 127/362/14.5 | 7.40 | 384 |
| 1977–78 | 36 | 158/401/11.1 | 7.54 | 422 |
| 1978–79 | 35 | 399/1018/29.1 | 9.22 | 468 |
| 1979–80 | 65 | 433/1034/15.9 | 6.45 | 499 |
| 1980–81 | 119 | 768/1740/14.6 | 7.42 | 537 |
| 1981–82 | 106 | 601/2337/22.1 | 4.66 | 560 |
| 1982–83 | 60 | 272/1221/20.4 | 7.62 | 598 |
| 1983–84 | 25 | 98/360/14.4 | 8.53 | 641 |

Total vaccinations: 125.11 millions

[a]In the 5-year period up to 1956, 3.1 million head had been vaccinated.
[b]Based on a constant population estimation of 20 million bovines.

be seen that in six important livestock-keeping states it took an average of around 13 years to reduce the annual level of rinderpest outbreaks to single figures. On the other hand, there can be no doubt that throughout this period the mass vaccination programme provided the majority of Indian livestock keepers with a considerable degree of surety against economic ruin. That said, by the

**Table 13.7** Number of years to reduce rinderpest endemic status[a] in various states

| State | No. of Years |
|---|---|
| Gujarat | 14 |
| Madhya Pradesh | 20 |
| Maharashtra | 16 |
| Orissa | 17 |
| Punjab | 5 |
| Rajasthan | 10 |

[a]Single figure outbreak returns for two consecutive years.

early 1980s it was clear that the National Rinderpest Eradication Programme was failing, and that there did not seem to be a managerial solution to its problems. Accordingly, in 1983 and with an element of impatience, the Government of India appointed a Task Force to recommend 'an action programme for the eradication of rinderpest from the country within a time-bound schedule'.

The Task Force report pointed out that sound strategies were in place, especially that based on village searches for rinderpest and when found, securing the outbreak site with a mix of sanitary and medical prophylaxis (ring vaccination, isolation of sick animals, segregation of in-contacts, disinfection, and provision of subsidized feeding). They also stated,

> lapses in the control of outbreaks is the premier factor responsible for perpetuation of infection year after year. Invariably the origin of rinderpest is linked with fresh ingress from an established outbreak. If the chances of seepage of infection from an outbreak are completely sealed there will be no spread of infection.

They then determined a conservative strategy, to be known as Operation Rinderpest Zero, within which it was recommended that states where the virus was still thought to be endemic (Andhra Pradesh, Karnantaka, Tamil Nadu, Maharashtra, Gujarat and Orissa) should re-embark on a mass vaccination programme aimed at providing a 90% immunity rate within a 3-year period.

# The second Indian elimination programme: the National Project for Rinderpest Eradication of 1989–2004

In late 1989 the Government of India entered into an agreement with the EU to support a time-bound, 6-year programme of rinderpest eradication based on the recommendations of the Task Force. The project was to be renamed the National Project for Rinderpest Eradication (NPRE).

In August 1989 the OIE had looked at core issues in relation to the formulation of surveillance strategies for declaring a country free from rinderpest and drawn up the various criteria for determining how a country, or a zone within a country, might gain international recognition as rinderpest-free – the 'OIE Pathway' (OIE, 1993; see also Chapter 15). The publication of these criteria had a profound effect on the design of the strategies to be followed by the NPRE, the more so as the Pathway has its own in-built time-bound framework that starts to run when a Declaration of Provisional Freedom from Rinderpest is made. Therefore there was no disparity between the objectives of the Government of India and requirements of the OIE Pathway.

While undertaking a preparatory phase, existing vaccination strategies were expected to continue while improvements were made to vaccine production capacity, vaccine quality control, cold chains, field mobility, disease reporting and disease diagnosis. Vaccination was still seen as the key component and during the eradication phase, the endemic areas were to be subjected to two rounds of 100% vaccination cover, including sheep and goats in the southern states.

Under the OIE Pathway, a Declaration of Provisional Freedom, although in the hands of the national authorities, is inappropriate until the lapse of 24 consecutive months without an outbreak and a concomitant willingness to abandon the use of rinderpest vaccination, the objective being to create a susceptible population in which meaningful disease surveillance can be undertaken. In India the main problem in progressing the NPRE lay with the introduction of the OIE Pathway in a country where the rinderpest situation varied enormously, some states being rinderpest-free and others endemically infected. Taking into account the Pathway's suggestion that zones within a country can make declarations of provisional freedom at different times and based on the national rinderpest reports for 1989–90, Taylor (1990) suggested a tentative schedule for introducing the concept of zonation within India. In effect it was possible to divide the country into zones according to the epidemiological situation. In the southern zone there were a number of states where rinderpest was clearly endemic (Andhra Pradesh, Karnataka, Tamil Nadu and parts of Maharashtra and Madhya Pradesh) while in the north-eastern zone (north-east states) it was not – and had not been for a long time.

In addition the north-central states had probably become rinderpest-free, but only recently so, and collectively were not therefore in a position to make a declaration of provisional freedom. It therefore appeared that the north-east part of the country might make immediate entry to the Pathway. The underlying purpose of demarcating zones was to allocate the available resources in a manner appropriate to the work to be done, with the endemic zone clearly requiring more attention than the rinderpest-free zone. The proposed 'roll-back' programme called for the three zones to proceed along the Pathway at times appropriate to their disease situation, coming together at the end with a final national declaration of freedom from infection.

Two years later, in 1992, the rinderpest situation was again reviewed and the same conclusion was reached: that rinderpest was endemic only in the southern states of the Deccan, essentially restricted to Karnataka and Tamil Nadu. At that point the zoning concept, developed and discussed over the previous two years, was finally incorporated in the first NPRE workplan (1993–94). Having rationalized the states of north-east India as a rinderpest-free zone (Zone A), where no mass vaccination would take place, and southern India as an endemically infected zone, where mass vaccination was still contemplated (Zone C), the problem was how to treat north-central India (Zone B). By this time the states of Zone B had enjoyed 2 years' freedom from rinderpest (Table 13.8) and, in keeping with the roll-back policy, should now have wished to declare provisional freedom. However, ending vaccination was regarded as a highly dangerous step, possibly leading to an upsurge of rinderpest outbreaks from hidden foci. In an attempt to manage this situation, an interim strategy was developed whereby a series of risk-containing boxes were proposed (the borders of individual states), the walls of which were made up of vaccinated cattle to a depth of 25 km; livestock in the interior were left unvaccinated. In theory then, the reappearance of rinderpest in one state would not automatically lead to the virus spreading out of control to neighbouring states, a strategy which allowed for the NPRE managers' mis-evaluation of the epidemiological situation. On the other hand, if successfully implemented, Zone B states were reducing the amount of vaccine used and beginning to position themselves to make a declaration of provisional freedom. In this respect this reduction was the pivotal point in the Zone B programme, eventually allowing it to continue within the time-bound framework. Nonetheless, this first step was regarded as highly dangerous and required considerable courage on the part of the relevant State Directors of Veterinary Services.

Two years later no disaster had befallen Zone B, outbreak levels in Zone C continued to decline and a decision was taken to end all rinderpest vaccination

**Table 13.8**  The decline of rinderpest outbreaks in Zone B states

| State | 1984 | 1985 | 1986 | 1987 | 1988 | 1989 | 1990 | 1991 | 1992 | 1993 |
|---|---|---|---|---|---|---|---|---|---|---|
| Bihar | 10 | 3 | 13 | 0 | 0 | 0 | 0 | 0 | 0 | 0 |
| Gujarat | 4 | 0 | 2 | 100 | 51 | 0 | 0 | 0 | 0 | 0 |
| Haryana | 0 | 0 | 13 | 9 | 18 | 0 | 0 | 0 | 0 | 0 |
| Himachal Pradesh | 0 | 0 | 0 | 0 | 1 | 0 | 0 | 0 | 0 | 0 |
| Jammu and Kashmir | 0 | 1 | 0 | 0 | 0 | 0 | 0 | 0 | 0 | 0 |
| Madhya Pradesh | 1 | 3 | 7 | 1 | 0 | 0 | 0 | 0 | 0 | 0 |
| Orissa | 2 | 1 | 9 | 2 | 12 | 3 | 0 | 0 | 0 | 1 |
| Punjab | 0 | 0 | 0 | 0 | 0 | 0 | 0 | 0 | 0 | 0 |
| Rajasthan | 0 | 2 | 0 | 0 | 3 | 0 | 0 | 0 | 0 | 0 |
| Uttar Pradesh | 2 | 3 | 1 | 3 | 0 | 0 | 0 | 0 | 0 | 0 |
| West Bengal | 6 | 8 | 25 | 1 | 2 | 0 | 0 | 0 | 0 | 0 |

along the Zone B inter-state borders and strengthen surveillance. Thus the livestock of the whole of north-central India became one enormous population of unvaccinated animals protected only by vaccine belts at the international borders and a buffer zone between Zones B and C. Zone B, by then adjusted to include the states of Goa and Maharashtra, advanced a declaration of provisional freedom in May 1996.

Up to 1992 the NPRE managers considered that for Zone C as a whole there was no alternative but to embark on the preparatory work required in order to increase freeze-drying capacity, improve cold chains, improve mobilization and introduce serosurveillance across the zone. These improvements were considered an essential prerequisite to the two rounds of mass vaccination in the 50 million bovines within the zone, for which the project was planning. For various reasons this preparatory work was delayed and within Zone C the state authorities were asked to devise and implement a strategy that would at least ensure no worsening of the epidemiological situation. Accordingly, from 1990 onwards the state veterinary services took it upon themselves to implement the mass vaccination schedule originally recommended by the Task Force, namely to vaccinate all bovines within the 3-year period 1990–91 to 1993–4. Taking Andhra Pradesh as an example, the proportion of the bovine population vaccinated was extremely high, as is demonstrated in Table 13.9. Even though only 11 districts reached their target proportion (1.0), this mini campaign was astonishingly effective and apparently succeeded in breaking the virus' endemic grip on the livestock population of the state. After the campaign there were only ever five more rinderpest outbreaks in Andhra Pradesh – one outbreak in 1993, three in 1994, one in 1995.

Similar results were forthcoming in neighbouring Karanataka and Tamil Nadu states, the other bastions of endemic rinderpest. Effectively then, thanks to the efforts of the state directors of veterinary services, rinderpest had been eliminated during the NPRE planning phase! The pipelined 2-year blanket vaccination campaign was therefore seen as unnecessary and abandoned, although the allocated resources were now used to provide an across-the-board strengthening of veterinary infrastructures. The project managers' function was to realize that rinderpest had in fact disappeared and to move the NPRE forward from that point. They might then, have taken exception to the remarks in Spinage (2003) relating to the situation in 1996, that 'the incidence of rinderpest in India has been declining steadily over the past five years but there is no conclusive evidence that this is due to vaccination or herd immunity'. In fact, there can be little doubt that Indian rinderpest was eliminated by introducing saturation vaccination of the livestock population of the areas of residual endemicity, a technique of which J.T. Edwards would have approved. The last case of rinderpest ever reported in India was in Tamil Nadu in September 1995. Nine years later, in May 2004, the General Session of the OIE accredited the rinderpest disease-free status of the Republic of India.

**Table 13.9**  Vaccination work in Andhra Pradesh 1990–1996

| District | Last reported case | Proportion vaccinated in mini campaign | | | |
|---|---|---|---|---|---|
| | | 1990–91 | 1991–92 | 1992–93 | Total |
| Adilabad | 1.2.81 | 0.45 | 0.43 | 0.33 | 1.21 |
| Vizianagaram | 1.9.86 | 0.67 | 0.45 | 0.38 | 1.50 |
| Warangal | 1.9.86 | 0.27 | 0.16 | 0.22 | 0.65 |
| Karimnagar | 1.11.87 | 0.42 | 0.38 | 0.12 | 0.92 |
| Nellore | 1.1.88 | 0.24 | 0.15 | 0.21 | 0.60 |
| Srikakulam | 1.1.89 | 0.55 | 0.48 | 0.49 | 1.52 |
| Prakasam | 1.1.89 | 0.22 | 0.30 | 0.17 | 0.69 |
| Nizamabad | 1.1.90 | 0.31 | 0.48 | 0.29 | 1.08 |
| West Godavari | 9.3.90 | 0.14 | 0.28 | 0.26 | 0.68 |
| Krishna | 1.6.90 | 0.53 | 0.30 | 0.37 | 1.20 |
| Anantapur | 1.7.90 | 0.71 | 0.72 | 0.57 | 2.00 |
| Mahaboobnagar | 17.7.90 | 0.33 | 0.60 | 0.52 | 1.45 |
| Kurnool | 5.9.90 | 0.68 | 0.69 | 0.53 | 1.90 |
| Guntur | 1.1.91 | 0.33 | 0.36 | 0.24 | 0.93 |
| Chittoor | 10.7.91 | 0.57 | .047 | 0.38 | 1.42 |
| Khammam | 19.7.91 | 0.36 | 0.44 | 0.43 | 1.23 |
| Medak | 27.7.91 | 0.45 | 0.18 | 0.05 | 0.68 |
| Nalgonda[a] | 11.9.92 | 0.31 | 0.23 | 0.22 | 0.76 |
| Hyderabad and Ranga Reddy | 16.7.93 | 0.46 | 0.29 | 0.22 | 0.97 |
| Cuddapah | 21.3.94 | 0.63 | 0.70 | 0.48 | 1.81 |
| East Godavari | 16.4.94 | 0.21 | 0.34 | 0.17 | 0.72 |
| Vishakapatanam | 7.2.95 | 0.20 | 0.26 | 0.16 | 0.62 |

[a]Non-border districts.

# Vaccine quality control

In 1986 FAO initiated a survey of rinderpest vaccine quality among African laboratories producing TCRV, the potency assessments being undertaken at the Institute for Animal Health, Pirbright. Most producers were unable to produce a uniformly potent vaccine and in a series of tests it was found that nearly half the vials did not contain the stated number of doses. This exercise demonstrated the vulnerability of the livestock owner in situations where the manufacturer was not subject to a secondary controller. Subsequently FAO established two Regional Vaccine Quality Control and Training Centres, one at the National Veterinary Institute, Debre Zeit, Ethiopia, and the other at the Laboratoire National d'Elevage et de Recherches Vétérinaires, Dakar, Senegal to provide PARC with a vaccine quality assurance facility and manufacturers with help in overcoming their problems. These units operated from 1989 to 1992 after which they were merged as the Pan African Veterinary Vaccine

Centre (PANVAC) hosted by the Ethiopian Government at the National Veterinary institute, Debre Zeit, with mandates to:

- perform quality controls on priority vaccines (rinderpest and CBPP primarily) according to international standards
- promote the adoption of biological standardization and control of veterinary vaccines in Africa through the establishment of a repository of characterized reference vaccine materials, the development of internationally recognizable quality control criteria and the promotion of the Principles of Good Manufacturing Practice.

With some interruptions in service, PANVAC functioned from 1993 until 2002. During the 1996 to 1998 period 193 rinderpest vaccine samples were submitted, representing a total of 55 million doses of which 47 million doses were certified for use. The quality of vaccines increased rapidly from an initially low pass rate of less than 60% in 1994 to over 90% by 1997. Availability of the assurance system enabled PARC managers to insist that only PANVAC-certified vaccines were to be used in national rinderpest eradication programmes and the same principle was applied by FAO and other international organizations involved in rinderpest control. The Quality Assurance procedures published by FAO (Rweyemamu et al., 1994) were applied widely and were a decisive factor in elimination of rinderpest from Iraq, Pakistan and Afghanistan, for example.

Quality assurance was also a problem for the eradication programme in India. A report by Ramachandran and Scott (1985), while concluding that rinderpest vaccine did not immunize cattle if held for more than one hour after reconstitution, failed to make the more valid point that the vaccine was probably of low potency in the first place. One of the problems facing State Biological Products laboratories was the poor control of tolerance levels during the manufacture of vials and stoppers, compounded by financial rules requiring purchase of the cheapest materials available. By developing a set of improved technical standards, the NPRE was able to make a considerable impact on the vial and stopper manufacturing industry and indirectly, on the quality of vaccines. In addition, paralleling the development of PANVAC, the NPRE also developed an independent rinderpest vaccine-testing laboratory at the Indian Veterinary Research Institute, Izatnagar.

# Quality assurance of vaccination programmes by seromonitoring

An inability to monitor herd immunity to judge the effectiveness of vaccination programmes can be seen as one deficit which compromised JP15. Under the PARC the Joint FAO/IAEA Division of Nuclear Techniques in Food and Agriculture, Animal Production and Health Section addressed this issue vigorously through providing and disseminating assay techniques by establishing in 1986 a coordinated research programme, the Seromonitoring of Rinderpest in

Africa, and maintaining this as a service to the PARC. A separate IAEA-funded Rinderpest Surveillance in West Asia project promoted similar activities in many countries of West Asia from 1995 to 2001. Fundamental to the concept was an understanding that if overall herd immunity levels could be raised above an arbitrarily selected 80%, rinderpest virus would cease to circulate in that population. Implicit was a related concept that if seromonitoring disclosed inadequately vaccinated populations, action would result to revaccinate those populations. It was an attractive and sound strategy but in practice it proved difficult to obtain the serological data in time to influence the conduct of vaccination programmes. Even in Ethiopia, where vaccination was conducted within a dynamically managed PARC national rinderpest eradication project, linking seromonitoring data to vaccination programmes provided little more than a retrospective analysis of vaccination efficacy (Gijs van't Klooster, personal communication). The principles were applied much more effectively outside Africa by the national authorities in Iran (Gholam Ali Kiani, personal communication), where seromonitoring was rigidly applied to assessing the efficacy of annual vaccination programmes and remedial action taken where necessary, and were effectively applied by FAO in dealing with rinderpest emergencies in Afghanistan and in Tanzania (Taylor et al., 2002a).

## The use of vaccine to build barriers against the movement of infection

Since live attenuated vaccines first became available, attempts have been made to prevent the spread of infection by the creation of belts of immunized livestock. Following the eradication of rinderpest from Russia in 1928, its subsequent invasion of Primorsky Kray from Manchuria in 1939, 1944 and 1945 and its invasion of Tajikistan from Afghanistan in 1944 prompted the development of measures designed to keep Russia free from rinderpest. In part, the solution lay in the development of the famous immune belt created by the immunization of livestock in a 30–50 km belt stretching along the Russian border from the Pacific Ocean to the Caspian Sea. After the last rinderpest invasions of the USSR, which occurred in Turkmenistan and the Far East of Russia in 1946 and 1950 respectively, rinderpest was never seen again apart from the enigmatic appearances in Georgia (1989–90), Tuva and Chitta (1991–93), and Amur Region (1998) (see Chapter 11). However, whilst concluding that the border vaccination buffer zone appears to have been very effective in controlling the risk of rinderpest invasion one must also realize that vaccination was combined with stringent border controls over livestock movement; for example, almost the entire length of the Sino-Russian border was fenced by 1960.

Vaccine belts were not included in the JP15 strategy. As discussed elsewhere (see Chapter 6), the successes of JP15 in Africa were temporary, and in the period 1975–83, rinderpest swept back across sub-Saharan Africa. The subsequent Pan African Rinderpest Campaign (PARC), launched in 1986, was expected to address methods of regaining control of the epidemiological situation. Through its coordination unit in Nairobi, PARC laid down strategy guidelines to be followed by individual National Veterinary Services, including reliance on vaccination as the principal weapon to be used. In addition to routine activities at national level, in its initial stages PARC conceptualized the development of inter-territorial vaccine belts as a means of preventing the likely spread of infection. The intention was to divide the endemic (sub-Saharan) region of Africa into a number of discrete, epidemiologically relevant 'cells', separated one from another by populations of well vaccinated cattle. Under these circumstances individual cells would be able to progress towards eradication at different speeds.

In 1988, and based on the, then, best estimate of the virus' distribution, with East Africa being more heavily contaminated than West, PARC proposed to use vaccine for the creation of a 'Central African Block (CAB)', consisting of highly immunized cattle populations in Chad and the Cameroons (Taylor, 1989). The intention of this block was to prevent the recontamination of West Africa from East Africa. Another concept was the 'West African Wall (WAW)', anchored at its eastern end in the CAB and running along the north of Nigeria, through southern Niger, Burkina Faso and Mali to Senegal. The objective here was to prevent transmission from the Sahelian region to the coastal region states. In reality, the improving situation in West Africa rendered the WAW concept redundant but elements of the CAB were later developed as '*cordons sanitaires*' in the east of the Central African Republic and Chad.

In practice it never proved possible to build a solid immune wall as a *cordon sanitaire* in Central Africa. This is clear from seromonitoring results obtained for the Chad *cordon sanitaire*, illustrated in Table 13.10, which fell far short of the 80% seropositivity intended. These results relate to eight annual vaccination campaigns conducted from 1989 to 1996 under PARC. The situation in the

**Table 13.10** Seromonitoring of the Chad *cordon sanitaire*

| Year(s) of Sampling | Sampling Basis | Mean Seropositive Rate (%)[a] | Comment |
|---|---|---|---|
| 1990–91 | 34 veterinary posts | 48 | |
| 1991 | 32 veterinary posts | 45 | Additional samples |
| 1992–93 | Not stated | 57 | |
| 1994 | 98 herds | 37 | |
| 1995 | 47 herds | 53 | Samples from the eastern part of the *cordon sanitaire* gave only 26% seropositivity |

[a]Using the OIE prescribed test – c-ELISA.
*Source:* Dr M. Saunders (1997) *Rapport d'une mission au Tchad* for AU–IBAR

Central African Republic, the other country which, with Chad, bore the burden of mounting the Central African *cordon sanitaire*, could hardly have been any better given the prevailing political and security environment.

Even so the presence of a nominal barrier to the movement of rinderpest into West Africa from the east provided a level of confidence of protection, however imperfect in practice, which was highly beneficial in reducing vaccine use in West Africa and pursuit of the OIE Pathway, enabling absence of rinderpest to be verified from 1999 under the Pan-African Control of Epizootics (PACE) programme.

Under the conditions discussed above, a rinderpest buffer zone becomes a strategic device to prevent the contact transmission of rinderpest from the livestock of an infected region or country to the livestock of an uninfected region or country. It is based on the premise that the licensed movement of stock out of the infected area is prohibited but that informal traditional movements will still occur. A process must therefore be devised to reduce the risk that infected animals entering this zone on foot could cross it and infect susceptible animals on the other side. Theoretically this reduction could be achieved by ensuring that animals remained within the buffer zone until they no longer excreted the virus. At the same time it would be impossible to ensure that the buffer zone cordon was free of resident local cattle and so, to prevent secondary infections and an increased risk of the virus entering the disease-free side of the buffer zone, the immunity level in this resident population needs to be maintained at a very high level and cattle entering need to be vaccinated.

It follows then that a buffer zone to prevent the contact transmission of rinderpest from an infected zone is, in fact, a precisely defined holding area within which animals excreting rinderpest must remain until they are no longer excreting it and in which they are prevented from transmitting infection. Therefore, to be effective a cordon must be sufficiently deep that an infected animal entering on foot from the infected zone is no longer excreting virus when it exits into the uninfected zone. This period can be taken as being 3 weeks.

It would obviously be nonsensical to escalate the risk of infection reaching the disease-free zone by failing to recognize the presence of clinically sick animals within the buffer zone and steps to avoid this risk must be taken, essentially by placing the entire zone under close clinical surveillance. In considering the width of the buffer zone, it is impractical to expect it to be so vast that no animal could walk through it in under 3 weeks – although a depth of between 50 and 100 km may be necessary. On the other hand, there has to be a means of ensuring that animals transiting the zone remain within it for the required period of time and again, surveillance and communications are necessary. While it is likely that one or more district administrations would be responsible for the day-to-day functioning of the cordon, it would be essential to ensure the existence of an enabling legislative environment and to have overall responsibility vested in a single national authority.

# Emergency vaccination

In the history of the battle against rinderpest there have been numerous occasions when the virus has suddenly appeared in a hitherto uninfected territory, usually when trade in infected animals has led to major epidemiological upheavals, as for example, when a number of West African states were reinfected during 1979–81. Experience has shown that at such time the virus will have increased in virulence and may be easily detected clinically and is also relatively easy to deal with by focused vaccination campaigns. The FAO has gained considerable experience in the delivery of 'Emergency Vaccination Campaigns' in response to such deteriorating situations. Essentially emergency vaccination campaigns deliver, with a minimum of bureaucracy, vaccine of attested quality along with funds for its administration by local staff according to agreed work plans. In the past this simple formula has worked extremely well. The rapid resolution of the West African emergency situation after 1980 was largely due to national initiatives supported by FAO ahead of PARC.

In 1982 rinderpest was diagnosed in Tanzania for the first time since 1966. Since 1980 abnormal mortality had been seen in eland and giraffe on the border with Kenya (Nyange *et al.*, 1983). The recorded signs were consistent with a rinderpest diagnosis (Kock *et al.*, 1999). Similar wildlife mortalities were reported in 1981 (now including buffalo and lesser kudu) but over a larger area until finally, after expanding further, the outbreak was diagnosed as rinderpest in 1982, when it reached Lobo in the Serengeti National Park (Rossiter *et al.*, 1983). Accepting that the 1980 wildlife reports represented the onset of the outbreak, it can be seen that the virus spread westwards within Tanzania for two years before a confirmed diagnosis was made.

The subsequent records suggest that the virus did not begin to transmit among cattle until 1982, however, once in cattle it spread rapidly southwards towards the Central Railway Line, killing thousands of head of animals in the process. Subsequent surveillance demonstrated that the virus was both virulent and extensively distributed across the north of the country, involving wildlife as well as cattle. For several months the situation in Tanzania looked extremely threatening, there being no apparent barrier to the southwards spread of the infection. Emergency vaccination campaigns initiated by FAO in 1983, and continued on a more long term basis by the EU, were successful in controlling and then eliminating the virus.

Apparent recapitulation of these events in 1987 stimulated Tanzania to seek international assistance for control. An emergency plan was formulated and implemented in which the extent to which the virus had penetrated the country was to be defined followed by elimination of the viral incursion by a focused vaccination campaign aimed at raising the level of immunity to an extent that the virus would no longer be able to transmit. The term 'immunosterilization' was coined for this technique to emphasize the use of immune cattle to create a sterile environment within which virus multiplication would be unsupportable (Taylor *et al.*, 2002a).

Unlike in the classical situation where an infected zone could be defined reliably by the presence of sick cattle, low virulence of the virus strain concerned in Tanzania was a complication requiring a combination of serological and clinical evidence to be used. Eventually, emergency vaccination was initiated both to control the outbreak and to develop standard procedures for the use of rinderpest vaccine in emergency situations. In the past much had been made of the lifelong immunity conferred by a single successful inoculation with a live attenuated rinderpest vaccine. However, it was felt that in an immunosterilization campaign the critical issue was to disrupt viral transmission through the short-term generation of a highly immunized population. Relative to the desired objective, it did not particularly matter if, in the succeeding months, the population remained cohesive and highly immune, or fragmentary and increasingly susceptible, provided that at the time a serviceable herd immunity had been generated.

Within the PARC programme seromonitoring was often used to obtain annual audits of the levels of population immunity despite reservations about the value of an audit taken several months after the completion of a routine vaccination campaign. In Tanzania two seromonitoring programmes, each conducted within 3–4 weeks of the end of the pulsed vaccination campaigns, tested these reservations. In this instance seromonitoring revealed the fact that the first campaign had failed to achieve the level of immunity (85%) considered essential to halt transmission and accordingly a second round of emergency vaccination was immediately organized. After the second round of seromonitoring the results were considered satisfactory, with a high prevalence of village cattle populations with antibody prevalences of over 85%. These populations were considered to have been 'immunosterilized'.

Within the same programme it was possible to monitor the immune status of the cattle of 25 districts, 3–4 months after the completion of vaccination. In a number of districts the immunity levels in yearlings, 2- to 3-year-olds and cattle more than 3 years old were unsatisfactorily low and would have called for further vaccination work if revealed by immediate post-campaign seromonitoring. On the other hand, as it was known that the livestock in these districts were being constantly traded, it was impossible to know whether the unsatisfactory immunity now seen was due to the introduction of susceptible animals, or to a low distribution of vaccine during the campaigns. The answer was that only immediate post-campaign seromonitoring would have resolved these questions, and that in any emergency vaccination campaign there should always be provision for such estimations to be made.

# Lessons to be learnt from the implementation of mass vaccination campaigns

In analysing the successes and failures of the mass vaccination campaigns described in this section a number of lessons have been learnt, some of them undoubtedly of generic importance being applicable to other similar campaigns. They are as follows:

- Vaccination was a very effective tool for disrupting the spread of rinderpest.
- Where mass vaccination is to be used, the more intensively it is applied, the more rapidly it achieves the objective desired.
- Vaccination campaigns require seromonitoring as an integral component to provide quality assurance of vaccination efficacy and that the results are used to generate remedial action; results must be available within two months if they are to provide a basis for action.
- Eradication programmes require careful management and work best when they are conceptualized within time-bound frameworks and managers are permitted to take risks.
- Eradication programmes require clear initial objectives and clear exit strategies.
- Eradication programmes should be designed around an understanding of the epidemiology of the pathogen involved; in India the epidemiology of rinderpest in small ruminants was not well understood and elucidating the role of PPR was an added difficulty.

# References

Datta, S. (1954) The national rinderpest eradication plan. *Ind. J. Vet. Sci. Anim. Husb.* **24**, 1–9.

Daubney, R. (1953) Rinderpest vaccination. *Bull. Epizoot. Dis. Afr.* **1**, 12–18.

Edwards, J.T. (1930) The problem of rinderpest in India. *Imp. Inst. Agr. Res. Pusa Bull.* **199**, 1–16.

Edwards, J.T. (1949) The uses and limitations of the caprinised virus in the control of rinderpest (cattle plague) among British and Near-Eastern cattle. *Br. Vet. J.* **105**, 209–53.

Khera, S.S. (1979) Rinderpest eradication program in India. In: W.A. Geering, R.T. Roe and L.A. Chapman (eds), *Proc. 2nd Int. Symp. Vet. Epidem. Econ.* (Canberra), pp. 581–6.

Kock, R.A., Wambua, J.M., Mwanzia, J., Wamwayi, H., Ndungu, E.K., Barrett, T., Kock, N.D. and Rossiter, P.B. (1999) Rinderpest epidemic in wild ruminants in Kenya 1993–97. *Vet. Rec.* **145**, 275–83.

Lepissier, H.E. (1971) General Technical Report on OAU/STRC Joint Campaign against Rinderpest in Central and West Africa, pp. 1–203.

Nyange, J.F.C., Mbise, A.N. and Ngereza, A.R.H. (1983) Reappearance of rinderpest in Tanzania. Tanzanian Veterinary Association Annual Conference, Morogoro.

OIE (World Organisation for Animal Health) (1993) Guidelines for the evaluation of veterinary services. In: Risk Analysis, Animal Health and Trade (R.S. Morley, ed.). *Rev. Sci. Tech. Off. Int. Epiz.* **12** (4), 1291–313.

Ramachandran, S. and Scott, G.R. (1985) Potency of reconstituted rinderpest vaccine. *Ind. Vet. J.* **62**, 335–6.

Rossiter, P.B., Jessett, D.M., Wafula, J.S., Karstad, L., Chema, S., Taylor, W.P., Rowe, L.W., Nyange, J.C., Otaru, M., Mumbala, M. and Scott, G.R. (1983) Re-emergence of rinderpest as a threat in East Africa since 1979. *Vet. Rec.* **113**, 459–61.

Rowe, L.W. (1966) A screening survey for rinderpest neutralising antibodies in cattle of Northern Nigeria. *Bull. Epizoot. Dis. Afr.* **14**, 49–52.

Rweyemamu, M.M., Sylla D., Palya, V. and Prandota, J. (1994) Quality control testing of rinderpest cell culture vaccine. FAO Animal Production and Health Paper No. 118. Rome: FAO.

Spinage C.A. (2003) *Cattle Plague: A History.* New York: Kluwer Academic/Plenum.

Taylor, W.P. (1989) Achievements, difficulties and future prospects for the control of rinderpest in Africa. In: *Livestock Production and Diseases in the Tropics. Proc. 6th. Int. Conf. Inst. Trop. Vet. Med.*, pp. 84–90.

Taylor, W.P. (1990) Operation Rinderpest Zero. The R.D. Nanjiah Endowment Lecture. Karnataka Veterinary Association Annual Meeting, Bangalore, 11 August 1990.

Taylor, W.P. and Ojeh, C.K. (1981) Rinderpest in Nigeria. *Vet. Rec.* **108**, 127.

Taylor, W.P., Diallo, A., Gopalakrishna, S., Sreeramalu, P., Wilsmore, A.J., Nanda, Y.P., Libeau, G., Rajasekhar, M. and Mukhopadhyay, A.K. (2002b) Peste des petits ruminants has been widely present in southern India since, if not before, the late 1980s. *Prev. Vet. Med.* **52**, 305–12.

Taylor, W.P., Roeder, P.L., Rweyemamu, M.M., Melewas, J.N., Majuva, P., Kimaro, R.T., Mollel, J.N., Mtei, B.J., Wambura, P., Anderson, J., Rossiter, P.B., Kock, R., Melengeya, T. and Van den Ende, R. (2002a) The control of rinderpest in Tanzania between 1997 and 1998. *Trop. Anim. Hlth Prod.* **34**, 471–87.

# Strategy for measles eradication

# 14

## BERTUS K. RIMA

*School of Biology and Biochemistry, Medical Biology Centre, The Queen's University, Belfast, UK*

## Introduction

Measles virus is a mainly human virus that can infect some primate species when these are in contact with humans but the susceptible primates act as 'dead end' hosts for the virus. It can only be successfully transmitted and create transmission chains between human beings. These facts, combined with the availability of an effective vaccine, should allow us to develop a vaccination strategy that could lead to the eradication of measles virus (MV). However, there are two complications that make this goal less than easy to attain. The first, which is multifaceted, consists of the lack of the necessary societal and political will to fully address the problem along with the lack of sufficient economic resources to fully implement current vaccination strategies in conflict-torn countries. A second derives from the existence of a window of opportunity for the virus to infect susceptible infants between the time of waning of the protection derived from their maternal antibody (MDA) and the time that the first vaccination against the virus is given. Because of the extraordinary infectious nature of the virus and its ability to seek out susceptible persons within a large population, this time window, though small, is potentially able to sustain a viral transmission chain.

Molecular aspects of the morbilliviruses were described in Chapter 3. This chapter describes measles virus and its clinical effects and complications using recent reviews (Griffin and Bellini, 2001; Rima, 1999), and approaches to eradication and vaccination using more primary research references.

ISBN-13: 978-0-12-88385-1
ISBN-10: 0-12-88385-6

# Clinical aspects

Measles virus causes a severe disease in childhood characterized by a maculopapular rash, dry cough, coryza, conjunctivitis and photophobia. This may be preceded by the appearance of Koplik spots in the mouth of the patient. Its incubation period is 10–14 days. It was not distinguished from infections caused by small poxvirus until the seventh century AD by the Arab physician Al Rhazes. In the developed world although 1 in 1000 cases has a fatal outcome, the infection is usually not life-threatening and apart from rare but severe sequelae, has usually no lasting after-effects. However, complications such as bronchiolitis and pneumonitis are more frequent and occur in up to 10% of the cases. In developing countries, however, the situation is very different. There the infection can have high mortality rates (5–10%) and severe morbidity is associated with the virus. The causes of these differences in clinical outcome of the infection are not well understood. Several hypotheses have been put forward to explain these differences, such as dose rate of infection, immunological challenge by other infections, vitamin status and strain differences. However, none of these offers a satisfactory explanation for the striking differences between countries in the clinical symptoms manifested in the infected child.

One of the main complications of measles is interstitial pneumonitis and mucosal inflammation in the respiratory tract. Giant cell pneumonia is much more clinically significant and is primarily a feature in immunocompromised people (see below). Another common occurrence in measles is diarrhoea although it is not clear whether this is caused by the virus infecting the gastrointestinal tract or a result of a virus-induced immunosuppression that allows secondary infections to become manifest. It is most common in the developing world where intercurrent bacterial and parasitic infections are frequent. Otitis media and laryngo-tracheo-bronchitis are possibly other manifestations of secondary infection associated with the virus-induced immunosuppression.

Delayed-type hypersensitivity responses to pre-existing antigens such as the tuberculin reaction may transiently disappear during acute measles infection and convalescence. Description of this phenomenon by von Pirquet in 1906 made measles virus the first recognized immunosuppressive agent. However, the immunosuppression does not appear to affect the development of an immune response to the virus itself or co-administered antigens. The mechanism by which this immunosuppression occurs is not clear but long-lived cytokine imbalances as well as direct effects on the proliferation of lymphocytes have been postulated. The latter are the probable cause of the marked lymphopenia associated with the disease.

Acute measles infection is associated with severe neurological symptoms in a very small minority of the cases. About 1:1000 cases will suffer a post infection encephalitis, which appears to be autoimmune in nature as no virus can be demonstrated in the brain of such patients. This is often fatal. An invariably fatal late complication of measles is subacute sclerosing panencephalitis (SSPE). It is rare, occurring in 1 in 10 000 cases between 2 and 30 years post infection, the average time to appearance of symptoms being 8 years after the acute infection. Infection below the age of 2 years is a risk factor in this disease. It predominates in males (2.5:1 sex ratio). The incidence of SSPE was severely reduced by measles vaccination campaigns that successfully controlled the disease. SSPE is caused by a persistent infection with measles virus, which finally manifests itself in demyelination and severe neuronal infection leading to neuronal death. Depending on the neural systems which are affected, severe neurological deficits and death of the patient occur between 3 months and 30 years after the onset of symptoms. The virus found in the brain is characterized by mutations, which render it defective. The mutations cause deletions in the cytoplasmic tail of the F protein and changes in sequence or the entire absence of the M protein. The gradient of gene expression is also altered so that only small amounts of the F and H proteins are produced (Chapter 3). This may aid the virus in escaping detection by the cellular immune system. SSPE patients also show a hyperimmune antibody response and oligoclonal measles-specific bands in the cerebrospinal fluid that recognize the N, P, F and H proteins of the virus, but even in this hyperimmune response antibodies to the M protein are scarce or absent.

In immunosuppressed patients measles can give rise to another CNS infection called measles inclusion body encephalitis (MIBE). In contrast to SSPE, MIBE is not associated with a hyperimmune antibody response to measles proteins but mutations in the M proteins are found similar to those in SSPE.

Other diseases have been suggested to be sequelae of measles virus infection. However, there is no confirmed evidence that the virus is associated with multiple sclerosis, Paget's disease, otosclerosis or the more recently suggested Crohn's disease and autism. No confirmed or robust evidence exists for a causative relationship between measles virus (or any vaccines derived from it) and any of these diseases.

## Immune responses

Antibody responses are detectable at the time of onset of rash 10–14 days after infection. The earliest are IgM responses, subsequently replaced by IgG1, IgG3 and IgA, the latter especially noted in mucous secretions and saliva. In the later convalescent phase IgG4 antibody levels increase (El Mubarak et al., 2004). The earliest antigens that are recognized by the humoral immune system are the N and P proteins of the virus and at the start of the acute phase these can be the only antigens to which antibody is demonstrable. Antibodies to the H and F protein develop later and as these include the main neutralizing antibodies, haemolysis inhibiting and neutralizing responses are thus delayed. Antibody responses to the M protein are difficult to demonstrate in most human infections and no immune response to the L protein has been observed. Antibody can protect against disease as witnessed by the protective effect of MDA in infants, but its role in the control of the virus infection is not clear as patients with dysgammaglobulinaemia usually overcome measles infection without problems. The cellular immune response is probably more important for protection as patients that are defective in this arm of the immune system are prone to suffer severe sequelae and widespread virus infection in many tissues. During the acute phase of the infection CD8+ T cells play an important role in clearance of infected cells, as is the case in most viral infections. The target antigens are probably the F protein and the N proteins of MV. Measles induces interferon-beta synthesis and in turn this up-regulates HLA class I expression *in vitro* so that infected cells are more easily recognized. However, differences exist between measles virus strains in their ability to induce the synthesis of type I interferons. Wild-type strains appear to induce much less interferon than the vaccine strains (Naniche *et al.*, 2000). In the later stages of infection CD4+ T cells predominate. The proliferation stimulating antigens appear to be the H, N, P, F and M proteins of the virus. A typical change from a Th1 to a Th2 response seems to occur in MV infection leading to early activation of cytolytic T cells followed by the later stimulation of Th2 cells which, through cytokine IL4, stimulate antibody production. The immune responses are very long-lived. Early island studies carried out by Panum in 1846 indicated that lifelong protection from disease follows after infection with 'wild-type' virus. After contact with wild-type virus the post vaccinal immune response to measles is boosted. The immune response to vaccination has been shown to wane and whether lifelong protection from disease can be elicited is an open question since those who have been vaccinated a long time ago in most cases have still been exposed to this boosting effect of circulating wild measles virus. The vaccine is unlikely to induce a sterilizing immune response.

## Transmission and molecular epidemiology

Measles virus used to give rise to seasonal 2-yearly epidemic patterns, presumably due to the need to accumulate sufficient numbers of susceptible individuals in the population whose maternal antibody levels had decreased sufficiently to allow infection and systemic virus replication to cause disease. In order to remain endemic, measles virus requires human populations in excess of 300 000 individuals so as to be supplied with adequate numbers of susceptible individuals to maintain the chain of transmission. Measles is transmitted by aerosol and is extremely infectious. One measure of transmissibility of a virus is the so-called $R_0$ value, which indicates the number of secondary cases that can occur from a single index case in a naive population. In the case of measles this is estimated to be about 400, one of the highest values reported for any virus. It has been estimated that one tissue culture infectious dose is sufficient to infect a rhesus monkey.

Measles virus is a monotypic virus. This means that there is only a single serotype and infection with one strain of measles appears to provide lifelong protection from a recurrence of measles disease. Nevertheless with the development of DNA sequencing techniques and reverse transcription polymerase chain reaction, it has become clear that strains vary in their nucleotide sequences, especially where it concerns the area of the genome encoding the last 150 amino acids of the N protein and the entire sequence of the H protein gene. Sequences for these variable regions of the genomes of over 250 strains and isolates have been determined during the past decade and these show that more than 21 different genotypes (see Table 14.1) exist which belong to eight different clades (see Figure 14.1). Some of these viral clades appear extinct (inactive: Table 14.1). They may have been geographically restricted in their distribution at an earlier time, for example before the increase in rapid, worldwide travel and global vaccination campaigns. In particular, the increase in travel by children, who are the prime reservoir for virus replication, has now allowed widespread distribution of some of the genotypes. The study of the

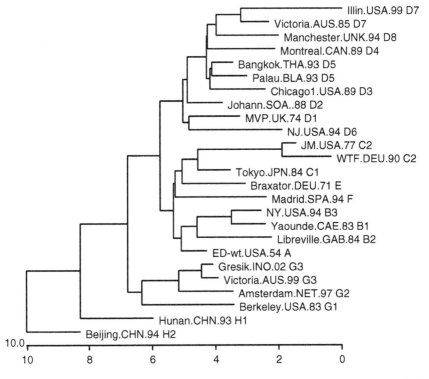

**Figure 14.1**   Phylogenetic analysis of 456 nucleotides of the variable region of the measles N gene sequences of the various clades and genotypes of wild-type strains listed in Table 14.1.

**Table 14.1**   Reference strains used for genetic analysis of wild-type measles viruses

| Genotype | Status[a] | Reference strains (MVi)[b] | H gene accession | N gene accession |
|---|---|---|---|---|
| A | Active | Edmonston-wt.USA/54 | U03669 | U01987 |
| B1 | Active | Yaounde.CAE/12.83 'Y-14' | AF079552 | U01998 |
| B2 | Active | Libreville.GAB/84 'R-96' | AF079551 | U01994 |
| B3 | Active | New York.USA/94 | L46752 | L46753 |
|  |  | Ibadan.Nie/97/1 | AJ239133 | AJ232203 |
| C1 | Active | Tokyo.JPN/84/K | AY047365 | AY043459 |
| C2 | Active | Maryland.USA/77 'JM' | M81898 | 89921 |
|  |  | Erlangen.DEU/90 'WTF' | Z80808 | X84872 |
| D1 | Inactive | Bristol.UNK/74 (MVP) | Z80805 | D01005 |
| D2 | Active | Johannesburg.SOA/88/1 | AF085198 | U64582 |
| D3 | Active | Illinois.USA/89/1 'Chicago1' | M81895 | U01977 |
| D4 | Active | Montreal.CAN/89 | AF079554 | U01976 |
| D5 | Active | Palau.BLA/93 | L46757 | L46758 |
|  |  | Bangkok.THA/93/1 | AF009575 | AF079555 |
| D6 | Active | New Jersey.USA/94/1 | L46749 | L46750 |
| D7 | Active | Victoria.AUS/16.85 | AF247202 | AF243450 |
|  |  | Illinois.USA/50.99 | AY043461 | AY037020 |
| D8 | Active | Manchester.UNK/30.94 | U29285 | AF280803 |
| D9 | Active | Victoria.AUS/12.99 | AY127853 | AF481485 |
| E | Inactive | Goettingen.DEU/71 'Braxator' | Z80797 | X84879 |
| F | Inactive | MVs/Madrid.SPA/94 SSPE | Z80830 | X84865 |
| G1 | Inactive | Berkeley.USA/83 | AF079553 | U01974 |
| G2 | Active | Amsterdam.NET/49.97 | AF171231 | AF171232 |
| G3 | Active | Gresik.INO/17.02 | AY184218 | AY184217 |
| H1 | Active | Hunan.CHN/93/7 | AF045201 | AF045212 |
| H2 | Active | Beijing.CHN/94/1 | AF045203 | AF045217 |

[a]Active genotypes have been isolated within the past 15 years.
[b]WHO name, other names that have been used in the literature appear in quotations.
*Source:* Modified from table in the *World Epidemiological Record* 78, 229–240

actual present day distribution of genotypes over the globe is hampered by the fact that surveillance is poor precisely in those countries in which the virus is endemic and in which specific, as yet undiscovered genotypes might exist.

In the USA and the UK mass measles vaccination campaigns have allowed transmission of the virus to be broken for short periods although the virus was quickly re-imported by infected children from other parts of the world. In the USA and UK it has been possible to link the origin of the imported strain with travel by specific index cases. Thus knowledge of the different genotypes has made it possible to establish transmission chains for a number of outbreaks. Knowledge and surveillance of the global distribution of measles genotypes is also important for future eradication campaigns.

# Vaccines

All viruses in the genus *Morbillivirus* display significant immunological cross-reactivity to such a high degree that the immune response to one virus protects from infection by the other viruses of the genus and in the past this has been used in emergency situations to control rinderpest by application of measles vaccines and a measles HI test has been used for estimating rinderpest antibodies. This indicates some level of shared receptor usage across the morbilliviruses and it has been suggested that the cell's signal lymphocyte activating molecule (SLAM) is a common morbillivirus receptor (Tatsuo and Yanagi, 2002).

Ever since it became clear in the mid-1960s that inactivated vaccines could lead to exacerbated disease (described below), only live-attenuated strains of measles virus have been used as vaccines (LAV). Though a number of different vaccine strains have been developed for commercial use they all are derived from the Edmonston strain, which was the first isolate of measles virus propagated by John Enders in 1954 from measles patient David Edmonston. Unfortunately the original wild type isolate has been lost and only a virus that has already undergone eight tissue culture passages in human embryo kidney cells is now available for study; it is known as the Edmonston wild-type strain. The loss of the original isolate has hampered studies on the identification of mutations in the genome responsible for attenuation though we slowly have come to recognize a number of changes in the genome that are associated with specific known phenotypic differences in the strain such as the ability to use and down-regulate CD46 and to interact with TLR receptors in the innate immune system. The change of one residue in the H protein of vaccine strains at position 481 from asparagine found in wild-type strains to tyrosine is sufficient to induce the ability of vaccine to interact with CD46. The effect of this *in vitro* is to make infected cells more susceptible to lysis by complement. CD46 can therefore act as an entry receptor for vaccine strains whilst all wild type (and vaccine) strains can use CD150 (SLAM) as an entry receptor. The effects that these changes have *in vivo* are not clear and one should be very careful in speculating about the significance of differences between vaccine viruses and wild-type strains as an explanation of human virulence and attenuation. Similarly, it is not clear what effect the better interferon-inducing ability of the vaccine strains have *in vivo* and again it is unwise to speculate about the link between interferon induction and attenuation.

The original Edmonston wild-type isolate has been attenuated by passage in non-human primate host cells or in embryonated chicken eggs. Currently, most vaccines are derived from culture *in ovo,* and administered by the subcutaneous injection of approximately 3000–5000 plaque-forming units of the virus.

Nowadays, measles virus vaccine in most developed countries has been incorporated into the trivalent measles–mumps–rubella (MMR) vaccine, which is a mixture of three live viruses. This vaccine is safe and efficacious and even though measles vaccine itself can have a slight immunosuppressive effect the combined vaccine elicits good protective responses to not only measles but the other two component viruses. It has been successfully used to control measles in developed countries using a two-dose schedule in which the first dose is given at 12–15 months of age and the second dose to children aged 4 or 5.

As described above there is substantial sequence variation, e.g. up to 12% in the H protein genes between the most divergent strains. Sequence variation in the proteins can be picked in neutralization tests not only with monoclonal antibody preparations but with human sera. These differences in humoral responses appear not to matter as vaccines derived from the Edmonston strain appear to protect from clinical symptoms of infection by all wild-type viruses.

# A window of opportunity for virus infection

The protection of Edmonston-derived vaccines against all currently circulating wild-type viruses in different clades provides an argument against the costly development of new live-attenuated vaccines. However, it has been argued that a new vaccine is necessary to close the window of opportunity for measles infection that results from the waning of the MDA response in infants and the time of first vaccination of a child. The current LAV does not lead to successful seroconversion and a protective immune response in the presence of maternal antibodies. Both the levels of MDA and the rate with which it decreases vary from one infant to another. Hence, in order for the LAV to be efficacious in a high proportion of the children, the first vaccination has to be programmed at a time when the MDA in most of the children has waned sufficiently for it not to interfere with replication of the vaccine virus necessary for the generation of an immune response. As a consequence a number of infants in whom the MDA has declined more rapidly are susceptible to infection by the wild-type virus between about 6 months of age (or even earlier when the starting level of MDA was low) and 12–15 months of age when the vaccine is given.

Attempts to solve this problem by the administration of high titre vaccines (a 10-fold higher dose) to children of 6–9 months of age were halted in 1992 when it became clear that this was statistically associated with a slightly increased mortality in girls (but not boys). This effect was observed in a number of studies carried out in African and South American countries in which the mortality caused by measles infection was high (about 10%). The mechanism by which this occurred has never been satisfactorily explained. The observed gender difference ran counter to the normal expectation that young boys are more susceptible to infectious disease than girls.

Another vaccination regimen could be to prime the immune response with an inactivated virus vaccine. However, inactivated measles virus has been shown to be unsafe. Formalin or tween-ether inactivated virus preparations derived from egg-adapted strains derived from measles virus Edmonston were introduced as a killed vaccine in 1964. However, these had to be withdrawn in 1967 as recipients of the formalin-inactivated vaccine suffered exacerbated disease when they contracted wild-type measles virus. A similar experience with another virus of the same family, e.g. human respiratory syncytial virus (hRSV), generated a move away from inactivated viral vaccines in this group of viruses and currently these are only in use for one member of the *Paramyxoviridae*, e.g. Newcastle disease virus in birds.

In hRSV the exacerbated disease after priming with inactivated vaccine is associated with severe eosinophilia. Early explanations for this effect centred on potentially inappropriate humoral immune responses to the F protein of the virus. Recently both the F and the G proteins of hRSV have been suggested to play a role. In the case of the G proteins this might occur via a CX3C motif and substance P induction (Haynes *et al.*, 2003). However, this is clearly not the sole cause of the enhanced disease. Although an experimental F vaccine with CpG oligonucleotides as adjuvant gave a good neutralizing antibody response and a reduction in viral load during challenge infection, there was still an enhanced pulmonary pathology (Prince *et al.*, 2003). In the case of measles even less is known about the cause of the exacerbation. There was some early evidence for inappropriate response to the haemolysis-inducing function of the virus (probably mediated by the F protein) but recent papers by the Griffin group have indicated that the formalin-inactivated vaccine failed to induce affinity maturation and probably led to the induction of a memory B cell response that had not undergone somatic hyper-mutation and selection in germinal centres. This has been proposed to result in an anamnestic production of non-protective, complement fixing antibodies, immune complexes in the tissues and atypical measles (Polack *et al.*, 1999, 2003a) by the formalin-treated vaccine. In contrast to the formalin-treated virus, Polack and co-workers found that the live-attenuated vaccine and a DNA vaccine against the H protein of MV elicited properly matured antibody responses and no atypical disease. If the lack of affinity maturation is indeed the sole mechanism of induction of exacerbated disease, it would become possible to predict or test for such reactions in macaque monkey models. This would allow a proper evaluation of new measles vaccines that could be useful in closing the window of opportunity for viral infection in infants.

## New measles vaccines?

As explained above the experience with inactivated vaccines has inhibited the development of measles sub-unit vaccines and vectors-based vaccines. Nevertheless, the need to close the window of opportunity has driven forward research in new generation measles vaccines other than LAV. However, the lack of understanding of the mechanisms involved in atypical measles has hampered their development into products for clinical trial.

Almost all current new approaches to viral vaccines have been tried, including vectored vaccines (including viral vectors and bacterial vectors such as BCG to express the N protein), subunit vaccines based on viral proteins included in ISCOMs, and peptide-based vaccines including B and T cell viral epitopes as well as DNA vaccines. An excellent and recent review of novel vaccines for measles in rodent and macaque models is that of Pütz and co-workers (Pütz et al., 2003). Vectored viruses expressing the N, F and H proteins of measles have been evaluated. Those based on replication-defective adenoviruses or poxviruses such as NYVAC and the avian poxvirus ALVAC required substantial doses in small animals (ferrets for the related canine distemper virus; cotton rats and mice for measles) to elicit an immune response. In a direct comparison of a replication competent vaccinia strain (WR) expressing the F and H proteins of measles virus with a replication defective Modified Vaccinia Ankara (MVA) expressing the same proteins, Zhu and co-workers (Zhu et al., 2000) showed that in the absence of MDA, neutralizing antibodies, CTL responses and protection from challenge can be induced. Lower titres were elicited by the replication-deficient MVA recombinant. The presence of MDA or passively transferred measles immunoglobulin prevented the development of a humoral response with both recombinant viruses and the frequency of CTLs was much lower under these conditions compared with the situation when no MDA was present (Zhu et al., 2000). The lower levels of CTLs were able to restrict the viraemia during challenge and also caused a reduction in rash. Thus, although these recombinant viruses appear able to modulate the infection by wild-type virus, they are not able to induce a strong immune response in the presence of high levels of MDA. Replication-defective adenovirus vectors have also been used and their immune responses have been evaluated in rodents. Adenovirus vectors, which express the N, F and H proteins of MV, all induced immune responses (Fooks et al., 1998; Sharpe et al., 2002 and references therein). The main problem for evaluation of the immune responses in mice and rats is that an appropriate challenge model is not available. The challenge infection in new-born animals involves intracerebral (i.c.) injection of the virus, but this is very different from the appropriate route of infection, e.g. intranasal challenge for a respiratory virus infection such as measles. Hence, the immune response necessary to control the i.c. challenge may be very different from that required in the protection from a respiratory infection. Only cotton rats (Wyde et al., 2000) and macaques can be used to evaluate the protective immune responses properly by natural routes of infection.

The use of other virus vectors such as HPIV3 (Skiadopolous et al., 2001) or other paramyxoviruses has been suggested and HPIV3 constructs expressing the H protein of measles have been found to induce a vigorous immune response of neutralizing antibodies to both measles and HPIV3 after intranasal inoculation in rhesus monkeys but although the protective response to HPIV3 was investigated, that to measles was not. The levels of neutralizing antibodies, however, were so high that a priori protection might have been expected to be achieved. Furthermore, the use of an intranasal route might allow the generation of these responses even in the presence of serum MDA.

Several groups of investigators have used DNA clones that can express the N, F and H proteins of MV to elicit immune responses in various animal species such as mice, cotton rats and rabbits. Some were protective, depending on the route and the challenge model. In monkey models Polack and co-workers (Polack et al., 2000) showed that DNA vaccines protected from challenge with wild-type measles virus. Protection correlated with levels of neutralizing antibody and not with cytotoxic T lymphocyte activity. They showed that the haemagglutinin protein primed for a type 2 cytokine response, with suppression of interleukin (IL)-12 and preferential production of IL-4 after MV challenge. The fusion protein primed for a type 1 response with preferential production of interferon-gamma (Polack et al., 2003b).

Isolated and purified viral glycoprotein preparations of measles virus similar to the inactivated influenza virus vaccines have not been evaluated for MV. Several groups have prepared ISCOMs and evaluated immune responses. In these, both glycoproteins from measles virus have been incorporated singly and in combination. MV-F containing ISCOMs were able to generate haemolysis-inhibiting and fusion-inhibiting antibodies, virus specific CTL and T helper cells and protection from encephalopathy by i.c. challenge. H containing ISCOMs were also able to protect against the injection of a neurotropic strain i.c. (Varsanyi et al., 1987). Hence it appears clear that ISCOMs are able to generate appropriate immune responses and protect in these artificial challenge systems. However, addition of measles immunoglobulin did prevent a proper development of a protective immune response to ISCOMs. In macaques, van Binnendijk and co-workers (1997) demonstrated that the ISCOM preparations containing H and F proteins of MV elicited excellent immune responses that were protective even in the presence of passively transferred MV specific antibodies. Further studies are required evaluating the toxicity issue with ISCOMs before these can progress to clinical evaluation.

Problems associated with the use of peptides as immunogens have been recognized for several decades now and generally the peptide vaccination approach will only be considered if these peptides are linked to carriers (reviewed in Pütz and Muller, 2002). Several epitopes have been identified in measles F and H proteins. When these were linked to universal T cell epitopes, H and F neutralizing antibodies were generated (El Kasmi et al., 2000); in addition, these experimental peptide vaccines induced protection. A multi-epitope conjugate vaccine may be possible but these have not yet been constructed or evaluated.

The above demonstrates that almost all currently contemplated vaccine development strategies have been applied to the problem of finding a vaccine against MV that can be used to close the window of susceptibility. However, to my knowledge no new experimental vaccines have proceeded to clinical trial as yet. The only area of vaccine trials for measles at present is studies applying the MR (measles/rubella) vaccine or monovalent LAV. These trials aim to compare the aerosolized vaccine with subcutaneous administration. Through both routes serum and nasal IgG and IgA were stimulated, but the responses by the aerosolized route were much higher than those obtained by subcutaneous administration of the vaccine (Bellanti *et al.*, 2004). The aerosol route was also found to be less reactogenic (Sepulveda-Amor *et al.*, 2002).

# Prospects for eradication

Theoretically the prospects for eradication of measles are good. Since there is no animal reservoir and transmission does not involve arthropod vectors, successful immunization of the human population should theoretically allow the chain of transmission to be broken. For this to be achieved over 95% of the susceptible population has to be effectively vaccinated, i.e. show seroconversion. This requires higher than 97% rates of uptake of the vaccines. These extraordinarily high percentages are derived from the highly infectious nature of the virus and this is one of the major obstacles for measles eradication. It requires a very highly developed level of organization of health care systems to administer and reach these percentages, if the vaccination of individual children is based on parental responsibility to present the children and have them vaccinated. Only in few developed countries has this been achieved, sometimes requiring mild levels of coercion based on access to schooling or compulsion, such as in the former German Democratic Republic. In these countries it has been possible to eradicate endemic measles. It is unlikely that the requirements for delivery of programmes such as these are fulfilled in many of the countries that are now forming the main reservoirs for measles. More successful have been programmes of mass immunization in which all children between the ages of 1 up to 14 years are immunized whether they have received previous vaccinations or not. This approach has been used in a number of Eastern European and Middle Eastern countries including Afghanistan under very difficult circumstances. A mass vaccination campaign achieved a temporary measles-free status for countries such as Brazil. Unfortunately this was followed a year later by a substantial outbreak which numbered over 50 000 cases probably due to re-importation of the virus.

One of the complications that provide a difficulty for the eradication campaign is that we are in a race against time to some degree. The current situation is that many mothers, especially in countries where there is endemic measles, have strong immune responses as a result of infection by wild-type strains. The immune responses in vaccinated mothers and hence those in their new-born offspring are much weaker (Pabst *et al.*, 1999). This leads to a situation where, unless we eradicate the virus soon, the background level of herd immunity of the overall population will fall and more viral transmission (even from baby to mother) may become an important problem. If this occurs eradication will become much more difficult.

The World Health Organization hopes to achieve control of the infection by the year 2007 and prospects for achieving this are to be re-evaluated in 2005.

Whether the programmatic ability to deliver such campaigns exists in those developing countries where they are most needed is a difficult issue. Kuroiwa and co-workers (Kuroiwa *et al.*, 2003) demonstrated the problems with a mass immunization campaign in Laos and this study indicated that difficulties to establish and maintain the cold chain as well as management difficulties of a mass vaccination campaign should not be underestimated. They concluded that after a mass vaccination campaign the routine vaccination service should be strengthened in order to maintain immunity especially in remote areas. On the other hand, the undoubted success of campaigns in the Americas (de Quadros, 2004) indicates that even under difficult circumstances it is possible to break endemic measles transmission by aggressive catch-up campaigns and extensive surveillance and investigation of imported index cases and their potential contacts. Whether the political will to spend the money required for such campaigns exists and whether our organizational capabilities are sufficient to run programmes of this kind, especially in those countries in Africa and Asia often under the threat of war, are open questions, especially as measles is very wrongly considered by some not to be a very serious disease.

# References

Bellanti, J.A., Zeligs, B.J. *et al.* (2004) Immunologic studies of specific mucosal and systemic immune responses in Mexican school children after booster aerosol or subcutaneous immunization with measles vaccine. *Vaccine* **22** (9–10), 1214–20.

de Quadros, C.A. (2004) Can measles be eradicated globally? *Bull. WHO* **82** (2), 134–8.

El Kasmi, K.C., Fillon, S. *et al.* (2000) Neutralization of measles virus wild-type isolates after immunization with a synthetic peptide vaccine which is not recognized by neutralizing passive antibodies. *J. Gen. Virol.* **81** (Pt 3), 729–35.

El Mubarak, H.S., Ibrahim, S.A. *et al.* (2004) Measles virus protein-specific IgM, IgA, and IgG subclass responses during the acute and convalescent phase of infection. *J. Med. Virol.* **72** (2), 290–8.

Fooks, A.R., Jeevarajah, D. *et al.* (1998) Oral or parenteral administration of replication-deficient adenoviruses expressing the measles virus haemagglutinin and fusion proteins: protective immune responses in rodents. *J. Gen. Virol.* **79**, 1027–31.

Griffin, D. and Bellini, W.J. (2001) Measles virus. In: D.M. Knipe *et al.* (eds), *Fields Virology*, 4th edn. Philadelphia, Lippincott-Williams & Wilkins, pp. 1401–42.

Haynes, L.M., Jones, L.P. *et al.* (2003) Enhanced disease and pulmonary eosinophilia associated with formalin-inactivated respiratory syncytial virus vaccination are linked to G glycoprotein CX3C-CX3CR1 interaction and expression of substance P. *J. Virol.* **77** (18), 9831–44.

Kuroiwa, C., Xayyavong, P. *et al.* (2003) Difficulties in measles elimination: prevalence of measles antibodies before and after mass vaccination campaign in Laos. *Vaccine* **21** (5–6), 479–84.

Naniche, D., Yeh, A. *et al.* (2000) Evasion of host defenses by measles virus: wild-type measles virus infection interferes with induction of Alpha/Beta interferon production. *J. Virol.* **74** (16), 7478–84.

Pabst, H.F., Spady, D.W. *et al.* (1999) Cell-mediated and antibody immune responses to AIK-C and Connaught monovalent measles vaccine given to 6 month old infants. *Vaccine* **17** (15–16), 1910–18.

Polack, F.P., Auwaerter, P.G. *et al.* (1999) Production of atypical measles in rhesus macaques: evidence for disease mediated by immune complex formation and eosinophils in the presence of fusion-inhibiting antibody. *Nat. Med.* **5** (6), 629–34.

Polack, F.P., Hoffman, S.J. *et al.* (2003a) A role for nonprotective complement-fixing antibodies with low avidity for measles virus in atypical measles. *Nat. Med.* **9** (9), 1209–13.

Polack, F.P., Hoffman, S.J. *et al.* (2003b) Differential effects of priming with DNA vaccines encoding the hemagglutinin and/or fusion proteins on cytokine responses after measles virus challenge. *J. Infect. Dis.* **187** (11), 1794–800.

Polack, F.P., Lee, S.H. *et al.* (2000) Successful DNA immunization against measles: neutralizing antibody against either the hemagglutinin or fusion glycoprotein protects rhesus macaques without evidence of atypical measles. *Nat. Med.* **6** (7), 776–81.

Prince, G.A., Mond, J.J. *et al.* (2003) Immunoprotective activity and safety of a respiratory syncytial virus vaccine: mucosal delivery of fusion glycoprotein with a CpG oligodeoxynucleotide adjuvant. *J. Virol.* **77** (24), 13156–60.

Pütz, M.M. and Muller, C.P. (2002) The rationale of a peptide-conjugate vaccine against measles. *Vaccine* **21** (7–8), 663–6.

Pütz, M.M., Bouche, F.B., de Swart, R.L. and Muller, C.P. (2003) Experimental vaccines against measles in a world of changing epidemiology. *Int. J. Parasitol.* **33** (5–6), 525–45.

Rima, B. (1999) Measles virus. Encyclopedia of the Life Sciences (CD ROM only). MR Ltd, Stockton Press. Article number 418.

Sepulveda-Amor, J., Valdespino-Gomez, J.L. *et al.* (2002) A randomized trial demonstrating successful boosting responses following simultaneous aerosols of measles and rubella (MR) vaccines in school age children. *Vaccine* **20** (21–22), 2790–5.

Sharpe, S., Fooks, A. *et al.* (2002) Single oral immunization with replication-deficient recombinant adenovirus elicits long-lived transgene-specific cellular and humoral immune responses. *Virology* **293** (2), 210–16.

Skiadopoulos, M.II., Surman, S.R. *et al.* (2001) A chimeric human-bovine parainfluenza virus type 3 expressing measles virus hemagglutinin is attenuated for replication but is still immunogenic in rhesus monkeys. *J. Virol.* **75** (21), 10498–504.

Tatsuo, H. and Yanagi, Y. (2002) The morbillivirus receptor SLAM (CD150). *Microbiol. Immunol.* **46** (3), 135–42.

van Binnendijk, R.S., Poelen, M.C. *et al.* (1997) Protective immunity in macaques vaccinated with live attenuated, recombinant, and subunit measles vaccines in the presence of passively acquired antibodies. *J. Infect. Dis.* **175** (3), 524–32.

Varsanyi, T.M., Morein, B. *et al.* (1987) Protection against lethal measles virus infection in mice by immune-stimulating complexes containing the hemagglutinin or fusion protein. *J. Virol.* **61** (12), 3896–901.

Wyde, P.R., Stittelaar, K.J. *et al.* (2000) Use of cotton rats for preclinical evaluation of measles vaccines. *Vaccine* **19** (1), 42–53.

Zhu, Y., Rota, P. *et al.* (2000) Evaluation of recombinant vaccinia virus–measles vaccines in infant rhesus macaques with preexisting measles antibody. *Virology* **276** (1), 202–13.

# Towards the global eradication of rinderpest

# 15

## MARK M. RWEYEMAMU,* PETER L. ROEDER† AND WILLIAM P. TAYLOR‡

*Woking, Surrey, UK
†Food and Agriculture Organization of the UN, Animal Health Service, Animal Production and Health Division, Rome, Italy
‡Littlehampton, Sussex, UK

## Introduction

Rinderpest has been described as the most dreaded of all animal diseases. In its classical, virulent form, it can result in more than 80% mortality of cattle, buffalo, yaks and many wildlife ungulate species (Scott, 1964; Rossiter, 1994). Wherever it has occurred, rinderpest has caused terrible destruction of cattle, adversely affecting livestock agriculture, rural livelihoods and food security, and impacting on urban nutrition bringing famine and starvation.

Chapter 5 traces the historical devastations of rinderpest, while Chapter 6 narrates the evolution of rinderpest in livestock and wildlife throughout the twentieth and twenty-first centuries, detailing its occurrence in both its virulent and mild forms. The present chapter traces the evolution of control strategies over the past nearly 300 years to the present state when there is a prospect of global eradication in the near future.

The presence of rinderpest virtually excludes sustainable bovine agriculture. Scott and Provost (1992) described rinderpest as an animal disease of unique historical impact, as:

> the most dreaded bovine plague known, belong[ing] to a select group of notorious infectious diseases that have changed the course of history. From its homeland around the Caspian Basin, rinderpest, century after century, swept west over and around Europe and east over and around Asia with every marauding army,

ISBN-13: 978-0-12-88385-1
ISBN-10: 0-12-88385-6

causing the disaster, death and devastation that preceded the fall of the Roman Empire, the conquest of Christian Europe by Charlemagne, the French Revolution, the impoverishment of Russia and the colonization of Africa.

So throughout the past 300 years the ultimate objective for rinderpest control has always been eradication. The early methods of prophylaxis have been detailed in Chapter 9 while in Chapter 11, the vaccine development milestones of the twentieth century have been described.

## Evolution of zoo-sanitary measures and a profession to control rinderpest

A seminal advance towards rinderpest eradication was in 1711 when Pope Clement XI ordered his physician, Dr Lancisi, to investigate the cause and prescribe measures for the control of the plague that had killed so many cattle in the papal herds (Lancisi, 1715; Scott, 2000; Blancou, 2003; Spinage, 2003). (See Chapter 9 for a detailed account of the methods recommended by Lancisi.)

In short, Lancisi's recommendations included: slaughter to reduce spread, restricted movement of cattle, burial of whole animals in lime, and inspection of meat. Their implementation was enforced rigorously by the papal edicts backed up by drastic penalties. This led to the first effective control of rinderpest in a country – Romagna (the equivalent of modern Lazio Province and the City of Rome of modern Italy).

The same measures were successfully applied to control an epidemic of rinderpest that had invaded England in 1714 in cattle shipped from the Netherlands. The rigorous application of the measures was recommended and advocated by Thomas Bates, surgeon to King George I. Bates, having been stationed as a naval surgeon in Sicily, was familiar with the edicts of Lancisi. In addition to following Lancisi's recommendations Bates also recommended the segregation of animals into small groups. Similarly enforced measures were successful in containing rinderpest in France and Germany through orders of the French Royal Council in 1714 and by Friedrich Wilhelm I in 1716, respectively, both of which included movement control measures. However, initially in other parts of Europe where the measures were not applied with the same rigour, rinderpest elimination was not possible.

It quickly became necessary to train a cadre of specialists to control rinderpest and other animal diseases, through the application of Lancisi's methods. Thus, the first veterinary school was founded in 1761 in Lyon under order of the French Comptroller-General of Finances. Over the next few years other European countries established veterinary schools. So, the control of rinderpest led to the beginning of the veterinary profession. This was followed by the establishment of State Veterinary Services in European countries to regulate and enforce the control of rinderpest.

During the second half of the eighteenth century and early nineteenth century incursions of rinderpest into England were less efficiently eliminated than in continental Europe. Each episode was very expensive and taking longer to eradicate than in France. This was attributed partly to an inadequate number of trained veterinarians and less vigour in the implementation of stamping-out and zoo-sanitary measures. Edwards, writing in 1928 (Edwards, 1930), observed that:

> this great expenditure was attributable most largely to the authorities paying heed to medical opinion and dallying with the disease initially by attempted treatment, instead of placing confidence at once in the methods recommended by the experienced veterinarians of the country. In France, where there already existed an organized veterinary service, the disease was exterminated at this time at relatively negligible cost.

This was recognized at the time and when, in 1865, the State Veterinary Service was established in England by Order of the Privy Council to deal with cattle plague, the epidemic was eliminated within 2 years (Pearce *et al.*, 1965). The control measures adopted in the eighteenth and nineteenth centuries comprised:

* quarantine measures to segregate infected from unaffected herds
* import restrictions
* movement restrictions for animals and people
* slaughter of all diseased and in contact animals
* safe carcass disposal – usually deep burial in lime
* prohibition of the sale of meat and milk from sick animals
* compulsory notification of disease to the authorities
* enabling legislation, enforcement and heavy penalties for offenders.

These measures remain valid to date and now form the core of the stamping-out policy for the control of highly contagious animal diseases, also referred to as transboundary animal diseases, which are of significant economic, trade and/or food security importance for a considerable number of countries and can easily spread between them reaching epizootic/panzootic proportions.

# The initial mandates of the OIE and FAO Animal Health Service

The inter-continental spread of rinderpest from India, via Europe to Brazil in 1920 and the constant disruption of agriculture and livestock trade in Europe led 28 states to obtain an 'international agreement' on 25 January 1924 to create, with the concurrence of the Secretary General of the League of Nations, the Office International des Epizooties (OIE), based in Paris, to coordinate scientific knowledge for the control of rinderpest. The OIE has now grown into a major inter-governmental organization of 167 countries with mandated obligations to facilitate transparent international exchange of information on the occurrence of animal diseases and to set international standards for the diagnosis and control of trade-limiting animal diseases (see www.oie.int).

In 1945 when the United Nations was established to succeed the League, the Food and Agriculture Organization (FAO) was one of the first specialized agencies to be set up. FAO held its inaugural conference in Quebec in October 1945 and, within a year, a meeting on animal health was convened in London to consider in what way the activities of veterinary organizations all over the world could be properly coordinated under the FAO umbrella, with particular attention being paid to mitigating the widespread ravages of animal plagues, especially rinderpest. In the ensuing year, the subcommittee on Animal Health of the FAO Standing Advisory Committee on Agriculture recommended that FAO should assist in the distribution and establishment of novel rinderpest vaccines (Hambidge, 1955; Rweyemamu et al., 1995). This was the beginning of the FAO Animal Health Service, which now covers the 188 Member Nations of the FAO. Right from its first year of existence FAO became heavily engaged in coordinated rinderpest control. Thus by 1947 FAO was already engaged in rinderpest vaccine development in China and in the succeeding years FAO was championing coordinated rinderpest control in East Asia (Chapter 6). In 1949 it convened a conference in Nairobi for stimulating the coordination of rinderpest control in Africa and in the early 1950s was organizing rinderpest training activities in India. Accordingly, the work of the Animal Health Service of FAO has always included a strong component of coordinating the control of rinderpest and other infectious animal diseases in terms of both progressive control and emergency response, especially in developing countries. This objective was further strengthened in 1994 with the approval by the 106th Council of FAO of a special programme, the Emergency Prevention System for Transboundary Animal and Plant Pests and Diseases, known by the acronym EMPRES, with a specific thrust on the coordination of the Global Rinderpest Eradication Programme (see www.fao.org/EMPRES).

Thus both the OIE and FAO Animal Health Service owe their origins to the coordinated international control of rinderpest. In 1952 the two organizations entered into a formal Agreement (see www.oie.int/eng/oie/accords/en_accord_fao .htm). To this day the two organizations have maintained the special agreement which governs their collaboration and synergy in animal health, including global initiatives such as the Global Rinderpest Eradication Programme (GREP).

# International rinderpest control during the first half of the twentieth century

While rinderpest was being successfully eradicated from Europe the disease was still causing untold misery in Asia and Africa. The first veterinary schools established in India and Africa were a consequence of rinderpest. The Lancisi method was proving unworkable in Asia and Africa. There were several reasons for this, including:

- The fact that rinderpest was becoming endemic in many parts of these regions, while the stamping-out and associated measures that had been developed in Europe were essentially for emergency response to rinderpest incursions and the eradication of rinderpest in its epidemic form. Thus the Lancisi edicts were for a quick intervention for disease elimination. By contrast, endemic disease demands a sustained, long-term, progressive control strategy.
- The economies of the affected countries of Africa and Asia were too weak to sustain a costly stamping-out strategy.
- Many countries lacked the necessary legislation and enforcement of strict animal movement control.
- In some areas, especially India, the mass slaughter of animals required by the stamping-out strategy would contravene social mores.
- This period was dominated by two world wars that both fuelled the spread of rinderpest and created a disincentive for collaboration on animal disease control among warring nations or colonial powers as well as economic ruination.

Accordingly, except for the activities of FAO in East Asia and rinderpest control in southern Africa, there was little international collaboration in rinderpest control during this period. Yet rinderpest was the most important and feared of all animal diseases in both Asia and Africa. It was the disease that most impeded livestock development. So research had to be undertaken *in situ* in Asia and Africa to seek alternative measures for the control of the disease. The most notable outcome of this research effort was the serum-virus immunization which was used to control rinderpest in southern Africa (Kolle and Turner, 1897; Anon, 1905; Turner, 1906; see Chapter 11), the caprinized vaccine which was to be the vehicle for mass vaccinations in South Asia and Tropical Africa (Edwards, 1930; 1949a, b) and lapinized or lapinized-avianized vaccines that were used in East Asia (Kesteven, 1949; Nakamura and Miyamoto, 1953; Nakamura, 1957). The details of the development of these vaccines and their application in the field are given by Taylor *et al.* in Chapter 11.

Thus although by about 1936 the main facts regarding rinderpest control had been worked out and the eradication of the disease from the country was considered a practical possibility the National Rinderpest Eradication Programme could not be launched until much later, i.e. 1954 (Khera, 1979; see Chapter 11).

The lesson from this period during the early twentieth century, just as in the eighteenth and nineteenth centuries, was that effective rinderpest control was not attainable merely through the application of technical methods (stamping-out, serum-virus or attenuated virus vaccination). It depended as much on the rigorous and concentrated application and implementation of all technical and zoo-sanitary measures to the entire target cattle population. Rinderpest control is clearly a public good which demands the cooperation of the entire community in the target areas/countries.

Edwards (1949a) cites Mr Brayne, the Secretary to the Government Development Department, Punjab, as stating:

> The number of inoculations and vaccinations of various kinds ran into many lakhs and demonstrates the growing popularity of modern methods of prophylaxis against disease. Until, however, it is possible to legislate against movement of diseased and suspected livestock, no amount of vaccination and inoculation will save the province from great and continuing loss from contagious diseases.

# International rinderpest control from 1950 to 1980

During the 1950s and 1960s individual countries in Africa, the Middle East and South Asia carried out national rinderpest control programmes based on the use of the goat-adapted vaccine while countries of East Asia preferred either lapinized or egg-adapted vaccines. These activities were based on individual country programmes, often with little coordination between neighbouring countries.

Even at this stage, it was accepted that the region that required greatest attention from the international community was Tropical Africa. This could be attributed to a variety of reasons including:

- The co-existence of other serious diseases with a very similar impact on productivity and animal survival. The most striking diseases were contagious bovine pleuropneumonia, tsetse fly-transmitted trypanosomosis and ticks and tick-borne diseases. Globally, it is worth noting that of the 15 OIE List A diseases, 12 are still endemic in sub-Saharan Africa.
- Animal movement on account of transhumance, traditional livestock farming and trade across national boundaries was often uncontrollable.
- The legislative framework was weak.
- The period of the late 1950s and early 1960s was dominated by the independence movements in most countries and therefore African societies were far more focused on gaining nationhood than enforcing zoo-sanitary measures, which sometimes were regarded as a colonial constraining tool.
- National economies were often too weak to bear a sustained rinderpest control campaign.
- The available vaccines (especially caprinized and lapinized rinderpest vaccines) were not produced in sufficient quantities to sustain major campaigns.

Accordingly, the seminal work by scientists working at the East African Veterinary Research Organization laboratories at Muguga, Kenya, which led to the adaptation of rinderpest virus to growth in cell culture in 1959 and its subsequent attenuation through serial passage in cell culture (Plowright, 1968), represented a major milestone for international rinderpest control. This work was the technological breakthrough that gave stimulus to the concept that rinderpest could be eradicated or at least brought under control cost-effectively in many parts of the world.

One could ask 'What were the virtues of the cell-culture rinderpest vaccine?'. The response given by Prof. Walter Plowright when he was designated the 1999 World Food Prize Laureate was:

- It was universally applicable – it was safe and effective in cattle of all breeds with widely differing levels of genetic susceptibility. It is also safe and effective in wildlife species.
- It could be used safely in animals of any age group or stage of pregnancy.
- It did not produce any significant clinical reaction or relapse to inter-current diseases such as babesiosis, anaplasmosis or trypanosomosis; it was not, in other words, immunosuppressive and did not interfere with other vaccines given simultaneously, such as that for bovine pleuropneumonia.
- Its immunizing potency could be accurately assessed by titration *in vitro*.
- It had been employed successfully for many years to protect small ruminants against PPR.
- 'Vaccine virus' could be used safely in serological tests for past exposure to infection or vaccination.
- The intensive use of cell-culture vaccine in cattle–game contact areas in the Serengeti–Mara region of Tanzania and Kenya not only eliminated cattle disease; it was a major factor in the 'explosion' of wildebeest and buffalo populations that ensued. The disappearance of rinderpest in 1961/62 heralded an increase in their population. The myth of 'game' animals maintaining rinderpest virus long term was finally exploded.

Consequently, in 1961, the Joint Campaign Against Rinderpest (JP15) was initiated at an inter-state conference held in Kano, northern Nigeria, under the aegis of the Inter-African Bureau for Animal Health (IBAH) of the then Commission for Technical Cooperation in Africa. The JP15 programme was launched with the support of the technical assistance and donor agencies. The objective of JP15 was 'to eradicate rinderpest from the region in question over a period of three consecutive dry seasons'. The campaign was run in three phases in West Africa between the end of 1961 and 1968 with a total vaccination of 81.5 million head of cattle. Between October 1968 and September 1971 JP15 was extended to eastern Africa to cover the areas comprising Kenya, southern Somalia to 5° north, Sudan, northern Tanzania and Uganda. The campaign was extended further to Ethiopia and northern Somalia from 1972 to 1975 (Lepissier, 1971; Macfarlane and Dahab, 1972; Macfarlane, 1976; a more detailed account of the JP15 campaign is given by Taylor *et al.* in Chapter 11).

This coordinated mass vaccination campaign was successful in drastically reducing the incidence of rinderpest in West and Central Africa. Extension of the campaign to eastern Africa was preceded by an epidemiological assessment by Atang and Plowright (1969). For East Africa (i.e. Uganda, Kenya and Tanzania), their analysis referred to two endemic ecosystems: the southern enzootic area comprising the Masailand of southern Kenya and northern Tanzania and the less well defined northern endemic area covering northern Uganda and northern Kenya and stretching into southern Sudan and parts of Ethiopia. Furthermore, they remarked that rinderpest was 'still more or less continuously present in the east and north-east provinces' of Kenya. This was the first signal of what has since come to be recognized as the southern Somali ecosystem covering southern Somalia and contiguous areas of Kenya and possibly Ethiopia, the primary endemic zone for lineage 2 rinderpest virus (Chamberlain *et al.*, 1993; Wamwayi *et al.*, 1995; Barrett, 1996; Rweyemamu, 1996; Roeder and Taylor, 2002; Mariner and Roeder, 2003).

With hindsight, it seems that the problem for rinderpest control was so enormous that the Joint Campaign planners and managers did not pay adequate attention to the epidemiological analysis of Atang and Plowright, in deciding on critical attack points for rinderpest eradication for eastern Africa. It appears that prior to JP15 Phase IV, national efforts in Kenya, Tanzania and Uganda may well have succeeded in eliminating endemic rinderpest from the Masailand ecosystem and the whole of central and southern Uganda. At any rate there was sufficient evidence to suggest that these areas were free of endemic rinderpest in both livestock and wildlife at the end of the JP15 Phase IV Programme in 1971 (see Taylor *et al.*, Chapter 11).

The JP15 campaign demonstrated that coordinated mass vaccination could reduce dramatically the incidence of disease. It also demonstrated that the international community would rally around such a well-coordinated campaign. Although the goal for JP15 had been stated as rinderpest eradication from sub-Saharan Africa, there was no clear definition of the benchmark for eradication and there was no mechanism in place for verification of such eradication other than through official national reports of disease incidence to the OIE. Furthermore, there was no preparedness put in place in case of a rinderpest resurgence or incursion into a rinderpest-free area.

At the end of the international vaccination campaign, countries were expected to maintain regular annual vaccination of yearling cattle without a clear indication of when such vaccination should cease. For example, in the final report for Phase IV JP15, Macfarlane and Dahab (1972) stated:

> More recently, in the case of Tanzania, with high vaccine coverage and high percentage of immunized livestock and absence of the disease in neighbouring countries, it might be thought that annual vaccination was not necessary. However, taking into account the recent outbreak of rinderpest in the Middle East, the meeting in Addis Ababa in December 1971 recommended that Tanzania should follow the general rule at present [i.e. annual vaccination] and that the position could be revised annually.

So at the end of JP15, it would appear, in retrospect, that there could have been as many as four residual endemic foci of rinderpest remaining, i.e. an area in the vicinity of the junction of Mauritania, Senegal and Mali in West Africa;

the southern Sudan ecosystem stretching into north-eastern Uganda, north-western Kenya and south-western Ethiopia; the Afar rangelands in Ethiopia; and the southern Somali ecosystem including southern Somalia, north-eastern Kenya and possibly south-eastern Ethiopia. Probably because the concept of residual areas of endemic persistence did not feature strongly in strategy setting, there were no specifically defined and internationally funded programmes for dealing with these reservoirs of infection nor were there specific contingency plans for rapid response should infection break out of these endemic areas.

Thus, the end of JP15 did not instil confidence in national veterinary services of countries from which rinderpest had been cleared to declare rinderpest freedom, regard rinderpest as exotic to such areas and adopt risk management strategies to ensure sustained rinderpest freedom.

## The international response to rinderpest resurgence in the 1980s

For five years between 1975 and 1980 there was a low global incidence of rinderpest. During the early 1980s significant outbreaks of rinderpest were encountered in several parts of Africa, the Middle East and South Asia, as a result of several factors which included the following:

- lack of sustained and targeted control activities in endemic areas
- a build-up of a susceptible bovine population
- long distance movement of trade cattle without adequate sanitary controls, e.g. influx of: trade cattle into the flourishing economy of Nigeria from as far east as Sudan; trade cattle from South Asia and the Horn of Africa into the Middle East
- complacency among both national governments and the international donor community
- diminished resources for national veterinary services for surveillance and disease control
- absence of a disease emergency response concept in developing countries.

Following the resurgence of rinderpest in many parts of Africa, the Near East and Asia during the early 1980s, FAO supported a series of emergency actions in most of the affected countries. These interventions resulted in a rapid reduction in the incidence and spread of rinderpest so that in Africa, for example, out of 18 affected countries only four were still reporting rinderpest by 1986, even if the number harbouring rinderpest was greater than this.

These emergency actions dovetailed with donor-supported programmes for long-term rinderpest control in Africa, the Middle East and India. In Africa the Pan African Rinderpest Campaign (PARC) started in 1986 in 35 countries through funding mainly by the European Union (Lepissier, 1983). The EU also supported a programme in India as a forerunner to a proposed coordinated programme in South Asia (South Asia Rinderpest Eradication Campaign – SAREC), while UNDP supported similar activities in the Middle East (the West Asia Rinderpest Eradication Campaign – WAREC) (Rweyemamu and Cheneau, 1995; see Chapter 12).

The rinderpest programmes up to 1993 were essentially for control, rather than eradication, and incorporated the following features:

- The use of only cell culture vaccine produced from the RBOK strain with quality independently assessed by a dedicated laboratory. In Africa, external quality control was provided by the Pan African Veterinary Vaccine Centre – PANVAC (Sylla *et al.*, 1995).
- Mass vaccination aiming at 100% coverage of the susceptible bovine population either throughout the country or within an epidemiologically defined zone.
- Ensuring a local diagnostic capability. The simplest and most widely used test throughout the three campaigns was the agar gel diffusion test.
- Seromonitoring to assess post vaccination herd immunity. This was based on an indirect ELISA later replaced by a competitive ELISA developed by the Institute for Animal Health, Pirbright and standardized for mass application by the Joint FAO/IAEA Division in Vienna.
- Epidemiological monitoring at both regional and national level. The intention had been to have a resident epidemiologist in each of the three regional campaigns. In practice, however, only the programme in Africa had a resident epidemiologist, although even in PARC this activity suffered several interruptions due to lack of continuity of donor funding.
- Using effective communication. This was found to be a valuable tool for securing the confidence of communities and involving them in the rinderpest campaign. It helped to foster a common strategy throughout the PARC area.

# The conception of a global rinderpest eradication programme coordinated by FAO

From 1984 and 1989, several specialists, at OIE and FAO, started to consider the need for and feasibility of a global rinderpest eradication campaign following the success of the smallpox eradication campaign (Fenner *et al.*, 1988). This culminated in FAO convening an Expert Consultation meeting in 1992:

> to examine the justification for and feasibility of global rinderpest eradication by the year 2010, having considered past and present campaigns against rinderpest as well as the experience of the WHO, particularly the global smallpox eradication programme. (FAO, 1992)

The FAO Expert Consultation identified the following factors as favouring global eradication of rinderpest:

- restricted geographical distribution of the disease
- availability of diagnostic tests
- transmission is by droplet, requiring relatively close contact between animals, indirect transmission being relatively insignificant
- short infectious period
- no latency or persistence except possibly aborted cows which may excrete virus for a few weeks
- excellent vaccine
- economic incentive.

Impeding factors were identified as:

- civil strife in areas of rinderpest endemicity
- social and religious attitudes
- weaknesses of veterinary services
- mild or subclinical disease which makes surveillance difficult.

The Expert Consultation concluded that:

global eradication of rinderpest was justified and feasible and that a *Global Rinderpest Eradication Programme (GREP)* should be launched. It was stressed that a global strategy could be successful only if based on viable and thoroughly executed national and regional campaigns. The meeting recognized that rinderpest was present in only 3 regions of the world: Africa, West Asia and South Asia. Therefore GREP should be planned to be executed through the programmes of 3 regional campaigns: Pan African Rinderpest Campaign (PARC), West Asia Rinderpest Eradication Campaign (WAREC) and South Asia Rinderpest Eradication Campaign (SAREC). A regional coordination unit is necessary for each of the 3 campaigns, with each unit covering the rinderpest control activities of all the countries in the region. At the global level, FAO should set up a *GREP Coordination Unit/Secretariat* within its Animal Health Service in order to link the activities of the regional programmes. Such a unit should be small, initially comprising one full time professional officer with supporting staff.

Furthermore, the Consultation recommended that FAO and OIE should collaborate in promoting the objective of rinderpest eradication throughout the world (Plate 8).

# The international rinderpest eradication standards established by the OIE

In 1989, the OIE adopted a three-stage pathway which a country needed to follow before it could be recognized by the OIE as free from rinderpest. Preceding these stages, mass vaccination campaigns were to be put in place leading to elimination of rinderpest from the country. After this the veterinary services were to strengthen surveillance systems which had to be demonstrably effective in their ability to detect rinderpest were it to be present. After 2 years without clinical rinderpest the country was to cease vaccination and declare itself *Provisionally Free from Rinderpest*. When a country that was provisionally free reported no clinical disease for at least 3 years from the initial declaration it could apply to OIE for recognition of the status of *Freedom from Rinderpest Disease*, which would be granted following external verification. A further 2 years after this, if recommended procedures had failed to detect any antibodies in unvaccinated livestock, and again following external verification, the country could apply for recognition of the status of *Freedom from Rinderpest Infection*. Two successive, annual rounds of sero-surveys were deemed necessary and if the first of these was performed in the year before application for Freedom from Disease, the pathway could be shortened by one year to 4 years from the declaration of provisional freedom. There were also two special procedures established to 'fast-track' countries which had been free from both vaccination and disease for 5 or 10 years. Thus, the OIE pathway provides operational targets for GREP. To clarify matters with regard to trade, the rinderpest chapter of the OIE International Terrestrial Animal Health Code was up-dated to define standards for safe trade with respect to rinderpest (see www.oie.int).

## The evolution of GREP between 1993 and 1996

The 1992 FAO Expert Consultation asserted the need for a globally coordinated programme linking regional campaigns in Africa (PARC), South Asia (SAREC) and West Asia (WAREC). The control strategy was still based on the concept of mass vaccination, which in many countries was interpreted as synonymous with vaccination of the entire national herd irrespective of epidemiological considerations, risk assessment or the desire to embark on the OIE Pathway. This process-orientated approach was exacerbated in some cases by the fact that there were delays between the conception of the enabling project and the release of donor funding. For example, although the last known outbreak in West Africa was in 1988, annual vaccination campaigns persisted until 1996. In Rwanda and Burundi vaccination of the entire herd was undertaken in 1992 and 1993 although rinderpest had not been diagnosed in these countries for over 50 years and there was no apparent immediate risk of disease. The experience of Tanzania, Ethiopia and India demonstrated further weaknesses in the policy of unqualified blanket vaccination (Rweyemamu *et al.*, 1997).

In the case of Tanzania, at least in retrospect, it seems that by 1986 there was no longer any evidence of viral activity in the previously affected areas. Nevertheless, when the coordinated programme started in 1992, it aimed at vaccinating all cattle north of the Central Railway Line. Only a shortage of financial resources, rather than an epidemiological evaluation, compelled the vaccination to be limited to a belt about 200 km wide, i.e. about two or three districts along the northern border with Kenya and Uganda. Essentially this was buffer vaccination.

In Ethiopia the task of vaccinating a cattle population of 30 million head proved to be a daunting one, even discounting the fact that during 1989 to 1991 there was an ongoing war in some parts of the country. The so-called blanket vaccination did succeed in reducing the frequency of epidemics but was having little effect on overall disease incidence. Consequently, between 1990 and 1992 Ethiopia deliberately undertook to study the epidemiological pattern of the disease resulting in a definition of areas of rinderpest endemicity in which vaccination could be concentrated. Consequently a new policy for target/strategic vaccination was pursued from the end of 1993 with the result that Ethiopia progressively reduced the incidence of disease and no outbreak has been recorded in Ethiopia since 1995.

In India two problems had to be overcome: differentiation of PPR from rinderpest and the concentration of rinderpest control activities to the rinderpest problem based on epidemiological assessment in the field. Thus India was able to forgo unqualified blanket vaccination in favour of a roll-back strategy based on clusters of states with a similar rinderpest epidemiological status. It is the latter policy that has propelled the unprecedented success in the long history of rinderpest control in India (see Chapter 13). Accordingly, India has not recorded a single outbreak of rinderpest since 1995 and the 72nd General Session of the OIE International Committee has recognized the whole of India as free from rinderpest disease (OIE, 2004a).

Thus, an important initial activity of the GREP Secretariat was to assess the global epidemiology of rinderpest. From this it became obvious that endemic rinderpest was confined to a few identifiable areas. On this basis FAO issued, in 1993, new operational and legal guidelines to national veterinary services and regional rinderpest campaign organizers urging them to focus the campaign towards eradication (Rweyemamu and Cheneau, 1995):

**GREP Guidelines – Eradication of Rinderpest**

1. Coordinated mass vaccination campaigns leading to a verifiable elimination of persistent endemicity.
2. The use of high quality vaccines, independently tested for efficacy and safety.
3. The proper management of a national veterinary services capable of organizing an intensive and sustained surveillance programme.
4. The development of a time-bound programme conforming to the relevant OIE guidelines for declaration of freedom from disease and from infection.
5. Providing a national laboratory service capable of providing or developing rapid and effective differential diagnosis results.
6. Articulating an effective strategy for prevention of the re-introduction of the aetiological agent.

7. Developing effective national/regional emergency plans including a pre-rehearsed action programme in case of an outbreak. This should include provision for a stamping-out policy.

**GREP Guidelines – Legal Powers**
National veterinary authorities should hold adequate legal powers which should include the following:

1. Compulsory notification of any suspected cases by the owner and/or relevant local authorities.
2. Authority to collect samples for laboratory investigation.
3. Powers of seizure, compulsory enforceable quarantines of infected premises, preferably with slaughter and destruction of infected animals, and ring vaccination.
4. Payment of compensation.
5. Zoo-sanitary and other procedures on infected premises.
6. Powers to stop vehicles and herds in order to inspect animals.
7. Powers to designate protection and surveillance zones for the purpose of implementing further intensive control measures.
8. Powers to implement emergency vaccination campaigns.

# The GREP strategy after 1996

In 1996, FAO convened two critical meetings to review in depth the GREP strategy and the priorities for the EMPRES programme, respectively the FAO Technical Consultation on GREP (FAO, 1996a) and the FAO Expert Consultation on EMPRES (FAO, 1996b). Rinderpest eradication was the central theme for both meetings.

The theme of the Technical Consultation was 'The World Without Rinderpest' and the Expert Consultation drew up a 'Blueprint for the Global Eradication of Rinderpest by the year 2010'. Crucially it was agreed that the EMPRES Expert Consultation would, during its annual meetings, review the technical progress on GREP and advise accordingly. Among the key recommendations and views of these consultations were the following:

- The consultation emphasized the continuing threat of rinderpest to world food security, commended the assistance by the EU to Africa and South Asia and noted with satisfaction the emphasis that was being placed on using rinderpest eradication programmes to strengthen the basic function of national veterinary services.
- They supported the adoption of the 'Blueprint'.
- All countries in GREP should be exhorted to adopt a time-bound programme leading to verified rinderpest eradication as enshrined in the OIE Pathway.

- All countries which have not experienced the disease for 2 years or more and for which there is not a serious risk of reinfection from neighbouring countries or trading partners should cease vaccination and enter the OIE Pathway.
- Any occurrence of rinderpest outside the currently known foci should be considered an international emergency.
- FAO should liaise with the OIE to establish verification procedures for regional and global rinderpest freedom.

So, the consultations emphasized the need for epidemiologically determined strategies, encouraged GREP to adopt the concepts of performance indicators, bench-marking and risk management and discouraged endless institutionalized vaccinations. These formed the guiding principles and challenges to the GREP Secretariat during the ensuing 4 years. Thus in all regional workshops and missions to GREP regions, the following four elements were emphasized (Roeder and Taylor, 2002):

- epidemiologically targeted approach for rinderpest control, where endemic rinderpest was still being suspected
- surveillance-based confidence in absence of rinderpest
- contingency planning and emergency rinderpest preparedness
- embarking on the OIE Pathway.

Therefore, the post-1996 GREP strategy was guided by two underlying thrusts: (a) time-bound milestones stipulated in the GREP Blueprint and (b) basic risk analysis principles. Accordingly:

- For **risk assessment** the GREP Secretariat at FAO collaborated with and encouraged regional organizations and Member countries in Asia and Africa to undertake epidemiological assessment of the rinderpest status, using conventional and participatory disease search techniques (Paskin, 1999; Mariner and Paskin, 2000). The GREP Secretariat started publishing rinderpest risk maps, instead of national incidence maps. The objective was to distinguish primary endemic areas from either epidemic or secondary endemic areas.
- At both the global and regional levels **risk communication** became an important element in the GREP strategy. A specific website was opened (http://www.fao.org/ag/AGA/AGAH/EMPRES/grep/e_rinder1.htm) and FAO started to issue specific GREP press releases at least twice a year. GREP became the principal topic of the FAO-EMPRES Quarterly Bulletin. Furthermore, FAO produced a series of manuals, pamphlets, posters and brochures as well as multi-media programs on rinderpest and GREP.
- **Risk management** was pursued through the following strategy:
  - The GREP Secretariat progressively encouraged countries to limit prophylactic vaccination only to areas identified by epidemiological results as high rinderpest risk areas, i.e. primary endemic areas. Elsewhere the

driving strategy became the withdrawal of vaccination and reliance on surveillance and rinderpest emergency preparedness. Chapter 11 details how this approach has been successfully and cost-effectively applied to eliminate rinderpest from such areas as the buffalo-rearing parts of southern Pakistan, the Kurdish Triangle in northern Iraq and the southern Sudan ecosystem. The strategy also quickly identified such areas as the rest of Pakistan, Afghanistan and the Middle East as epidemic (or at worst, secondary endemic) areas which were periodically being infected from the primary endemic areas. The elimination of rinderpest from the primary endemic areas quickly released the rest of the region from the menace of constant threat from rinderpest.

- Specific manuals and guidelines for rinderpest contingency planning and emergency preparedness, including multi-media programs were produced to help GREP countries develop confidence in a risk management-based strategy rather than perpetual blind vaccination.
- A vaccination emergency response strategy termed immunosterilization for peri-focal vaccination around a rinderpest outbreak was devised and successfully field-tested in Tanzania in 1997 (Taylor *et al.*, 2002).
- A continuing active surveillance involving village searches through organized participatory epidemiology techniques and sero-surveillance.

In 1996, the problem of a lineage 2 endemic focus in the southern Somali ecosystem was already being flagged as a likely stumbling block for the GREP Blueprint. The Technical Consultation (FAO, 1996a) observed:

> In view of the possible existence of a cryptic endemic focus of rinderpest in Kenya, southern Somalia and southern Ethiopia caused by a virus strain of unusual mildness in cattle, participants stressed the importance of continuing intensive investigations in these areas until the issue is resolved. Recognising that such a strain might be maintained in a transmission chain involving cattle, wildlife and small ruminants, and that in cattle clinical disease might not be always apparent, all available investigation methods, including participatory community dialogue, should be applied to defining its possible existence and territorial range.

This issue is discussed more fully by Mariner and Roeder (2003) and by Roeder *et al.* in Chapter 11.

# Planning for the end game

The GREP Expert Consultation meeting in May 2000 (FAO, 2000) emphasized the continuing need for countries to embark on the OIE Pathway. Furthermore, it envisaged the possibility of a regional, i.e. ecosystem-based, surveillance programme as a component of enhancing global verification of rinderpest freedom. Such a scheme was to be complementary to the existing OIE Pathway.

## The proposed OIE/GREP Pathway
## to Global Rinderpest Freedom

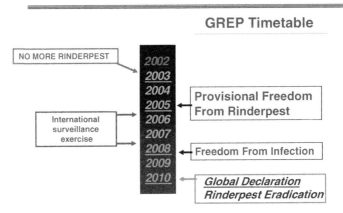

Figure 15.1   The GREP timetable conceived in 2000.

Roeder (2000) revised the GREP Blueprint and charted out a strategy towards verified global rinderpest freedom with a timetable to be adhered to (Figure 15.1). The Consultation emphasized that:

> For global eradication of freedom to be confirmed and announced in 2010 it is critical that there should be no more rinderpest occurring by the end of 2002. This sets the timeline for GREP.
> The process of proving the world free from rinderpest cannot commence until there is a reasonable assurance that the last reservoir of rinderpest infection has been eliminated.

So far the greatest threat to this timetable is the possible persistence of rinderpest risk in one ecosystem, namely the southern Somali ecosystem, apparently with the epicentre in southern Somalia with some spillover into the contiguous parts of north-eastern Kenya and south-eastern Ethiopia. The culprit virus in this ecosystem, rinderpest lineage 2, seems to be characterized by causing mild to subclinical infection in cattle but severe disease in certain wildlife species, especially the Cape buffalo. The virus seems to cause intermittent viraemia in cattle and has proven difficult to isolate in the laboratory (Dr Henry Wamwayi, personal communication). According to the OIE data, the last time rinderpest was confirmed in Kenya was in 2001 in buffalo in Meru National Park, north-east Kenya and in 2003 in cattle in Garissa district, also in north-east Kenya.

However, recent surveillance employing participatory disease search techniques and serological surveys in cattle and wildlife have indicated that a syndrome compatible with descriptions of mild rinderpest is still to be found in the southern Somali pastoral ecosystem which transcends southern Somalia, south-east Ethiopia and north-east Kenya (PACE, 2004). Whether the symptoms of disease seen are caused by rinderpest virus has yet to be proved.

# Verification and accreditation of rinderpest freedom – the 'OIE Pathway'

Accreditation of rinderpest freedom is a 5-year process which is overseen by the Office International des Epizooties (OIE). As mentioned above, currently it is a three-stage process of, progressively, self-declaration of Provisional Freedom from Rinderpest; recognition by OIE of Freedom from Rinderpest Disease and subsequent recognition of Freedom from Rinderpest Infection. The procedures are outlined in the OIE Terrestrial Animal Health Code (OIE, 2004b) with guidelines and laboratory tests prescribed for use in surveillance are described in the OIE *Manual of Diagnostic Tests and Vaccines for Terrestrial Animals* (OIE, 2004c). The whole system is strongly surveillance-based and proving rinderpest freedom has evolved to come to depend on applying a portfolio of surveillance techniques which include:

- routine and animal disease reporting and follow-up
- emergency reporting with follow-up
- village disease searching
- risk-focused (on prior knowledge) and random serosurveillance studies
- wildlife surveillance where sufficient numbers of susceptible wild species make this appropriate.

Disease searching methodology has been strengthened considerably in recent years by the application of participatory rural appraisal methods to devise a system now referred to as participatory disease searching as a tool within participatory epidemiology (Catley, 1997). For verification of rinderpest freedom surveillance should actually target detection of a 'stomatitis-enteritis' syndrome; the performance of the surveillance system is ideally assessed and monitored by the use of performance indicators (Mariner and Roeder, 2003).

Accreditation of rinderpest by the 'OIE Pathway' is progressing reasonably well in Asia and in Africa in areas where proximity to the suspected reservoir of infection in the Somali pastoral ecosystem is not a constraint (Plate 9). This is a dynamic field and the figure inevitably lags behind the actual state of accreditation. Russia and China are known to be progressing well and another 13 countries in Africa and Asia are in the process of being accredited as free from rinderpest disease or infection. Areas of particular concern remaining are the central Asian countries of Turkmenistan, Uzbekistan, Kazakhstan, Kyrgyzstan and Tajikistan, of which at least two continue to vaccinate against rinderpest. The major constraint to progress is the persisting suspicion concerning the rinderpest status of the Somali pastoral ecosystem. Neighbouring countries which share populations of livestock in border areas, and countries in the Middle East trading in livestock from the Somali pastoral ecosystem who seek to protect themselves against risk by vaccinating the traded cattle, can make little progress as matters stand. Breaking this impasse by resolving the uncertainty over rinderpest in the Somali pastoral ecosystem is an important element of the challenge facing GREP.

## The verification and certification process

To date, rinderpest is the only animal disease for which there exists a global programme with the aim of worldwide eradication. During the next 6 years, FAO and OIE will need to ensure that all the five stages defined for the eradication of an infectious disease (Dowdle and Hopkins, 1998; Dowdle, 1999) have been satisfied:

- **Control:** reduction of disease incidence, prevalence, morbidity and mortality to acceptable levels
- **Elimination of disease:** reduction to zero of incidences of disease in a defined geographical area
- **Elimination of infection:** reduction to zero of incidences of infection caused by a specific agent in a defined geographical area
- **Eradication:** permanent reduction to zero of worldwide incidences of infection caused by a specific agent
- **Extinction:** the specific agent no longer exists in nature or the laboratory.

The efforts that are being made by the partners in the Global Rinderpest Eradication Programme have been summarized in Chapter 6. All available evidence points to the southern Somali ecosystem as being the only focus in the world where, in 2004, there is still reason to suspect the presence of cryptic rinderpest infection. This area requires special attention by the partners in GREP. FAO through its GREP Secretariat, and in close collaboration with the Inter-African Bureau for Animal Resources of the African Union (AU–IBAR) and OIE, needs to galvanize the activities of all key players in this ecosystem into one coherent strategy agreed to by the major stakeholders and donors. An approach along these lines has already been successful in establishing the rinderpest status of the southern Sudan ecosystem (see Chapter 6). The central immediate issue for the Somali ecosystem concerns surveillance in order to assess the risk as to whether rinderpest virus is still active in this ecosystem and if so to try to map the geographical area affected and at immediate risk. Only from such specific knowledge will it be possible to devise the most appropriate means for squeezing the virus out of this ecosystem. The surveillance would need to dispassionately reassess, on one hand, the clinical criteria for establishing a presumptive rinderpest diagnosis and, on the other hand, the criteria for serological and virus/antigen/nucleic acid detection tests that are most likely to establish unequivocally whether or not there is still viral activity in the livestock and wildlife populations of this challenging ecosystem.

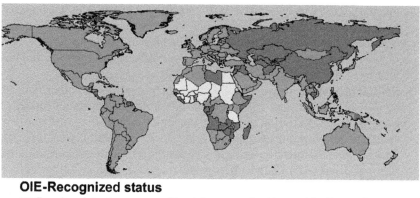

**OIE-Recognized status**

■ Free from infection
□ Free from disease
■ Provisionally free
■ No declaration

The status recognized is zonal for Kenya, Ethiopia, Sudan, Chad and Congo Democratic Republic.

**Figure 15.2** Accreditation of rinderpest freedom by the OIE Pathway as of August 2005.

Otherwise the accreditation through the OIE Pathway system seems to be proceeding well (see Figure 15.2 and Plate 9). Nevertheless, privileged funding for the final verification of global freedom from rinderpest infection by programmed international surveillance of the critical ecosystems, so far, does not seem to have been secured by the partners in GREP coordination. Another issue which has yet to be addressed is the fate of the different strains of rinderpest virus that are held in various laboratories around the world. This is a serious shortcoming bearing in mind the contemporary concern for bioterrorism. By contrast, in 1999 the polio eradication programme issued its first guidelines to minimize the risk of reintroduction of wild polioviruses from the laboratory into the community. In 2002 this was revised and was issued as the WHO global action plan for laboratory containment of wild polioviruses.

# Lessons from smallpox, polio and measles global programmes

From the outset in 1992, GREP sought constantly to take lessons from the successful eradication programmes coordinated by the WHO. Nevertheless GREP has differed from these programmes in the following manner:

- **Smallpox** was eradicated on the basis of a global campaign that was centrally funded and tightly controlled (Fenner *et al.*, 1988). Right from the outset, GREP was conceived as a programme rather than a campaign, with the FAO-based global coordination unit of the secretariat fulfilling primarily a normative rather than an operational role. The effectiveness of GREP, therefore, ultimately relies on national and regional funding whether from local or donor sources.

- **Polio initiative:** This has been a partnership programme jointly promoted by WHO–CDC–Rotary International. The initiative enjoys a centralized system for the definition of targets, strategies and funding, and for constantly renewed political support (http://www.polioeradication.org). The Global Polio Eradication Initiative is the largest public health initiative the world has ever known. It is well and comprehensively funded. It occupies a prominent position within the structure of the WHO both at its headquarters and in the regions. A single agency is responsible for defining and coordinating all strategic issues including field operations, vaccinations, surveillance, a global laboratory network, and regional and global certification. The programme is subject to regular review by the highest governing body of WHO, namely the World Health Assembly. The programme enjoys political support at the highest level, often not only at ministerial but at head of state/government level. For example, in January 2004 the ministers of the six countries where polio transmission was still considered possible reaffirmed their national commitment through a common declaration called the Geneva Declaration for the Eradication of Poliomyelitis. Although GREP coordination is a prominent component of the FAO Special Programme, EMPRES, it comprises of only a small secretariat within a unit for all animal health issues and does not enjoy privileged funding that can be deployed at point of need in accordance with epidemiological determinants. GREP does not enjoy the same level of political support as polio eradication. This may be a reflection of the contrast that when the programme for the global eradication of poliomyelitis was launched by WHO in 1988 the disease was affecting both developed and developing countries and even where it had been eliminated, there were still fresh memories of polio. By contrast when FAO launched GREP in 1994, the rinderpest was being regarded by many as essentially a problem of the developing countries of Africa and Asia.
- **Measles:** The pace of progress towards global measles eradication has probably been slower than that for rinderpest. There seems to be a robust regional programme for the western hemisphere but a variable one for Europe and a weak one for developing countries. Measles control is generally taken to be part of a wider child health immunization programme. As the risk of disease in industrialized countries has receded there has been increasingly far greater concern for absolute safety than for the efficacy of vaccines (Davey, 2001).

## Lessons for future global animal disease control programmes

In recent years there have been serious epidemics of animal diseases other than rinderpest in both industrialized and developing countries. Examples include foot-and-mouth, classical swine fever and highly pathogenic avian influenza. There is an increasing awareness that, with globalization, the most effective way to deal with such diseases is to develop an international initiative for controlling such diseases at their source, where they are endemic (Cheneau, 2002; Rweyemamu and Astudillo, 2002). In general, this means paying particular attention to controlling the disease in developing countries.

Accordingly, FAO and OIE have embarked on a joint initiative for the Global Framework for the Progressive Control of Foot and Mouth Disease and other Transboundary Animal Diseases (GF-TADs). Lessons from GREP have been used to formulate GF-TADs to incorporate the following elements:

- GF-TADs is to be a partnership approach with a jointly funded FAO–OIE Secretariat.
- GF–TADs is to provide emphasis on epidemiological definition first before vaccination campaigns. The objective is initially to target international funding at controlling disease in areas epidemiologically defined (or at least suspected) to be primary endemic areas. GREP has shown that targeting primary endemic areas is a more cost-effective way to tackle the regional elimination of transboundary animal diseases than undefined nation-wide mass vaccination.
- There is a need for effective global funding for a central coordination secretariat separate from regional and national programmes.
- Milestones are to include funded verification and certification process.
- There is a need for international early response to target disease emergency as part of eradication planning.
- Parallel coordinated funding for enabling research is required.

The FAO and OIE now face three key challenges, namely (a) the completion of GREP without loss of momentum, (b) convincing the international development community to fund new coordinated programmes for progressive control of key transboundary animal diseases as an international public good in which both developing and developed countries have a stake in their success, (c) determining with regional organizations and member countries the priority disease (or a small set of diseases) of common strategic importance without embarking on a long list of diseases for progressive, coordinated control.

# References

Anon (1905) The danger of the simultaneous immunisation with serum and virulent blood for rinderpest in cattle not immune against redwater. *Report of the Transvaal Department of Agriculture*, 1 July 1903 – 30 June 1904, pp. 166–9.

Atang, P. and Plowright, W. (1969) Extension of the JP-15 rinderpest control campaign to Eastern Africa: the epizootiological background. *Bull. Epizoot. Dis. Afr.* **17**, 161–70.

Barrett, T. (1996) Morbilliviruses into the twenty first century. In: *The World without Rinderpest*. Proceedings of the FAO Technical Consultation on the Global Rinderpest Eradication Programme, Rome, 22–24 July 1996. FAO Animal Production and Health Paper 129, Annex 3. FAO, Rome. http://www.fao.org/docrep/003/w3246e/W3246E00.htm.

Blancou, J. (2003) Rinderpest. In: *History of Surveillance and Control of Transmissible Animal Diseases*. Paris: OIE, pp. 161–92.

Catley, A. (1997) Adapting participatory appraisal (PA) for the veterinary epidemiologist: PA tools for use in livestock disease data collection. Proceedings of the Society for Veterinary Epidemiology and Preventive Medicine, April 1997, Chester.

Chamberlain, R.W., Wamwayi, H.M., Hockley, E., Shaila, M.S., Goatley, L., Knowles, N.J and Barrett, T. (1993) Evidence for different lineages of rinderpest virus reflecting their geographic isolation. *J. Gen. Virol.* **74**, 2775–80.

Cheneau, Y. (2002) The FAO concept: global initiatives for the progressive control and eradication of FMD. In: *Foot and Mouth Disease Control Strategies*. Lyons: Fondation Marcel Merieux.

Davey, S. (2001) Measles eradication still a long way off. *Bull. WHO* **79**, 584–5.

Dowdle, W.R. (1999) *The Principles of Disease Elimination and Eradication*. MMWR Supplement. http://www.cdc.gov/epo/mmwr/preview/mmwrhtml/su48a7.htm.

Dowdle, W.R. and Hopkins, D.R. (eds) (1998) *The Eradication of Infectious Diseases*. Report of the Dahlem Workshop on the Eradication of Infections Diseases. Chichester: John Wiley & Sons.

Edwards, J.T. (1930) The problem of rinderpest in India. *Imp. Inst. Agr. Res. Pusa Bull.* **199**, 1–16.

Edwards, J.T. (1949a) The uses and limitations of the caprinised virus in the control of rinderpest (cattle plague) among British and Near-Eastern cattle. *Br. Vet. J.* **105**, 209–53.

Edwards, J.T. (1949b) Uses and limitations of the caprinized virus in the control of rinderpest (cattle plague) in Near Eastern and British cattle. 14th International Veterinary Congress. London, 8–13 August 1949, **2**, 440–3.

FAO (1992) Report of the FAO Expert Consultation on the Strategy for Global Rinderpest Eradication. Held at FAO Headquarters, Rome, 27–29 October 1992. Rome: FAO.

FAO (1996a). The world without rinderpest. Proceedings of the FAO Technical Consultation on the Global Rinderpest Eradication Programme, Rome, 22–24 July 1996. FAO Animal Production and Health Paper No. 129. http://www.fao.org/docrep/003/w3246e/W3246E00.htm.

FAO (1996b) Prevention and control of transboundary animal diseases. Report of the FAO Expert Consultation on the Emergency Prevention System (EMPRES) for Transboundary Animal and Plant Pests and Diseases (Livestock Diseases Programme) including the Blueprint for Global Rinderpest Eradication. Rome, 24–26 July 1996. FAO Animal Production and Health Paper No. 133. Rome: FAO.

FAO (2000) Verification of rinderpest freedom. FAO-EMPRES Technical Consultation on the Global Rinderpest Eradication Programme, Rome, 29–30 May 2000. Rome: FAO.

Fenner, F., Henderson, D.A, Arita, I., Jezek, Z. and Ladnyi, I.D. (1988) Smallpox and its eradication. Geneva: WHO. http://www.who.int/emc/diseases/smallpox/Smallpoxeradication.html.

Hambidge, G. (1955) *The Story of FAO*. New York: D. Van Nostrand Co./London: Macmillan.

Kesteven, K.V.L. (1949) Lapinized rinderpest vaccine. In: 14th International Veterinary Congress, London, 8–13 August 1949, **2**, 427–9.

Khera, S.S. (1979) Rinderpest eradication program in India. In: W.A. Geering, R.T. Roe and L.A. Chapman (eds), *Proc. 2nd Int. Symp. Vet. Epidem. Econ.* Canberra, pp. 581–6.

Kolle, W. and Turner, G. (1897) Über den Fortgang der Rinderpestforschungen in Koch's Versuchestation in Kimberley. Mit spezieller Berücksichtigung einer Immunisierungs methode durch gleichzeitige Applikation von virulentem Infektionsstoff (Blut kranker Tiere) und Serum hochimmunisierter Tiere. *Dtsch. Med. Wochenschr.* **23**, 793–5.

Lancisi, J.M. (1715) *Dissetatio de bovilla peste. Ex Campaniae finibus anno MDCCXIII Latio importata Ex Typographie.* Rome: J.M. Salvoni.

Lepissier, H.E. (1971) General Technical Report on OAU/STRC Joint Campaign against Rinderpest in Central and West Africa, pp. 1–203.

Lepissier, H.E. (1983) *Pan-African Campaign against Rinderpest: Organization and Logistics.* Nairobi: Organization of African Unity – Inter-African Bureau for Animal Resources.

Macfarlane, I.M. (1976) A general technical report on the OAU/STRC Joint Campaign against rinderpest in Eastern Africa, 1 October 1968–30 June 1973. OAU/STRC, PMB 2359, Lagos, Nigeria.

Macfarlane, I. and Dahab, A.M. (1972) Final report of the Joint Campaign against Rinderpest Phase IV. 1 October – 30 September.

Mariner, J.C. and Paskin, R. (2000) *FAO Animal Health Manual 10 – Manual on Participatory Epidemiology: Method for the Collection of Action-Oriented Epidemiological Intelligence.* FAO: Rome.

Mariner, J. and Roeder, P.L. (2003) The use of participatory epidemiology in studies of the persistence of lineage 2 rinderpest virus in East Africa. *Vet. Rec.* **152**, 641–7.

Nakamura, J. (1957) Peste bovine. *Bull. Off. Int. Epizoot.* **47**, 542–54.

Nakamura, J. and Miyamoto, T. (1953) Avianisation of lapinized rinderpest virus. *Am. J. Vet. Res.* **14**, 307–17.

OIE (2004a) Resolution XXII of the 72nd General Session of the OIE International Committee: Recognition of Member Countries Free from Rinderpest Infection and Rinderpest Disease, Paris, May 2004.

OIE (2004b) *Terrestrial Animal Health Code.* www.oie.int/eng/normes/mcode/en_sommaire.htm.

OIE (2004c) *Manual of Diagnostic Tests and Vaccines for Terrestrial Animals.* www.oie.int/eng/normes/mmanual/A_summry.htm.

PACE (2004) Proceedings of the Workshop on the Eradication of Mild Rinderpest from the Somali Ecosystem, 18–20 February 2004. Held at Kenya Wildlife Services Headquarters, Langata Road, Nairobi. Pan-African Programme for the Control of Epizootics (PACE), AU-IBAR, Nairobi, Kenya.

Paskin, R (1999) *Manual on Livestock Disease Surveillance and Information Systems.* FAO Animal Health Manual No. 8. Rome: FAO.

Pearce, J.W.R., Pugh, L.P. and Ritchie, J. (1965) *Animal Health: A Centenary, 1865–1965.* London: HMSO.

Plowright, W. (1968) Rinderpest virus. *Monogr. Virol.* **3**, 25–110.

Roeder, P.L. (2000) Future prospects for verification of rinderpest freedom. In: *Verification of Rinderpest Freedom.* FAO–EMPRES Technical Consultation on the Global Rinderpest Eradication Programme, Rome, 29–30 May.

Roeder, P.L. and Taylor, W.P. (2002) Rinderpest. *Vet. Clin. Food Anim.* **18**, 515–47.

Rossiter, P.B (1994) Rinderpest. In: J.A. Coetzer, G.R. Thomson, R.C. Tustin and N.P.J. Knriek (eds), *Infectious Diseases of Livestock with Special Reference to Southern Africa*, Vol. 2, pp. 735–57.

Rweyemamu, M.M. (1996). The global rinderpest status in 1996. In: The world without rinderpest. Proceedings of the FAO Technical Consultation on the Global Rinderpest Eradication Programme, Rome, Italy, 22–24 July 1996. FAO Animal Production and Health Paper 129. FAO, Rome. http://www.fao.org/docrep/003/w3246e/W3246E00.htm.

Rweyemamu, M.M. and Astudillo, V.M. (2002) Global perspective for foot-and-mouth disease control. *Rev. Sci. Tech. Off. Int. Epizoot.* **21**, 765–73.

Rweyemamu, M.M. and Cheneau, Y. (1995) Strategy for the global rinderpest eradication programme. *Vet. Microbiol.* **44**, 369–76.

Rweyemamu, M.M., Roeder, P.L, Benkirane, A., Wojciechowski, K. and Kamata, A. (1995) Emergency prevention system for transboundary animal and plant pests and diseases: The livestock diseases component. In: *World Animal Review 50 years*, a Quarterly Journal on Animal Health, Production and Products. Rome: FAO. http://www.fao.org/ag/againfo/resources/documents/WAR/war/V8180B/V8180B00.htm.

Rweyemamu, M., Roeder, P. and Cheneau, Y. (1997) Lessons on animal disease eradication from the global rinderpest eradication programme. In: S. More (ed.), Proceedings of the 10th FAVA Congress, Cairns, 24–28 August, 1997, Cairns, Australia. University of Queensland, Brisbane.

Scott, G.R. (1964) Rinderpest. *Adv. Vet. Sci.* **9**, 113–224.

Scott, G.R. (2000) The Murrain now known as rinderpest. *Newsletter of the Tropical Agriculture Association, UK* **20**, 14–16.

Scott, G.R. and Provost, A. (1992) Global eradication of rinderpest. Background paper prepared for the FAO Expert Consultation on the Strategy for Global Rinderpest Eradication. Rome, October.

Spinage, C.A. (2003) *Cattle Plague: A History.* New York: Kluwer Academic/Plenum.

Sylla, D., Rweyemamu, M.M. and Palya, V.J. (1995) Regulatory framework and requirements for managing risks associated with veterinary biological products in Africa: present systems and future needs. *Rev. Sci. Tech.* **14**, 1171–84.

Taylor, W.P., Roeder, P.L., Rweyemamu, M.M., Melewas, J.N., Majuva, P., Kimaro, Mollel, J.N., Mtei, B.J., Wambura, P., Anderson, J., Rossiter, P.B., Koch, R., Mlengeya, T. and Van den Ende, R. (2002) The control of rinderpest in Tanzania between 1997 and 1998. *Trop. Anim. Hlth Prod.* **34**, 471–87.

Turner, G. (1906) Rinderpest: its prevention and cure. Report of the British Association for the Advancement of Science, 1905, p. 552.

Wamwayi, H.M., Fleming, M. and Barrett, T. (1995) Characterisation of African isolates of rinderpest virus. *Vet. Microbiol.* **44**, 151–63.

# Conclusions

# 16

## THOMAS BARRETT,* PAUL-PIERRE PASTORET† AND WILLIAM P. TAYLOR‡

*Institute for Animal Health, Pirbright Laboratory, Surrey, UK
†Biotechnological and Biological Sciences Research Council, UK
‡Littlehampton, Sussex, UK

Throughout history, the social, economic and ecological consequences of morbillivirus infections have been severe and they continue to this day, despite the availability of modern vaccines and diagnostic tools. This is in part due to the difficulties in transferring the technology to laboratories in countries where rinderpest and PPR remain a problem but also the reluctance by manufacturers to incur the expense of licensing new genetically engineered vaccines, particularly where there is a very limited market for the vaccine. Given that rinderpest is likely to be eradicated in the near future we may ask, therefore, what can the modern molecular sciences contribute to improving our knowledge and control of morbillivirus infections? It is clear that research must continue to try to develop and improve morbillivirus vaccines, almost certainly with genetically defined versions of the viruses using reverse genetics so that they are as safe and effective as the rinderpest TCRV vaccine. This need is illustrated by the fact that the current CDV vaccines are not suitable for use in wildlife species and so susceptible zoo animals (among them pinnipeds, large cats, bears and pandas) cannot be very effectively protected against distemper infection. Another weakness is that the current live attenuated morbillivirus vaccines cannot be administered before 6–9 months of age due to interference with maternal antibodies. New types of vaccine are required that can protect children and young animals from morbillivirus infections in the presence of passive maternal immunity. Other problems to be solved relate to the immunosuppressive nature of some morbillivirus vaccines, and the measles vaccine, unlike the rinderpest vaccine, has some immunosuppressive effects and the gene(s) that determine this characteristic have not yet been identified.

ISBN-13: 978-0-12-88385-1
ISBN-10: 0-12-88385-6

Another tool that would greatly benefit control and eradication programmes for rinderpest and PPR would be genetically marked vaccines (see Chapter 12). The use of these so-called DIVA vaccines, allows the **D**ifferentiation of **I**nfected from **V**accinated **A**nimals by serology. This very issue is a problem for the control of PPR in West Africa, and in some regions of Asia, where reaching all the animals that require vaccination is a very difficult and expensive task. As a result the disease can remain in a less visible form since the high death rate is prevented by the resulting partial immunity of herds or flocks. It is therefore difficult to identify where the problem areas are located as the current vaccine does not allow differentiating serologically between vaccinated animals from naturally infected animals.

A better understanding of the epidemiology of morbillivirus diseases could be gained using the latest mathematical modelling techniques, combined with spatial epidemiology using GPS, to predict the spread of infection in different ecosystems. Diagnostic tests that are highly sensitive and specific and which are easy and rapid to use in the field would make it easier for veterinarians and stockmen to stop the spread of rinderpest and PPR once an outbreak had occurred. New technologies such as microarray analysis of infected cells from diseased animals could be used to detect a spectrum of diseases and give a rapid and more useful differential diagnosis and perhaps answer the question 'if it is not rinderpest what is it?' It would also be easier, using this knowledge, to devise new therapies or antiviral drugs.

The underlying features of virus–cell interactions in response to infection that define rinderpest species barriers, breed differences and host cell restrictions within a particular host are still poorly understood but with reverse genetics and post-genomics technologies these questions can now begin to be addressed in a more scientifically meaningful way. This will be important if in future measles and rinderpest virus are eradicated globally. This could potentially permit other morbilliviruses like canine distemper virus to occupy vacant niches in the absence of cross-protective responses, giving rise to new zoonoses. The same applies to other morbilliviruses with the potential for disastrous ecological and economic consequences, particularly if PPR virus, which is considered the most serious threat to small ruminant production in many parts of Asia and Africa, were to gain the ability to cause disease in cattle and other large ruminants. Another alarming prospect is the potential of virulent rinderpest strains as agents of agroterrorism and in a post-rinderpest era an agreed international policy will need to be established to ensure that the virus is withdrawn from all but a few very secure laboratories.

Two morbillivirus-induced diseases are currently targeted for global eradication, measles by WHO and rinderpest by OIE and FAO. Already there are signs that measles is not considered a serious disease in parts of Western Europe and vaccination levels are dropping in many countries (see Chapter 14). This is partly due to worries about vaccine safety, but complacency about the seriousness of the disease could mean that measles again becomes a significant cause of childhood mortality in developed countries. Similarly, the lack of significant mortality in domestic cattle with the current lineage 2 strain of rinderpest virus in eastern Africa could lead to a situation where the virus is no longer considered a threat, with potentially disastrous consequences. Given the mutability of RNA viruses and the relatively few changes in the genome sequence that can significantly affect pathogenesis, a currently circulating mild strain might revert to virulence if passaged in enough susceptible hosts – the ideal scenario for this now exists in Africa where almost all herds lack antibodies to rinderpest as a result of the efforts of the Global Rinderpest Eradication Programme (Plate 10). If rinderpest becomes a disease of the past, PPR is certainly a disease of the future. PPR is set to expand its geographical distribution dramatically and has recently spread into one of the Central Asian countries and all are potentially contaminated. It will require strong determination to continue the fight to eradicate measles and rinderpest and not to relax vigilance under economic or social pressures when it appears that these viruses no longer pose a threat or that the goal of eradication has been achieved without rigorous surveillance to confirm that this is in fact the case.

# Biographical notes on key players in rinderpest study and control

**ADIL-BEY Mustafa (1871–1904)**
Turkish veterinary bacteriologist
Together with Maurice Nicolle in 1902 discovered the virus responsible for rinderpest at the Imperial Institute for Bacteriology, Constantinople.

**BATES Thomas (c.1760)**
Surgeon to King George I of Great Britain
Bates was familiar with Lancisi's edicts having been stationed as a naval surgeon in Sicily and he applied them successfully without the draconian penalties prescribed by Lancisi, introducing instead a policy of indemnities. Bates's campaign eradicated the disease within three months.

**BORDET Jules (1870–1961)**
Belgian physician and medical bacteriologist-immunologist
Assistant to Elie Metchnikoff (1845–1916; Nobel Prize in 1908) at the Pasteur Institute in Paris. Studied rinderpest in South Africa during the great epizootics and proposed serumization. Nobel Prize for Physiology and Medicine in 1919 for his work on humoral immunity.

**BOULEY Henri (1814–1885)**
French veterinary professor (Maisons-Alfort)
Friend of Louis Pasteur (1822–1895). Demonstrated that vaccination of cattle with vaccinia virus does not protect against rinderpest.

**BOURGELAT Claude (1712–1779)**
French advocate and horseman
Founded the two first veterinary schools, in Lyon (1761) and Paris (Maisons-Alfort) in 1766.

ISBN-13: 978-0-12-88385-1
ISBN-10: 0-12-88385-6

### CARRÉ Henri (1870–1938)
French veterinarian
Discovered the virus responsible for canine distemper, later called in French 'maladie de Carré'.

### DANYSZ Jan (1860–1928)
Polish bacteriologist
Worked in France at Pasteur Institute of Paris and collaborated with Jules Bordet in South Africa during the great rinderpest epizootic.

### EDWARDS James (1889–1953)
British bacteriologist
Developed the first caprinized vaccine against rinderpest working at the Indian Veterinary Research Institute at Mukteswar.

### GALEN Claudius (131–201)
Greek physician
Defined the main characteristics of a pest (plague).

### JENNER Edward (1749–1823)
British physician and naturalist
Discovered in 1796 vaccination against smallpox. Described the neurological clinical signs of dog distemper.

### KAKIZAKI Chiharu
Japanese veterinarian
Developed a rinderpest vaccine in 1917, which was successfully used in the control of rinderpest in Korea from 1924 and lead to the establishment of an immune belt on the border between China and Korea.

### KITASATO Shibasaburo (1852–1931)
Japanese physician
Co-discovered with Alexandre Yersin the bacterium responsible for human plague. Worked in collaboration with Robert Koch

### KOCH Robert (1843–1910)
German physician and bacteriologist
Discovered the bacterium responsible for tuberculosis. Together with Friedrich Henle (1809–1885), issued what is known as the Koch's postulate. Worked on rinderpest with Paul Kohlstock during the great rinderpest epizootic in South Africa, where they developed the bile vaccine. Was awarded the Nobel Prize for Physiology and Medicine in 1905.

### KOHLSTOCK Paul (1861–1900)
German physician and bacteriologist
Worked together with Robert Koch during the great rinderpest epizootics in South Africa where they developed the bile vaccine.

**LANCISI Giovanni (1654–1720)**
Italian physician
Medical Doctor to Pope Clément XI. He was the first to propose effective sanitary prophylactic measures to control rinderpest.

**NAKAMURA Junji**
Japanese microbiologist
Working in Korea in the 1930s and inspired by Edwards's success with the caprinized vaccine he developed a lapinized rinderpest vaccine by multiple passage in rabbits. This vaccine was used widely in Asia and in parts of Africa to control rinderpest before the availability of the Plowright TCRV.

**NICOLLE Maurice (1862–1932)**
French physician and medical bacteriologist
Together with Mustafa Adil Bey, he discovered the virus responsible for rinderpest at the Imperial Institute for Bacteriology, Constantinople. Brother of Charles Nicolle (1866–1936; Nobel Prize in 1928).

**OZAWA Yoshihiro (1931– )**
Japanese veterinarian
As Chief of the Animal Health Service of the Animal Production and Health Division at the FAO he oversaw the organization's dynamic respose to the deteriorating rinderpest situation in Africa in the early 1980s. Out of this grew his conviction that such events much not be repeated and that, as all the technical requirements for eradication were in place, a final solution was necessary. He oversaw the FAO Expert Consultation on global strategy for control and eradication of rinderpest (1987) at which 'the veterinary profession is firmly of the opinion that a final internationally-coordinated assault on rinderpest should be made with global eradication as its target'. Dr Ozawa took a leading role in expanding the compaign in two other regions; the West Asia Rinderpest Campaign (WAREC) and the South Asian Rinderpest Eradication Campaign (SAREC). These campaigns were financially and technically supported by the UNDP and EEC, and successfully achieved the objective of eradication of rinderpest in these regions.

**PLOWRIGHT Walter (1923– )**
British veterinarian and virologist
Working in the East African Veterinary Organization's Muguga Laboratory in Kenya, together with R.D. Ferris, he developed the first attenuated vaccine against rinderpest in cell culture, largely used during the eradication campaigns. He is fellow of the Royal Society, London; in 1984 he received the King Baudouin Award from Belgium and in 1999 he received the World Food Prize – often described as the Nobel Prize for food research – from the FAO.

**PROVOST Alain (1930–2002)**
French veterinary virologist
Together with Gordon Scott was instrumental in implementing the eradication campaign against rinderpest under the auspices of the Food and Agriculture Organization (FAO).

**RAMAZZINI Bernardino (1633–1714)**
Italian physician
Was the first to give a clear clinical description of rinderpest.

**REINDERS Geert (1737–1815)**
Dutch farmer
Carried out inoculation experiments against rinderpest in the Netherlands and discovered the maternal transmission of acquired immunity.

**SCOTT Gordon (1923–2004)**
British veterinary virologist
Together with Alain Provost, was instrumental in implementing the global eradication campaign against rinderpest under the auspices of the Food and Agriculture Organization (FAO).

**THEILER Arnold (1867–1936)**
Swiss veterinary bacteriologist and parasitologist
Founded and Directed the Onderstepoort veterinary laboratory in South Africa. Worked on Rinderpest together with Jules Bordet and Jan Danysz during the great epizootic. His son Max Theiler (1899–1972) was awarded the Nobel Prize for Physiology and Medicine in 1951.

**VEGETIUS** (Flavius Vegetius Renatus) (end of the fourth century, beginning of the fifth)
Latin writer, the first to relate an epizootic of rinderpest.

**VICQ d'AZYR Félix (1748–1794)**
French physician
Wrote a treatise *Médecine des bêtes à cornes* (1781), and investigated measures to control rinderpest in France.

**YERSIN Alexandre (1863–1943)**
French (from Swiss origin) physician and bacteriologist
Assistant to Emile Roux (1853–1933) and Louis Pasteur (1822–1895) in Paris. Discovered, independently from Shibasaburo Kitasato, the bacterium responsible for human plague (*Yersinia pestis*). Worked on the transmission of rinderpest.

# Index